Memory and the Brain

CW01084992

Memory and the Brain explores the fascinating psychology and neuroscience of human memory.

Written by a world expert in the field, John P. Aggleton, this book covers learning and memory from the very beginning of life to its end, with an emphasis on real-world applications throughout. Aggleton begins by considering the fallibility of long-term memory and explores the many reasons why we forget. He goes on to contrast this with superior memory and examines what, if anything, is special about individuals with remarkable memory powers, and how might we improve our own memory. The significance of sleep, our ability to 'remember' the future, the various brief memory stores, and the multiple forms of amnesia are also covered, as well as the most common forms of dementia – including Alzheimer's disease. The book concludes with an Alphabet of Memory Curiosities, which showcases a diverse range of topics: from aphantasia to zebrafish, stopping off at topics such as Jennifer Aniston neurons, bilingualism, and neuromyths in education.

Drawing on classic studies alongside many discoveries from contemporary research, this book is written for anyone curious about how our memory works and will appeal to students and general readers alike.

John P. Aggleton is an Emeritus Professor of Psychology at Cardiff University, Wales. In recent years he was President of the British Neuroscience Association and in 2012 he was made a Fellow of the Royal Society in recognition of his discoveries concerning the brain and memory.

Memory and the Brain
Using, Losing, and Improving

John P. Aggleton

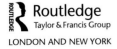

LONDON AND NEW YORK

Designed cover image: Getty Images via DrAfter123

First published 2025
by Routledge
4 Park Square, Milton Park, Abingdon, Oxon OX14 4RN

and by Routledge
605 Third Avenue, New York, NY 10158

Routledge is an imprint of the Taylor & Francis Group, an informa business

© 2025 John P. Aggleton

The right of John P. Aggleton to be identified as author of this work has been asserted
in accordance with sections 77 and 78 of the Copyright, Designs and Patents Act 1988.

All rights reserved. No part of this book may be reprinted or reproduced or utilised in
any form or by any electronic, mechanical, or other means, now known or hereafter
invented, including photocopying and recording, or in any information storage or
retrieval system, without permission in writing from the publishers.

Trademark notice: Product or corporate names may be trademarks or registered
trademarks, and are used only for identification and explanation without intent to
infringe.

British Library Cataloguing-in-Publication Data
A catalogue record for this book is available from the British Library

Library of Congress Cataloging-in-Publication Data
Names: Aggleton, John P., author.
Title: Memory and the brain : using, losing, and improving / John P. Aggleton.
Description: Abingdon, Oxon ; New York, NY : Routledge, 2025. |
Includes bibliographical references and index.
Identifiers: LCCN 2024030795 (print) | LCCN 2024030796 (ebook) |
ISBN 9781032884141 (hardback) | ISBN 9781032826592 (paperback) |
ISBN 9781003537649 (ebook)
Subjects: LCSH: Memory.
Classification: LCC BF371 .A37 2025 (print) | LCC BF371 (ebook) |
DDC 153.1/2--dc23/eng/20240807
LC record available at https://lccn.loc.gov/2024030795
LC ebook record available at https://lccn.loc.gov/2024030796

ISBN: 978-1-032-88414-1 (hbk)
ISBN: 978-1-032-82659-2 (pbk)
ISBN: 978-1-003-53764-9 (ebk)

DOI: 10.4324/9781003537649

Typeset in Times New Roman
by SPi Technologies India Pvt Ltd (Straive)

In memory of Hugh Aggleton 1984-2022
(All author royalties to the charity Brain Tumour Research)

Contents

Acknowledgements   *ix*
Preface   *x*

1 Memories make us who we are   1

2 From before birth to adolescence   8

3 Adulthood, aging, and superaging   30

4 How accurate and durable are our adult memories?   39

5 Comprehension, encoding, and recall   52

6 Why do we forget?   66

7 Context and memory   78

8 Superior memory in individuals: Mnemonists, memory champions,
   and savants   84

9 Superior memory for all: Mnemonics, imagery, and skilled performance   95

10 'Smart drugs', supplements, and self-brain stimulation   106

11 The value of sleep   121

12 Imagination, future memory, and prospective memory   128

13 Recognition memory and illusions of familiarity   139

14 Brief memory stores: Sensory memory   145

15 Brief memory stores: Short-term memory   151

16 Brief memory stores: Working memory   156

17 Losing memory: Real amnesias and simulated amnesias   166

18 Losing memory: Alzheimer's disease and other dementias   198

19 An alphabet of memory curiosities   212

    A Aphantasia: People who lack imagery   *212*
    B Bilingualism: Does it aid memory?   *213*
    C Computerised brain training: Does it work?   *215*
    D Duplicates, delusions, and familiarity disorders   *216*
    E Exercise: Is it worth it?   *217*
    F Food preferences and learnt taste aversions   *219*
    G The 'generation effect', the Aha! moment, and memory   *221*
    H Hypnosis, memory, and the law   *223*
    I Illusions of learning and illuminating text   *223*
    J Jennifer Aniston neurons   *225*
    K Knowing your own memory: Metacognition and metamemory   *226*
    L L learners: Spaced versus massed practice   *228*
    M Mozart, music, and memory   *231*
    N Neuromyths in education: Eight seductive ideas   *233*
    O Openness and the three Rs (reproducibility, robustness,
       and replicability)   *236*
    P Parrot learning: Learning by rote   *238*
  QI Quite interesting and quite curious   *240*
    R Return trip effect   *241*
    S Surprise and memory   *242*
    T Truth serums   *243*
    U Unconscious learning: Can you learn when anaesthetised?   *246*
    V Vegetative brain state, awareness, and new learning   *246*
    W White matter learning   *247*
 XX XY Sex differences and memory   *249*
    Y Y is money called money? The worship of memory   *251*
    Z Being at the end of the alphabet: Good or bad? (not to forget zebrafish) *251*

20 Naming the brain   253

21 Twenty (plus one) ways to improve your memory   256

   References   *258*
   Index   *265*

Acknowledgements

First and foremost, Jane, without whom none of this would have been possible. Huge thanks to Frank Sengpiel and Andrew Holmes for their wildlife photos. I must also thank the friends who bravely read earlier drafts.

Preface

Memories matter – they make us who we are and who we will become. Despite a career spent studying memory, I never imagined writing a book on the subject. Everything changed following the death of our son. I frequently think about Hugh and about my memories of him. Those thoughts led to the writing of this book. Don't worry, this book is not about grief. Rather, it is a celebration of memory.

The book describes the very many facets of memory. How they work, what happens when they don't work, and how best to maintain and improve your memory. No technical expertise is required to enjoy this book, just a curious mind. (The state of being curious helps the brain to engage in more effective learning.)

Memory affects just about everything in our lives. A glance at the Contents shows the breadth of topics covered. Some of the topics you might anticipate, others will undoubtedly surprise you. The book combines real-world memory experiences with experimental findings that explain these phenomena. The resulting insights are especially relevant if you are a student, a teacher, a parent, or are concerned about your memory – which is just about everyone.

1 Memories make us who we are

Lest we forget.

Rudyard Kipling ('Recessional', 1897)

Let me begin with an ancient Greek paradox and a classic TV comedy series. There is a brain teaser called 'the ship of Theseus'. It goes like this. If the pieces of a ship are replaced bit by bit, when does it stop being the original ship? Only a fifth of Nelson's HMS Victory is original, so is the ship in Portsmouth just a replica? You might also recognise this paradox as 'Trigger's Broom' from the BBC comedy series 'Only Fools and Horses'. Trigger received an award from the council for keeping the same broom for 20 years: "*This old broom has had 17 new heads, and 14 new handles in its time*", boasts Trigger.

Why is this paradox so relevant for memory? The reason is that when we retrieve an old memory we may inadvertently replace part of that memory – so which part of the memory is the original and which part is the replacement? Likewise, new memories are often a mixture of what really happened and what we expected to happen. These intrusions pervade even our most precious memories.

Despite a career studying memory, I never imagined writing a book on the subject. Everything changed following the death of our son. I frequently think about Hugh, dwelling on my treasured memories. I am, however, deeply concerned that my memories of Hugh are being replaced bit by bit, like HMS Victory or Trigger's broom. This very personal example reflects the much wider concern that many of our memories are part illusion. Much more about that later.

Memory capacity: Let's start with some good news. Human memory is phenomenal. Imagine being shown 2,500 different pictures of objects in a single sitting lasting several hours. How many of these pictures might you later recognise? Astonishingly, people correctly identified over 90% when each picture was later paired with a novel image (Brady et al., 2008). Even more impressive, accuracy scarcely dropped when people had to distinguish between the picture previously seen and a different picture of the *same* object. Clearly our brains can readily store highly accurate representations of thousands of images.

For those who try to sharpen their memory, the results can be amazing. Competitors at the World Memory Championships have to memorise successive packs of 52 playing cards. The current record stands at 2530 cards memorised within an hour. We might also remind ourselves that countless people around the world can recite the 77,430 words of the Quran.

Given these achievements we might reasonably ask what is the brain's capacity for storing information? Estimates start with the number of nerve cells (neurons) in our brain as they are the principal carriers of information. The adult brain contains around 85 billion

DOI: 10.4324/9781003537649-1

neurons. Each neuron may directly interact with ~1000 other neurons. These interactions create innumerable patterns of different brain activity that can be modified by experience. Calculations of the memory capacity of the human brain have come in at around a million gigabytes. Helpfully, this has been equated to three million hours of TV programmes. In fact, these eye-watering numbers may be an underestimate. Recent evidence suggests that each information point in a key brain structure called the hippocampus, might carry four or five bits of information, rather than just the one used for earlier calculations. Counteracting this gain is the fascinating claim that the brain contains many 'dark neurons' that remain surprisingly silent – a topic for later.

The bad news is that our memory is also very fallible, despite its enormous capacity. Names that make the news headlines are rapidly lost – why, for example, did Margaret Keenan become famous worldwide in 2020? Why can I never remember whether I have just locked the front door? Why is it so difficult to remember people's names? The disparity between our potential storage capacity and our woeful memory lapses gives oxygen to the neuromyth that we only use ~10% of our brains, along with the idea that we should somehow release the remainder to gain our full potential. Rather alarmingly, a recent survey found that over a third of Australian school teachers still believed the myth that we only use 10% of our brains (Hughes et al., 2020), possibly reflecting a jaundiced disillusionment with their pupils.

There is an urgent need is to understand what happens when memory systems are damaged by disease. This issue has profound clinical implications, not least for the 57 million people worldwide with dementia – a number predicted to rise to a terrifying 152 million by 2050. Clearly, we need to understand how memory works and why it fails. (By the way, Margaret Keenan from Northern Ireland was the first person in the world to receive a COVID-19 vaccination, excluding those volunteers in clinical trials.)

A fundamental distinction: Much of this book is about long-term memory – our remembrance of information for minutes, hours, days, or years. It might come as a surprise to discover that our long-term memories can be divided between two super-categories, often labelled 'explicit' and 'implicit'. When people discuss their memory they almost always refer to explicit memory. This category of memory equates to the 'bright side of the moon'.

Explicit memories are consciously accessed. For that reason, they can be mentally viewed and described. At this point you might choose to recall what you had for breakfast this morning (a question popular with sound recording engineers). Your description will require explicit memory, as will any description of past events.

In addition to individual experiences, explicit memory also contains shared factual knowledge. If you know that Nassau, Brasilia, Bern, Tbilisi, Bangui, and Suva are all capital cities then you are accessing explicit memory. Indeed, reading this sentence relies on explicit memory, as its understanding requires conscious knowledge about the meaning of each word. For this reason, any acquired information that can be brought to mind is 'explicit'.

Reflecting these different aspects of explicit long-term memory (personal and factual), psychologists talk about episodic memory and semantic memory. Episodic memory contains unique, personal events (episodes). Recalling the details of last night's TV programmes would be an example of episodic memory as the information is date and location specific. Meanwhile, semantic memory concerns factual knowledge that is not specific to a given time or place. For example, 'Friends' was a TV comedy based around six flatmates.

The relationship between episodic and semantic memory can be explained by looking at the photograph of an almost invisible moth (Figure 1.1). If you are a lepidopterist you

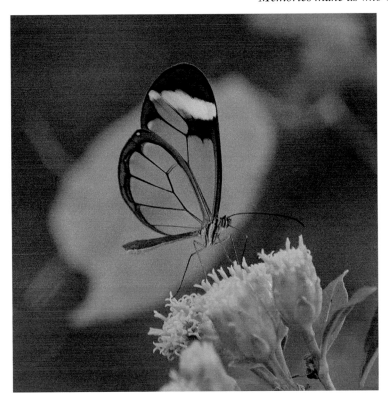

Figure 1.1 Glasswing moth.

will know that you are looking at a Glasswing moth. For such an expert, that piece of factual information comes from your semantic memory as it has been repeatedly acquired, detaching it from any individual experience. But, if this is the first time you have come across a Glasswing, the moth will be unique to this current experience – placing that information in episodic memory. Should you subsequently learn more about Glasswing moths, then the name may occupy semantic memory as it becomes increasingly removed from this specific episode.

If explicit memory is the bright side of the moon, then implicit memory represents the dark side. We constantly rely on implicit memories, but we cannot bring them into our conscious awareness. Just like the dark side of the moon, they cannot be directly 'viewed', leaving them invisible. This description makes implicit memory sound incredibly mysterious. To dispel the mystery, it is often easiest to give examples that illustrate implicit memory.

Consider riding a bike. We have no conscious insight into the motor memories that allow us to master the art of cycling. You cannot tell a child how to stay upright on a bicycle, other than shouting unhelpful instructions like 'keep pedalling' and 'don't fall off!' While I can explicitly recall and describe passing a full-size model of a Dalek just near Pontypridd on a recent bike ride (apologies if you have never seen *Dr Who*), I cannot tell you how I balance on a bike – I just do.

All skilled sensorimotor actions become implicit with sufficient practice, enabling us to perform them automatically. In this way, implicit memory is accessed effortlessly. The countless examples of implicit memory include learning to walk, driving a car, writing with pen and paper, surfing, playing a musical instrument, and riding a bicycle. Should you ever try to ride a tricycle, you will discover how these same implicit skills can suddenly let you down because they have become automatic. It turns out that when steering a tricycle, you use a completely different set of bodily actions from those used on a bicycle, something I discovered after crashing into a Norfolk ditch (Figure 1.2). As will become clearer, implicit memories and explicit memories are stored differently within the brain, resulting in very different reactions to brain injury or drugs.

As I write these very words I am employing an implicit motor skill, touch-typing. I have the explicit memory of first learning to type using a flat card on which the typewriter keys were printed. I touched the card while being tutored by a tape cassette. (I could not afford a typewriter and personal computers did not exist.) What I cannot now bring to mind are the implicit memories that help me to place the correct finger on the correct letter without looking. Explicit and implicit memory are not, however, completely divorced. Music teachers and sport's coaches rely on the ability of explicit instructions to help shape and refine implicit actions. Driving a car depends on the integration of explicit memory and implicit skills. Just consider Sweden on the 3rd September 1967. On that day (called 'Dagen H'), all car drivers made the permanent switch from the left to the right side of the road.

Overview of the book: The opening chapters chart the rise and fall of our many memory abilities, beginning with learning by the unborn baby and ending with old age. Consideration is given to that special group of elderly individuals known as 'super-agers'. Next, is the contentious issue of whether our autobiographical memories are accurate and permanent. As you may recall, it was this issue, and how it relates to my memories of Hugh, that set this book in motion.

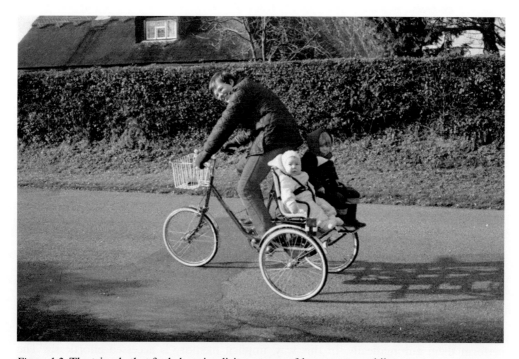

Figure 1.2 The tricycle that fooled my implicit memory of how to steer a bike.

The many reasons why we forget come next. Superior memory follows – what, if anything, is special about individuals with remarkable memory powers? Closely related is the question of how, by fair means or foul, we might improve our own memory abilities. Then comes sleep. We spend a third of our lives sleeping, yet its importance for learning and memory is only now emerging. Along with remembering the past, our ability to remember the future is then examined – some experts now suggest that this might paradoxically be the most valuable function of our memory machinery. Next, our brief memory stores are compared. These stores capture our sensory experiences and then transiently hold them for on-line mental processing. The cruel face of memory loss is next explored. The many forms of amnesia are described, including the deliberate feigning of amnesia as it is probably a lot commoner than you might think. Finally, age-related dementia comes under the microscope. The three commonest forms of dementia, which include Alzheimer's disease, are considered in detail.

Not all aspects of memory fit neatly into the above categories. To remedy this problem, Chapter 19 provides of an alphabet of 26 memory phenomena. Many of the topics bring memory from the laboratory to the real world, with direct implications for education. Topics include whether 'brain training' really helps, how learner car drivers should space their lessons, does highlighting text help revision, 'Jennifer Aniston neurons', bizarre delusions of familiarity, whether truth serums work, why the return trip seems to take less time than the same outward trip, if being bilingual gives you a better memory, how surprise affects memory, whether it matters for education and work if your surname is near the end of the alphabet, and much more.

To meaningfully discuss topics such as amnesia and dementia, it is necessary to incorporate the brain. I know from years of teaching that brain names are often a source of bewilderment and mystery. I fully sympathise. A glossary (Chapter 20, *Naming the brain*) at the end of the book is there to help. I have included the origins of many of the brain names, hopefully appealing to your curiosity while also making the terms feel more concrete. A second glossary (Chapter 21, *Twenty ways to improve your memory*) gives practical advice on ways to assist and protect your memory.

> *A myriad of memories* – Many animals have wonderful collective nouns; examples include a bloat of hippos, an exultation of larks, a murder of crows, and, not to forget, a memory of elephants. If there were a collective noun for the many types of human memory, I feel it should be 'a myriad of memories'. Implicit memory and explicit long-term memory have already been singled out, but as Figure 1.3 shows, there are finer divisions of memory. These various forms of memory are gradually introduced in the book but, to help, the following section briefly explains each of these memory types along with some useful terms. It is a lot to take in at this stage, so you may want to skip this section and refer back if needed.
>
> *Autobiographical memory* – contains those long-term memory experiences that directly relate to the individual, in other words, your personal history. These personal memories help to create and maintain a coherent self-identity over time. This form of memory contains both general (semantic) and specific (episodic) events. *Example*, remembering I had driving lessons in Cambridge and my inability to do hill starts, even in such a flat city.
>
> *Classical conditioning* – occurs when two stimuli are repeatedly paired. If one stimulus elicits an automatic response, by association the second stimulus may acquire that same response. *Example*, Pavlov's famous dogs learnt to salivate to a sound

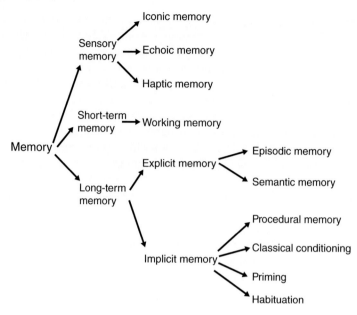

Figure 1.3 Divisions of memory.

associated with food. Closer to home, consider the Christmas music played for months in shops designed to raise your spirits (and willingness to spend) because of its association with the festival, though my conditioned reaction is mild panic.

Consolidation – the storing of received information.

Encoding – the initial representation of information by the brain.

Episodic memory – our memory for individual day-to-day events, containing what, where, and when information about that experience. Recalling episodic memories involves the conscious sense of travelling back in time to retrieve a personal experience. *Example*, recalling what you were doing just before you started reading this book, or my recollection of seeing a model Dalek near Pontypridd.

Explicit memory – is the division of long-term memory that holds information for which we have conscious access and insight, hence, 'explicit'. Our ability to declare or describe this information means that the term encompasses both shared factual knowledge about the world (Cardiff is the capital of Wales) as well as our individual life experiences (this morning's breakfast).

Habituation – the decrease in response over time to a repeated stimulus. This decrease is not a result of sensory or motor fatigue. We often think of habituation as becoming accustomed to a situation or stimulus. *Example*, when visiting a house close to busy traffic, the car sounds gradually become less intrusive.

Implicit memory – refers to the wide array of learning (classical conditioning, priming, habituation, perceptual-motor skills) that can operate below the radar of consciousness. Such learning lacks conscious insight into the precise nature of the learning, even though implicit memories produce changes in behaviour. *Example*, learning to stay upright when ice skating or skiing.

Long-term memory – refers to all forms of memory, verbal and non-verbal, with the potential to be long lasting. The principal division within long-term memory is between explicit and implicit memory. Separate brain systems help to support these two classes of memory.

Priming – occurs when exposure to a stimulus alters how we later detect or respond to that same or a related stimulus, without conscious guidance or intention. There are many different forms of priming. *Example*, give the first five-letter word that comes into your mind that begins with the letters **Dal.**. Hopefully, you will be word 'primed' by a recent word, rather than give the only other five letter word that matches dal.. Other examples of priming include how the meaning of the word 'swallow' changes dramatically if previously primed by the word 'bird' or by 'throat'.

Procedural memory – concerns the acquisition of perceptual and motor skills. With practice these skills become automatic, not requiring conscious supervision. *Examples*, driving a motorbike, playing the piano, and knitting.

Retrieval – the resurrecting of stored information. Encoding, consolidation, and retrieval are so fundamental that the term 'memory' has sometimes been defined by reference to them – memory being the psychological process that ensures the acquisition, storage, and subsequent retrieval of information.

Semantic memory – the name for our mental thesaurus, containing our acquired knowledge about words and other verbal symbols, including their meaning and relationships, along with other factual information (verbal or non-verbal). Its contents are often thought to be compiled from repeated episodic memories that share the same semantic fact. *Examples*, that the Tan Hill Inn is the highest pub in England, West Bromwich Albion have the highest football ground in the English Football Leagues, and Daleks come from the planet Skaro.

Sensory memory – comprises separate stores that briefly hold visual (iconic), auditory (echoic), and tactile (haptic) information. This information may persist for up to 1-2 sec. *Example*, the brief trail of light you see following a moving sparkler (iconic memory).

Short-term memory – maintains a small amount of information in an active, available state for a short duration (typically just seconds). This store helps us to hold sensory events, such as numbers, words, spatial cues, and visual objects, long enough to allow further cognitive processing. *Example*, holding a car registration in your head when using a car parking machine.

Working memory – like short-term memory, working memory holds limited information in an active available state. Unlike short-term memory, the term 'working memory' emphasises the ability to control and consciously manipulate the contents of this mental blackboard, hence, 'working'. *Example*, any complex multiplication carried out in your head, such as 17 x 12.

2   From before birth to adolescence

Mothers and unborn babies

Greatness from small beginnings.

Sir Francis Drake (1540–1596)

Pregnancy and memory: The very beginning is the pregnant mother and the foetus. Mothers often report a loss of memory during pregnancy. One of the first studies into this 'pregnancy brain fog' reported that nearly half of the professional women surveyed believed that their memory had deteriorated during pregnancy. The researchers coined the unfortunate term 'benign encephalopathy of pregnancy', stating that this syndrome should be recognised so that precautions might be taken to prevent its interference with professional or other activities. Put more simply, pregnant women should be given tasks that make fewer demands on memory.

Unsurprisingly, such statements were seen as scare-mongering and derogatory, even though subsequent surveys have repeatedly described the same subjective feeling of memory loss during pregnancy, with reported rates reaching up to 80%. For many pregnant mothers there is a real sense that their memory has deteriorated.

But, just thinking that your memory has deteriorated is a far cry from suffering a genuine loss of memory. Indeed, complaints of memory loss during pregnancy are likely to have been exaggerated as they increase when women are directly asked to report any lapses. In other words, spontaneous (unprompted) complaints of memory problems are less frequent than those reported in surveys. To find out what is really going on we need to give objective memory tests.

Pregnancy does not affect recognition memory, the ability to tell apart familiar from a novel experience, such as recognising a face or a picture. After that, the story becomes more complicated. Some, but not all, studies find a reduction during pregnancy in the ability to recall recently learnt information, such as passages of prose or sets of words. Likewise, being able to plan future actions is sometimes affected. This inconsistent pattern of results prompted the need for what is called a meta-analysis. This technique combines the findings from different studies and examines this larger pool of results with more powerful statistics.

Meta-analyses have shown that it is during the last three months of pregnancy that memory problems are most likely to be experienced (Davies et al., 2018). Of the various types of memory, it is the recall of individual events and conversations (episodic memory), along with working memory, that are most often affected. (Working memory actively holds information in mind to help us solve ongoing cognitive challenges.) There may also be

DOI: 10.4324/9781003537649-2

broader disruptions to wider aspects of cognition. One example concerns what are called 'executive functions' which, together with working memory, help us to focus attention, plan, and juggle multiple tasks in our head.

Fewer studies have looked at memory in women shortly after giving birth but, rather unsurprisingly, current evidence points to a rapid recovery in any aspects that might have been affected. There is, however, an important qualification. There is a well-documented increased risk for depression and anxiety after giving birth. Over 10% of women experience an extended period of depression after giving birth, while close to 10% experience anxiety disorders. Depression is associated with difficulties in the immediate recall of information, difficulties that are made all the worse when also suffering from an anxiety disorder.

So, what does this all mean? As mentioned, while some pregnant women believe that their memory is suffering, the extent of this belief is exaggerated by directly asking pregnant women to self-assess their memory. When cognitive changes do occur, they are often only evident in the later stages of pregnancy. It is also the case that only after the results from many women are combined, such as in a meta-analysis, that any consistent memory changes emerge. This need for large sample sizes reflects the considerable individual variation from pregnant mother to pregnant mother, as well as the modest size of any genuine memory losses. Put simply, for some pregnant mothers there is no evidence of a disruption in memory, yet for others it is a reality, though the impact is typically modest. Of more concern is that for some women any loss of memory may be accentuated by depression or anxiety, which may occur both before and after giving birth.

Given that pregnancy can sometimes affect memory, it is worth considering why this may happen. Obvious explanations include sleep disruption and lifestyle adjustments, alongside more specific factors such as anaemia or morning sickness. As it has proved difficult to identify individual culprits from this list, attention has shifted to the role of hormones. It is suspected that rapidly changing levels of hormones in the pregnant mother can affect neuronal plasticity and neuroinflammation, contributing to any negative impact on memory caused by a lack of sleep, for example.

A complementary approach is to look at the brains of pregnant mothers using magnetic resonance imaging (MRI). An MRI makes it possible to look at the details of someone's brain, but from the outside, making MRI non-invasive. To almost everyone's surprise, brain MRI measurements show that pregnancy is often accompanied by pronounced decreases in the volumes of multiple brain areas (Hoekzema et al., 2017). Figure 2.1, a schematic view of the brain from the midline, depicts the location of some of those areas.

Areas of tissue shrinkage were found in regions associated with episodic memory (the hippocampus and retrosplenial cortex) and with social empathy (the medial prefrontal cortex, upper parts of the temporal cortex, and posterior cingulate area). While this initial study reported that the shrinkage may persist for up to two years after giving birth, others have found a much more rapid return to previous brain volume levels. An important point is that a decrease in volume does not necessarily mean a decrease in effective function. Indeed, it can sometimes mean the very opposite. It has, for example, been suggested that a reduction in the volume of a brain structure called the striatum may help promote the sensitivity of the mother's reward circuits to signals from her baby.

What of memory for labour and labour pains? In most mothers there is a slow decline in the remembered intensity of labour pain over subsequent years, though this decline is mainly seen in those with a positive, overall experience of childbirth. Meanwhile, those first-time mothers who subsequently recall labour as a negative, painful experience tend to have fewer subsequent children with a longer interval to their next pregnancy.

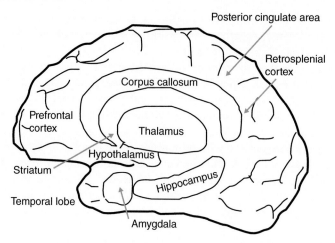

Figure 2.1 Medial view of the cerebral cortex and some subcortical structures. (Front of brain to the left.)

Foetal learning and memory: Studies beginning in the 1930s asked a simple but profound question. Is the unborn baby capable of learning? A prerequisite is the presence of modifiable synapses in the foetal brain. (A synapse is not only the junction point between two neurons, but also the principal site of neuronal plasticity and learning.) Pregnancy typically lasts around 40 weeks, but cortical synapses can appear as early as week ten. The formation of these synapses ramps up dramatically from around week 28. The presence of so many synapses means that foetal learning becomes a realistic possibility.

At first glance, testing this question might seem impossible, but ingenious solutions have been found. The realisation that some stimuli, such as vibrations and sounds, can travel through the mother's body to the unborn baby, made it possible to ask whether an unborn baby can learn about these same stimuli while still in the womb.

Studies from the 1940s found that in the last two months of gestation the unborn baby could demonstrate classical conditioning when vibration of the mother's tummy was repeatedly paired with a loud noise. In other words, the unborn baby learnt that these two events were associated. Subsequent replications have demonstrated classical conditioning in foetuses as young as 32 weeks. Equally remarkable is that a foetus as young as 22–23 weeks can show habituation to a specific auditory tone. Habituation, arguably the most universal form of learning, is the reduction in reaction to a repeated, neutral stimulus that has no particular biological significance.

"Neighbours: Everybody needs good neighbours ......" Those worlds will be instantly familiar to the many millions who watched the popular Australian TV soap 'Neighbours' as they are the opening lines of the theme music. The show was broadcast in more than 60 countries around the world.

In a wonderfully inventive experiment from 1988 titled 'fetal soap addiction', Peter Hepper studied the newborn infants of mothers who, when pregnant, had regularly watched the TV soap 'Neighbours'. Just a few days after birth the theme to Neighbours caused the babies to become more alert and their heart-rate decreased. These responses were selective as they were not found for unfamiliar tunes nor were these same reactions seen in the newborn babies of mothers who did not watch Neighbours. This preference learning appears to begin after 30 weeks of gestation. Probably of more biological relevance, an unborn baby can learn the vocal characteristics of its mother and then display a preference for its mother's voice shortly after birth. This learning helps the newborn infant to establish a familiar, safe environment.

The potential to learn preferences before birth applies to tastes as well as sounds. Foetal taste receptors start to mature around week 17, followed by olfactory receptors in week 24. Consequently, there is the possibility of acquiring pre-natal food preferences through ingested chemical signals in the amniotic fluid. When mothers repeatedly drank carrot juice during the last three months of pregnancy, their babies showed a greater acceptance of a carrot flavoured cereal. Similar evidence comes from mothers who ingested garlic pre-natally. When tested shortly after birth, these babies showed no apparent aversion to garlic, unlike babies not pre-natally exposed to garlic. Likewise, a preference for the smell of anise can be acquired pre-natally. Evidently, mothers can influence the taste and smell preference of their babies even before birth.

Foetal brain development: The demonstration of classical conditioning around week 32 raises questions about the status of the brain in the unborn baby. We now know that the brain develops at an astonishing rate. By the time of our birth (around week 40), the brain contains around 100 billion neurons, which equates to the generation of about 250,000 new neurons each minute throughout pregnancy. It is worth pausing for a moment to appreciate these truly astonishing numbers. For example, the number of new nerve cells *each minute* (250,000) corresponds to the entire population of Wolverhampton. In reality, the rate of neuron production varies during gestation. Consequently, at times it is more like the population of Liverpool being born every minute (~500,000). Just as astonishing is the degree of apparent overproduction, we may be born with 100 billion neurons, but lose many billions by adulthood.

The foetal period of most neuronal birth is from week five to week 25. By week 33 the main features of the cortex are apparent. Pathways connecting adjacent brain areas begin to appear by week 12, while long-range pathways start to become established in months seven to nine (weeks 30-40). At the time of birth, much of the architecture of the adult brain is present, but there is still a lot more to complete.

To appreciate what and when a foetus might be able to learn we need to look more closely at the developing brain. Not only must the brain generate vast numbers of neurons, but these same neurons also need to migrate and end up in the right place. This migration slows down appreciably by around week 30 as neurons find their resting place. It is around then that learning, such as classical conditioning, becomes possible. Neuron birth and migration is followed by a lengthy period when nerve cells try to establish the connections that will ultimately allow the transmission of information. This process of connection forming, which starts as early as foetal week ten, continues throughout our lives.

One of the most surprising aspects of foetal brain development is the programmed *death* of neurons, which begins even before the baby's birth. Just as there is a burst of new neurons during early gestation, so there is a planned elimination of many of these same neurons (called 'apoptosis'). This programmed cell death, which controls the final numbers of neurons in the baby's brain, starts as early as foetal week seven and continues throughout gestation. One of the many harmful effects of foetal exposure to alcohol is the disruption of this programmed cell death.

Not all brain areas develop at the same rate. One example is the cerebellum, which sits at the back of the brain, tucked under the cerebral cortex. This structure is full of surprises. For instance, it contains many more neurons than the rest of the brain. Also, its development is unusually protracted so that the birth of new cells, their migration and maturation all extend into the first few months after birth. Historically, the cerebellum was thought to support skilled motor movements, but is now also implicated in many aspects of cognition. The cerebellum seems particularly vulnerable to developmental challenges, and alterations to this structure are associated with conditions such as autism and attention deficit hyperactivity disorder (ADHD).

Infant and children's memories

> I can never remember if it snowed for six days and six nights when I was 12 or whether it snowed for 12 days and 12 nights when I was six.
>
> A Child's Christmas in Wales. Dylan Thomas (1952)

Memory development is like a three-legged race. During our early lives, memory progression is tied to the rate of brain development. At the same time, brain development is tied by our learning experiences. This relationship creates a shared dependency. Each holds the other in check, but each holds the key to further advances. With this partnership in mind, I will describe memory advances over the first few years of life, followed by the parallel brain developments.

But first, it is important to appreciate that rates of cognitive development in young children show considerable individual variation, making it dangerous to jump to conclusions about any particular child. Famously, it is claimed that Albert Einstein did not start to speak until the age of three, or four, or five years old (depending on the biographer), and that his worried parents consulted specialists about his apparent language problems. They need not have worried. But, as a result, the term 'Einstein syndrome' is used for those children who seem late in starting to speak yet are gifted in other cognitive domains. The critical point is that there are no hard and fast rules for rates of development, but there are typical trajectories. For example, at birth our brains are usually about a quarter of adult size, doubling in size over the first year.

The first three years – memory: Immediately, following birth, an infant begins to master an astonishing repertoire of vital information. For example, newborn babies prefer to look at their mother rather than a stranger after as little as two days. During that same time, babies continue to learn their mother's voice. For example, newborn babies will alter their sucking patterns when hearing their mother's voice, showing how they can distinguish her voice from other female voices.

You may have heard that newborn babies will also readily copy the facial expressions of adults. Famously, it was reported that babies will imitate tongue protrusions, even in the first few days of life. The remarkable nature of these findings prompted many follow-up studies, but these studies sometimes failed to replicate the imitation findings. As a result, there has been a 40-year controversy over whether neonates will imitate (Slaughter, 2021). One concern is that babies are aroused when tested, causing them to make more expressions. As a result, they might increase the number of times they make the target response, such as mouth opening, while also making more additional expressions. Tongue protrusion can be especially difficult to interpret as rates of this behaviour seem to go up whenever a baby is stimulated. Imitation is clearly a vital element of human development, but it remains questionable whether neonates already have this ability. Less controversial is the belief that imitating facial expressions and hand gestures emerges between four and seven months of age.

You might be wondering how it is possible to discover what very young children can remember when there are so many practical obstacles. The most obvious difficulty stems from our frequent reliance on language when studying memory, both for giving task instructions and when using verbal material to be remembered. Clearly this creates impossible problems for the pre-verbal infant. As a result, it is often easier to test for implicit rather than explicit memory skills. There are also motor and sensory constraints that limit how young children can demonstrate their growing memory capabilities.

Arguably the simplest form of learning and, hence, memory, is habituation. One example is the reduced responses babies show when the same, initially unexpected, stimulus is repeated. This form of learning is found across the animal kingdom. Its universality is explained by how habituation helps the animal to reduce its reactions to a repeated stimulus that proves to have no negative consequences. In this way, habituation helps you to ignore and filter out stimuli that prove to be unimportant or uninformative, allowing you to devote more resources to other things, including those that might signal danger or food. As habituation is an automatic process, lacking conscious oversight, it is an example of implicit memory.

Rather than play a loud, unexpected noise to a baby (not always a good idea), researchers have often looked at habituation to visual stimuli. When a novel visual image is first presented, the baby is likely to view it, but then look away. With repetition of the same image, viewing times diminish as habituation occurs. Babies just one or two days old show this form of habituation when repeatedly shown the same visual pattern. This technique has helped to show that newborn babies just a couple of days old can distinguish between two distinct patterns presented at the same time. The same babies struggle, however, to make this discrimination when there is an interval of a few seconds between the presentation of the familiar and the novel stimulus, pointing to the impact of the greater memory load. But, by five weeks of age, babies show enhanced interest for new patterns when displayed sequentially, now being able to bridge that same short gap. By three months, babies viewing preferences show that they can retain an image in their minds for at least two hours.

Because babies will look at a novel image in preference to a habituated, familiar image when the two are presented together, this form of testing is sometimes called 'preferred viewing' or 'visual-paired comparison'. The same methods can also be used for familiar versus unfamiliar sounds. The great advantage is that preferential choice tasks rely on spontaneous behaviour and require no verbal instructions. Consequently, they have been adopted and refined to ask many questions about sensory and cognitive development. The same methodology has even been used to ask questions about the emergence of complex cognitive abilities, including numerical concepts. One study found evidence that five-month-old babies can appreciate that one doll added to another doll makes two dolls, while one doll removed from two dolls leaves just one doll. This imaginative study, which implies that we possess some innate mathematical abilities, has since received general support.

Other tests of learning for newborn children include classical conditioning, another form of implicit memory. For example, five-month-old babies learnt to blink to the sound of a tone that was associated with a puff of air into the eye. Infants also display memory by learning to perform an operant learning task. The term 'operant' refers to an action that operates on the environment to gain a reward. The frequency of that action increases when it is positively reinforced. Examples of operant learning include increasing the frequency of kicking (the operant) by a baby in order to see a mobile above the cot (the reward). Other operant tasks include training older infants to press a lever that makes a miniature train move. (Some adults retain this particular operant training.) In this way, action-outcome associations are learnt from a very early age.

As already mentioned, tasks involving habituation and classical conditioning tax implicit memory, as most likely do operant tasks and preferential viewing. We can come to this conclusion because animals, such as rats, are very adept at performing all of these types of memory task, despite presumably lacking the conscious control that is a hallmark of explicit memory. In other words, we can be confident that some types of implicit memory are effective from a very early age, but identifying the emergence of explicit memory in babies is far more challenging.

It has been suggested that deferred imitation taps into the rudiments of episodic memory (our explicit memory for unique day-to-day events). Here, an infant repeats an action it had previously seen. After watching hand puppets, nine-month infants showed better deferred imitation of their actions if their state at encoding (calm or animated) was the same as their state at retrieval (Seehagen et al., 2021). This result has clear parallels with a phenomenon in episodic memory called state-dependent learning (see *Context and memory*). By 18 months, verbal cues at both learning and subsequent testing further extend the retention of imitation learning, which can by then persist for a month.

Another approach to testing pre-verbal memory is via signing. Here, babies learn hand gestures associated with specific objects. This ability can be trained in infants from under a year old, potentially giving access to pre-verbal memories. The approach has, however, been somewhat hijacked by claims that teaching sign language in hearing infants can advance their cognition, including their communication skills. This is not a straightforward issue as there is much commercial hype about the potential benefits of signing for accelerating infant skills. Careful reviews find that any benefits of signing for promoting cognitive development are at best modest and often undetectable. Put another way, there is no convincing evidence that signing interventions are associated with benefits in language acquisition for typically developing children. At the same time, there is no evidence that the practice is harmful.

Despite these side-issues, signing can provide fascinating insights into infant memory. Anecdotal reports point to the beginnings of episodic memory from early in the second year of life. For example, Angie (13 months) used the gesture for 'fish' and pointed to a door. When taken through the door she gave further 'fish' gestures and directions to obtain fish crackers (Vallotton, 2011). Meanwhile, Glenna (16 months) signed 'butterfly' and pointed to the location where she had seen a butterfly a week before. At the same time, infants start to develop a sense of self, beginning with physical self-recognition. This process may then take another two years to become more fully formed. The development of self-awareness is significant as it promotes episodic memory. This promotion occurs because episodic memory centres around oneself – what happened to me today, to me yesterday, and so on.

For most infants, it is the development of spoken language that provides the first opportunity to unambiguously test episodic memory. Give or take, by about 18 months, most infants can use simple words and point to named objects or parts of the body. This same ability highlights the beginnings of semantic memory, the knowledge base for concepts, word meaning, and shared facts. In their second year, many infants can string together a few words, and by three years of age new words are learnt rapidly, including abstract ideas and spatial concepts.

Even though it is often risky to draw general conclusions from descriptions of a single individual, it is difficult to ignore the delightful study of Emily, by her mother Katherine Nelson. Before sleeping at night, Emily would talk to herself in her cot. Her monologues were recorded when she was aged 21 to 36 months. It is probably fair to say that Emily was rather precocious, but her reminiscences remain fascinating. She often talked about the previous day but could also talk about events from months ago. There is little doubt that she retained episodic memories as a two-year old (Nelson, 2006).

The findings from other studies that questioned children about significant past events again show that two- and three-year-olds can retain personal memories, including memories for events occurring some months previously. Indeed, as most parents will testify, toddlers (between 24 and 30 months) can have a lot to say for themselves, and this will include references to past experiences. By the age of three, children can sometimes describe a particularly notable event. Examples include medical procedures that may have happened up to a year before. This emergence of episodic memory, points to the growing maturation and communication between key brain sites.

The first three years – brain development: The large majority of our neurons are produced before birth. Astonishingly, at around 350–400g, the weight of the brain at birth is already around 25% of its adult weight, even though the baby may be only 6% of its full adult weight (Figure 2.2). The infant brain then undergoes many further changes, some of which are very protracted. Consequently, despite being born with almost all our neurons (and more), full maturation may take another 20 years. This means that when an adult is interacting with a child, the child might simply not have the neuronal equipment in place to react and learn as an adult might.

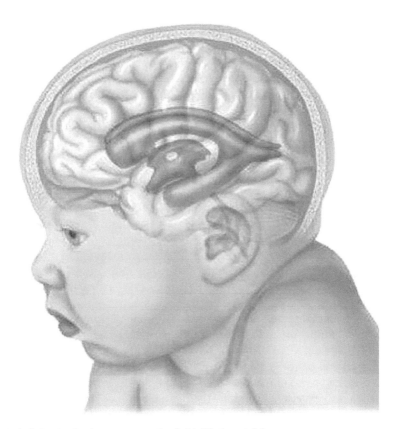

Figure 2.2 Baby's brain. In the centre are the fluid-filled ventricles.

Following birth, the production of new neurons rapidly diminishes. Although neuron numbers largely stabilise, the brain continues to enlarge. Over the first year, neurons grow longer and make more connections. By 18 months, different brain regions are well demarcated in ways that resemble an adult brain. In the first two years of life, cortical volume, surface area, and cortical thickness all increase. By the age of three, our brains reach about 80% of adult volume, at a time when our bodies are only around 15% of adult weight. Clearly, brain development is fast tracked. This rapid, early development then slows down in later childhood years, so that adult brain weight is reached around the age of ten.

In these early years, the brain continues to form innumerable new synapses. As already mentioned, synapses allow neurons to communicate with each other, and because synapses can be modified by experience they are regarded as the principal site of memory storage.

The rate of synapse formation differs enormously across different brain sites as we develop. In other words, different brain sites mature at different rates. In some cortical brain sites, such as the auditory cortex, the highest levels of synaptic density occur within the first few years of life, and then stabilise at that level. In other cortical areas it may take many years to reach the highest levels of synaptic density. For example, the density of synapses in some parts of the prefrontal cortex does not peak until adolescence.

As a rule-of-thumb, sensory processing areas mature rapidly while those engaged in higher-level cognitive tasks take appreciably longer. This means that children's ability to learn will have changing bottlenecks that vary with increasing age. It is also the case that we do not simply amass more and more synapses as we progress through life, instead their density typically peaks before declining as the brain helps to unclutter and streamline processing. This process continues through adolescence, when overall cortical volumes decrease.

Particular interest has focussed on the early development of the hippocampus, a brain structure closely linked with memory for places, context, and episodes. Recent MRI studies show that hippocampal volumes increase very rapidly during the third trimester of pregnancy and during the first year of life, only to slow at around two years. It is in their second year that toddlers begin to solve spatial problems that require the hippocampus, also corresponding with the emergence of more lasting episodic memories. The implication is that for the first two years of life children are often reliant on non-hippocampal forms of learning. During this time, the immature hippocampus may encode information in toddlers, but it is prone to rapid forgetting.

It is easy, however, to become rather fixated on the hippocampus as this brain structure has been intensively studied, often at the expense of other brain areas. It is important to see the bigger picture. For instance, recent analyses of the adult mouse brain found changes in more than a hundred different sites associated with a single memory. In other words, a great many brain sites contribute to the same act of learning, although some sites will be especially significant. Consequently, it may take many years for our memory machinery to reach full maturity.

You may well read that there are critical periods for childhood development. The problem is that different authorities give different time periods. These include the first three, the first five, or the first eight years. To make sense of this apparent confusion it is helpful to realise that any critical period depends on several phases of brain plasticity. First, the key neuronal circuits need to be in place, which is then followed by an increase in plasticity as those circuits react to experience. Finally, there is a closure of the critical period as those same circuits now show decreased plasticity to the same experiences. In the human brain, there are different critical periods for different brain functions. For example, we acquire effective binocular vision well before any critical period for language acquisition. As a result, the notion of any critical period must include its function and appreciate the need to have already formed the right brain architecture as well as experiencing the appropriate stimulation.

From four to adolescence – memory development: In parallel with the neurological findings, different aspects of memory develop at different rates. For example, when three-year-old and five-year-old children were first shown pictures from a story book, their ability to recognise those same pictures after three months was at chance for the younger children but much better for the five-year-olds. In contrast, there was no developmental difference between the three and five-year-olds on an implicit memory task (perceptual priming). The belief is that the neural systems for implicit learning mature far more rapidly than those for effective explicit learning, which may need five or more years.

Episodic memory: By its nature, episodic memory is complex. Episodic memory involves bringing together the different elements of a unique event (what? where? when?) to form a memory that involves a sense of self. It is this latter element that helps to explain why those with autism may struggle with episodic memory.

At retrieval, control processes search back to time to locate the correct episodic memory, another complex process that involves a sense of self, along with the ability to distinguish our inner thoughts from external events. Other control processes involve inhibiting interruptions to our passage of thoughts and discarding competing memories. These same control processes partly rely on our prefrontal cortex, a brain area that does not fully mature until we reach our 20s.

Given the many subskills involved in episodic memory formation and retrieval, it is perhaps not surprising that young children tend to retain more schematic, general knowledge at the expense of learning and recollecting individual, specific events. With ageing, the gradual switch from more generalised information learning to acquiring more specific experiences seems to be associated with maturation of the hippocampus and prefrontal cortex. By neuroimaging people aged between six and 27 years it has emerged that some areas within the hippocampus and its neighbouring cortex continue to enlarge across this same time period, while other areas remain at the same size or even shrink slightly. Those hippocampal areas thought to help distinguish similar experiences and so ensure distinct memories (a process called 'pattern separation'), seem to be the same areas that take the longest to mature. In other words, this ability can take decades before it its optimised.

There are also cognitive factors that delay effective episodic memory, our store of individual day-to-day events. As will become clear in later chapters, information that is understood and can be integrated with prior knowledge is far more likely to be subsequently remembered. A key part of this process is the development of 'schemas'. A schema is a structured, mental model of how related events go together. For a child, different schemas could relate to what typically happens at nursery, lunchtime, bedtime, in the park's play area, or when in the car. Given this acquired array of supporting factors, it should be no surprise that episodic memory takes many years to become fully effective.

Developing sophisticated models of aspects of the world (schemas) takes time, putting children at a disadvantage because they have yet to acquire a sufficient depth of related information. There can, however, be exceptions. Children may sometimes outperform adults when the memory test concerns a subject in which the child, but not the adult, is an expert. While nine-year-olds might recall more items relating to children's cartoons than 20-year-olds, the 20-year-olds will outperform the nine-year-olds on most other tests of episodic memory. As a rule-of-thumb, when children possess considerable knowledge about a particular subject, they process information from that same domain more effectively. This means that a group of nine-year-olds with a keen interest in baseball will recall more baseball terms from a list than other, non-expert nine-year-olds. Acquiring a strong knowledge-base, which takes time, is seen as one of the most important factors in the development and refinement of memory.

From this increasing knowledge-base two seemingly opposite effects can happen – we can create more unique memories, but we can also create more fuzzy memories. Going from the ages of five to ten years there is a sharpening of memory content, making each event more discriminable from similar, but different, instances. At the same time, we can also acquire a vaguer 'gist' of what happened. These gist memories contain core factual information but lack individual depth and detail. Consequently, gist more reflects your compilation of similar, past experiences, while verbatim traces reflect the actual, individual occurrences. My memories of past Christmas's contain both generic gist (last-minute wrapping of presents) and unique, individual memories (overdoing the brandy when trying to ignite a Christmas pudding). Because gist derives from your conceptual knowledge of the information to be remembered, we might predict that as children age and acquire more semantic knowledge, they can form more gist-based memories. This prediction is supported by experimental evidence.

Working memory: An aspect of children's memory that has received considerable attention is working memory. This form of memory provides a temporary store for on-line thinking. Rather than being a single store, it consists of different stores for different kinds of information, along with executive functions that handle and control that information (see *Chapter 16*). The various components of working memory are in place by around the age of five but are yet to reach their final capacity. In a detailed analysis, focussed around three components of working memory (the phonological loop, the central executive, and the visuospatial sketchpad), boys and girls aged from four to 15 performed a variety of memory tasks. The children showed a year-on-year improvement in all three components of working memory, only reaching adult levels by around the age of 14 (Gathercole et al., 2004).

One test of working memory capacity is digit span backwards. For this, you are required to repeat back a sequence of numbers, but in the reverse order (Figure 2.3). This is a 'complex' span task as it requires mental manipulation as well as the storage of the serial digits. U.S. children aged five have an average digit span backwards of around two, rising to just over four by the age of ten. Performance on this same task continues to improve with age until around 14 years, when it slows down as children reach the adult digit span backwards of around five numbers. One limiting factor for children is the speed of saying words in

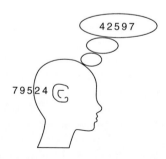

Figure 2.3 Digit span backwards.

their head, an ability that increases with age. It is believed that subvocal rehearsal is important for maintaining information in parts of working memory, helping to extend span tasks. This method of holding information is, however, time limited, so the quicker you can say the words the more you can hold in mind. This form of storage benefits older children.

Interest in children's working memory is understandably high given how this type of memory is closely associated with current and future levels of school performance. For example, children with working memory deficits often exhibit current difficulties with reading and mathematics. In a similar vein, working memory performance can predict future mathematical achievements. Even more striking, is how the working memory capacity of children aged 2.5 and 3.5 years can predict the future risk of dropping out of high school by the age of 13 (Fitzpatrick et al., 2015).

Perhaps unsurprisingly, testable models support the idea that working memory capacity is a key driver of mathematical abilities. To test this link further, children have been trained to increase their working memory skills using computer-based programmes. Their subsequent school performance was then examined. Current evidence is that working memory capacity training can be effective in aiding children's performance, with some improvements transferring to novel working memory tasks. In one study, training working memory in children aged between nine and 11 years led to subsequent greater success across the academic year in mathematics and English (Holmes & Gathercole, 2014). In other words, working memory capacity directly affects a broad range of scholastic achievements.

From infancy to adolescence, our memory skills improve across a wide range of fronts for multiple reasons. The encoding of information speeds up with increasing age, while rates of forgetting decrease, and a wider range of retrieval strategies become available to older infants, including the more flexible use of contextual cues. With development, virtuous circles are created. As we learn more about a topic, we can more effectively process additional material about that same topic, e.g., dinosaurs. In addition, the repeated, successful retrieval of a memory prolongs its subsequent retention. What is perhaps surprising is just how long it takes for the brain to finally mature. In adolescence (ages ten-19), those parts of the brain involved in aspects of working memory and memory retrieval, along with planning and social interactions, are still maturing, helping to make this lengthy period of our lives unusually challenging.

From four to adolescence – brain development: Between the ages of one to five years the density of synapses (connections) between neurons appears largely stable in most cortical areas, but thereafter it often declines. The cause is a lengthy period of synapse elimination. The drive for synapse elimination stems from the competition between the innumerable neuronal interconnections, creating the need to stabilize those favoured connections while discarding those not wanted. This removal process, which is called 'synaptic pruning', follows the earlier period of neuronal pruning (Figure 2.4). In other words, after having put so much effort into creating astronomical numbers of synapses, our infant brains then set about eliminating huge numbers.

The term 'pruning' is helpful as it captures the idea that this process is beneficial. Synaptic pruning, which can begin a couple of years after birth, continues throughout childhood creating a lengthy period of extensive synaptic elimination. This period of active pruning operates at a far higher rate compared with the slower loss of synapses that follows throughout adulthood and ageing. For the auditory cortex this period of active synaptic pruning is completed by around the age of 12, but for the prefrontal cortex it continues into later adolescence and beyond.

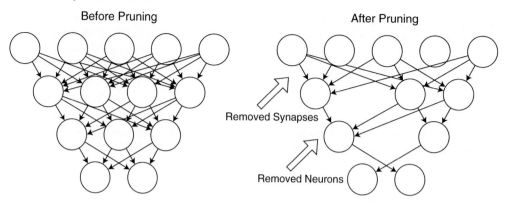

Figure 2.4 Neuronal and synaptic pruning are major features of brain development across the first few years.

In childhood, brain volume continues to increase so that by the age of six the brain has quadrupled in size from birth and has reached roughly 90% of overall adult volume. This continued enlargement is not due to the production of new neurons. Instead, the volume increase largely reflects the coating of nerve axons with an insulating sheath (myelination), a process that raises the speed of information transfer in the brain, while also benefiting favoured synapses. Myelination continues through childhood and beyond such that the amount of white matter in our brains does not peak until around our mid-20s. This long period of maturation can be especially true for brain pathways involved in cognition and memory (Figure 2.5). Axon diameter also appears to increase, which again aids information transfer and contributes to overall brain volume.

Brain volume changes are not uniform, as increases occur at different rates in different areas. For example, from the ages of five to ten, those prefrontal cortical regions associated with language continue to develop, showing a greater increase in thickness than adjacent cortical areas. In contrast, many other brain structures reach their full volume by the age of six.

More surprising is what happens next. Across the adolescent years and beyond (ages ten-25) there is a year-on-year *reduction* in cortical volume. This volume loss is largely due to a decrease in cortical thickness. This thinning process is seen across the cerebral cortex, although it varies between regions, so that the parietal lobe may show the greatest thinning during these years. It is not yet certain what drives this cortical thinning, but candidates include continued synaptic pruning as well as increases in the underlying white matter, which then stretch the cortex. It is presumed that these same changes help the cortex to operate optimally. Meanwhile, some subcortical sites, such as the putamen and caudate may reach their peak volume as early as the age of six, beginning to decline thereafter.

Another subcortical structure is the cerebellum. As already mentioned, the cerebellum has many extraordinary properties. Despite occupying around 10% of the brain's mass, it contains around 80% of all our neurons, around 70 billion. (I am tempted to repeat that sentence as it is so utterly astonishing.) As well as continuing to produce new neurons after birth, the cerebellum shows a protracted development period thereafter. Its volume does not peak until around the age of around 12 for females and 16 for males.

Again and again, the message is that brain development occurs at different rates in different sites. It can be surprisingly protracted, extending well past adolescence. This lengthy development seems to be especially true for regions involved in cognition, emotion, and

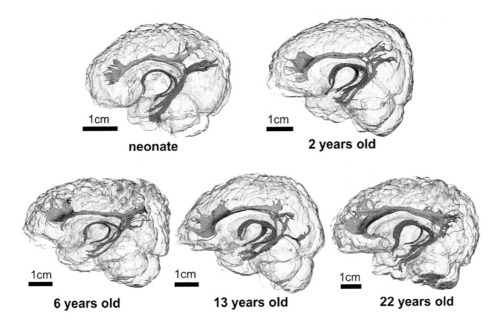

1cm
neonate

1cm
2 years old

1cm
6 years old

1cm
13 years old

1cm
22 years old

Figure 2.5 The continued development with age of two key tracts required for cognition, the cingulum bundle and the fornix.

social interactions. It is clear that adolescents do not have the same neuronal equipment as either children or adults, and so it should come as no surprise that they have their own cognitive attributes.

Childhood amnesia

> What I have in mind is the particular amnesia which, in most people, though by no means all, hides the earliest beginnings of their childhood up to their sixth or eighth year.
>
> Sigmund Freud (1905)

There is one form of amnesia to which we all succumb. It is called 'infantile amnesia' or 'childhood amnesia'. Both terms describe our inability to recall any episodes from the first few years of life. Sigmund Freud was fascinated by this phenomenon as he presumed that these memories were repressed in later life. He used the term 'repression' to describe the active removal of past memories that are uncomfortable or traumatic, largely due to their supposed sexual content. However, this explanation for childhood amnesia is now dismissed. This is not to say that memory repression cannot exist, it is just that there are far more persuasive explanations for this universal amnesic condition.

Age of first memory: In 1893, Caroline Miles, an instructor at Wellesley College, asked 100 female students for the age of their earliest memory. A few years later in 1898, the husband-and-wife team of Victor Henri and Catherine Henri asked the same question of students in several different European countries. In both cases the average age for their first memory was around three years. My first memory is of seeing a stag beetle in the garden of my nursery school at the age of four (Figure 2.6). Other estimates come from large internet surveys. In one, adults dated their first memory to around four years of age. A second, larger survey from 2018 recruited adults via the BBC. These people reported their first memory at around three years.

We have to be slightly careful with these ages as the precise definition of an 'earliest memory' can have a big effect. For example, how much detail is required to constitute a first memory? Another problem is that people sometimes describe a different 'earliest memory' when interviewed in separate sessions. On top of this, the episode might be a false memory, acquired later in life from family anecdotes and photographs.

One possible solution is to ask adults about a time-stamped event from their early childhood. Even better is to find an event that is experienced by many but, nevertheless, is individual. One example is the birth a younger brother or sister. The age gap between you and your sibling gives your age at the time of this notable event. Any memories can then be verified with parents' accounts.

Young adults often describe such memories from the ages of two or three years. There are, however, some concerns. As already noted, how detailed does a description need to be to constitute a memory? Furthermore, are these childhood memories real or were they subsequently created when these major family events were described by their parents or elder siblings in later years? As we will see later, it is possible to plant in adults the description of a past childhood event that had never happened, thereby, creating a false memory. To combat these problems, researchers have compared memories about the birth of a younger sibling with the knowledge of an older sibling's birth (which could not be a 'memory'). Their conclusion remained that genuine memories from the ages of two or three years can occasionally persist. Such memories remain a rarity, however, when set against the backdrop of so many lost childhood experiences.

So, why does childhood amnesia happen? Multiple explanations exist, both cognitive and neurological, and it is safe to conclude that there is no single cause. Any account not only needs to explain the absolute amnesia that blankets the first few years of life, but also

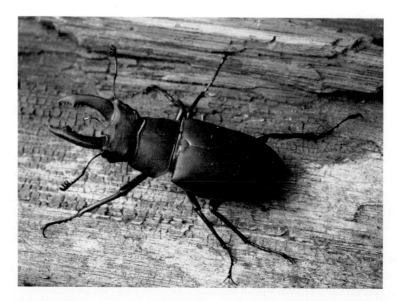

Figure 2.6 My first episodic memory – a stag beetle.

our poor memory for individual events over the following years of childhood. Consequently, the date of our earliest memory does not mark the beginning of a sudden transition to adult memory. As we develop through childhood, our subsequent memories remain patchy, though key events, such as our first day at school, start to be retained with increasing frequency as adults. For this reason, childhood amnesia should really be seen as a two-stage phenomenon. There is an early period of absolute amnesia up to around two or three years of age. This is followed by a relative amnesia that lasts until at least six years of age.

Changing perspective: One intriguing explanation for childhood amnesia is offered by the 'ecological model'. This explanation focusses on the different demands and experiences of infants and adults. Instead of there being a marked change in the way we learn as we grow, it is the world that we inhabit (our ecological niche) as infants and then later as adults that dramatically changes. To make the point, I cannot do better than borrow from one of the greatest children's books of all time, 'The Phantom Tollbooth' by Norton Juster (1961). In a chapter aptly called 'It all depends how you look at things', our hero Milo meets the feet of Alec Bings. (I say feet as Alec is floating in mid-air). Alec explains how his point of view never changes because his feet grow down to the ground and his head stays at the same height.

> *"Oh no" said Milo seriously. "In my family we all start on the ground and grow up, and we never know how far until we actually get there."*
>
> *"What a silly system." The boy laughed. "Then your head keeps changing its height and you always see things in a different way. Why, when you're fifteen things won't look at all the way they did when you were ten, and at twenty everything will change again."*

The ecological model supposes that what we perceive, learn, and remember about the same event differs as we age. On looking back from adulthood, we simply cannot reconstruct that very different infant learning experience. Part of this effect stems from how contextual cues that normally aid autobiographical retrieval will have a diminishing effect as our adult perspective becomes increasingly far removed from that of a child. An obvious example concerns remembering our school days. These changes become immediately apparent should you sit down in a child's classroom (Figure 2.7). You will be struck by the low chairs, the sense of looking up, as well as the absence of your schoolmates. Everything feels changed.

Language and memory skills: Perhaps the most obvious cognitive explanation for childhood amnesia is the lack of language. The period of childhood amnesia coincides with when our ability to use language to support memory is either absent or much restricted. Furthermore, the rapid increase in new vocabulary between 2½ years and 4½ years, coincides with our earliest memories as adults. Perhaps the dense amnesia for events experienced before the ages of two or three years reflects the challenge of gaining later verbal access to memories that were encoded before we had language. This explanation assumes that we struggle to superimpose language on pre-existing non-verbal representations. As we develop, the growing ability to encode information linguistically helps to increase the durability of a representation, with language sophistication offering an increasing range of retrieval cues to access a particular memory.

With the further development of language and knowledge, additional factors such as depth of semantic processing and better use of imagery help consolidation and, thereby, aid our release from childhood amnesia. While such explanations emphasise the importance of effective encoding, factors such as rapid rates of forgetting in early childhood will add to the mix. When children of different ages are interviewed, the age of their earliest

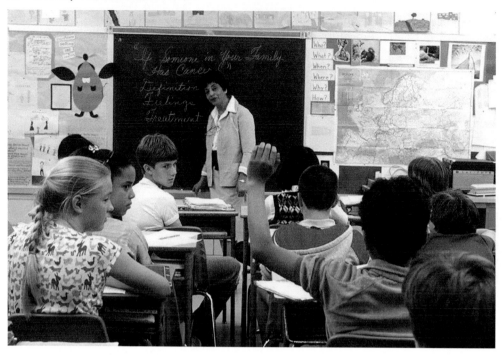

Figure 2.7 It all depends on how you look at things. The changing perspective as we grow.

memories increases with the age of the child. In other words, some early autobiographical memories are encoded but subsequently forgotten as we age. If these memories are forgotten within months it is inevitable that those same memories will be lost when we try to access them in later years.

Self-awareness: Another potential contributor to childhood amnesia concerns how and when we develop self-awareness. This ability, which begins around the age of two, allows you to position yourself within your own life events. This cognitive skill is especially relevant for episodic memory, the store of those things that happen to and around you. The personal perspective requires the development of a distinct sense of 'self'. This explanation is appealing as there is evidence that children struggle to fully encode events as self-experienced before four or five years. The maturation of this ability would then explain the further increase in available childhood memories at around that age.

Tests of reflective self-awareness famously include the realisation that the image in the mirror is yourself and not a copy (Figure 2.8). Most children pass the mirror test by the age of two. One classic way to measure this ability is to place a mark, such as a red spot, on the subject's forehead and see if they touch their forehead after looking in the mirror, rather than the forehead image in the mirror. Very few other animal species can pass the mirror test – great apes can but monkeys cannot. However, this version of the mirror test only captures a stage of self-awareness. It is not until four or five years that a child can also see themselves from the perspective of others, in other words, how they appear in the mind of others.

Neurobiological explanations: As attractive as these cognitive accounts are, we should ask whether childhood amnesia occurs in other mammals. In which case, explanations based on language, or a sense of self, are probably not sufficient. This turns out to be the

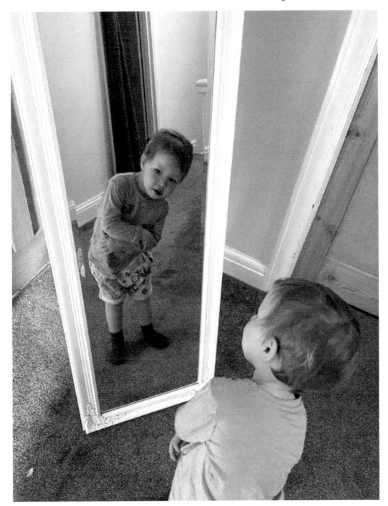

Figure 2.8 The beginnings of self-awareness.

case. Research show that young animals often show a much faster rate of forgetting than adults, appearing to mirror childhood amnesia. In one famous study, rats ranging in age from 18 days (infants) to 100 days (adults) learnt to avoid a signal associated with an unpleasant experience, an example of classical conditioning (Campbell & Campbell, 1962). Immediate learning was shown by both infants and adults. But, marked differences emerged as the retention interval increased. While the infant rats showed almost complete forgetting of the fear-inducing signal after 21 days, the adult rats showed excellent retention for twice that number of days.

Neurobiological explanations of childhood amnesia often centre on the development of the hippocampus (Figure 2.9). The hippocampus is one of several brain sites vital for the long-term retention of episodic memory – the very thing lost in childhood amnesia. The human hippocampus has a lengthy maturation period that matches the amnesic period. Attention has also focused on the prefrontal cortex, a structure that functions closely with the hippocampus to support memory. As already observed, the prefrontal cortex is one of

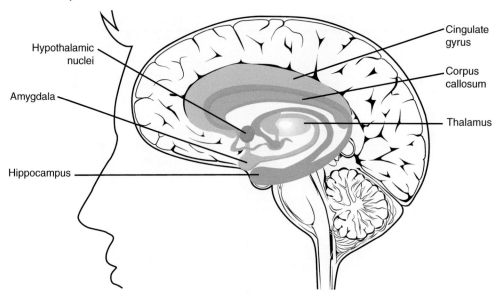

Figure 2.9 The location of the hippocampus (H) and its relationship with brain structures supporting memory and emotion.

the last brain areas to mature fully. The protracted development of these same brain areas (hippocampus and prefrontal cortex) parallels the gradual release from childhood amnesia over many years. Indeed, the very slow maturation of prefrontal cortex also predicts a partial 'amnesia' affecting our ability to recall our teenage years when we are middle-aged or older.

A different neurobiological explanation centres on a highly unusual property of the hippocampus. When I began studying neuroscience it was agreed that the human brain stopped producing new neurons at or shortly after birth. It is now clear that this general principle has a couple of exceptions. One demonstration came from terminally ill patients who selflessly agreed to take a drug that would label any new neurons in their brains. After the patients died, days or years later, their brains were removed and examined. One of the very few brain sites able to produce new neurons in adulthood was found to be the hippocampus. In fact, it is only one part of the hippocampus, called the dentate gyrus, that continues to produce new neurons (Figure 2.10).

The rate of hippocampal neurogenesis is high at birth but declines rapidly over the first few years of life, so that in human adults the levels of hippocampal neurogenesis are relatively low. It has been argued that this change in the physical make-up of the hippocampus (neurons being replaced in early life but less so in later life) means that as adults we cannot access our infantile hippocampus and its memories because the structure has rebuilt itself. This explanation takes us back to the Ship of Theseus and Trigger's Broom in the opening paragraph of this book.

While fascinating, this explanation is not without its limitations. One issue is that much of the supporting evidence comes from animal learning tasks that do not require episodic memory. Instead, many of the behavioural tests, such as fear conditioning, tax rodent implicit memory. This is clearly a problem as childhood amnesia is principally a failure of explicit memory. A further issue is the debate over the extent of hippocampal neurogenesis

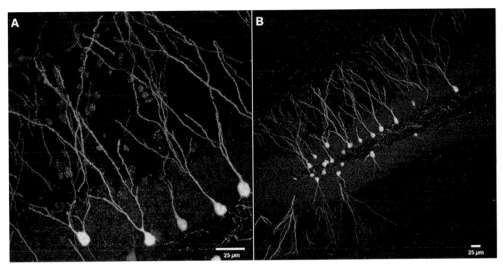

Figure 2.10 Photographs of new, fluorescent neurons in the dentate gyrus of the mouse hippocampus (neurogenesis). The image on the left is at higher magnification.

in later life. If neurogenesis persists across our lifetime, then we would expect to see 'childhood amnesia' being replayed over and over again as we age.

A word about hypnotic regression: During age-regression under hypnosis, seemingly lost memories from early childhood may be recalled. At first sight, some claims seem impressive, such as becoming non-verbal when regressed to six months. The implication is that childhood memories are not lost but just require the right retrieval conditions, as predicted by the ecological model of childhood amnesia. Unfortunately, what hypnotised subjects 'remember' during age regression typically fails to match the memory characteristics of real children of the suggested age. Rather, age-regressed memories often reflect mistaken assumptions of childhood and age-appropriate abilities.

Claims of memories from the womb or from when being born only further undermine the validity of these reports of hypnotic regression. One famous (infamous) example concerns Virginia who was repeatedly hypnotised by Morey Bernstein. Under hypnotic regression, Virginia recalled being Bridey Murphy (1798–1864), a housewife from Ireland. As Bridey, she detailed events in her 'life' from the age of eight to her death, caused by falling from a horse at 66. She then went on to describe aspects of her (Bridey's) funeral. Alas, past life experiences under hypnosis reflect expectations, fantasies, and beliefs regarding a given historical period rather than any miraculous transportation back in time.

Getting a bad start to life

Equality may perhaps be a right, but no power on earth can ever turn it into a fact.

Honoré de Balzac (1834)

There is a truly appalling statistic from the year 2007 that is every bit as relevant today. It was estimated that 200 million children under five years of age are not fulfilling their cognitive development potential. The causes are many, some are unsurprising, others less so. Culprits include malnutrition in both mother and baby, a lack of cognitive stimulation including limited education, malaria, environmental toxins and pollution, maternal stress, depression, not to mention iodine deficiency and iron-deficiency anaemia. Their damaging effects, singly and together, are all closely linked with poverty. The consequences include changes to the architecture and functions of the developing brain, many of which are lifelong.

To appreciate just one factor, the extent of education, it is helpful to consult the World Inequality Database on Education (WIDE). This database, supported by UNESCO, is currently based on statistics going back to 2018. The headline conclusion is that there are unacceptable levels of education inequality across countries and between groups within countries. The data in WIDE include age span at school, years attended, levels of absenteeism, and how these key measures are impacted by gender, location across the world, wealth, ethnicity, and religion. For example, while the average years of education in Mali is just over three years, for the U.K. and U.S. it is around 13 years. We do not live in an equal world, and countless children suffer as a consequence.

Environmental stimulation matters. It has long been known that being raised in an impoverished environment is bad for the brain and, hence, cognition. For understandable ethical reasons, much of the carefully controlled evidence comes from animal studies. These studies consistently show that being reared in an enriched environment is hugely beneficial for those brain structures required for learning and memory. In addition, the ability of animals to combat brain injury and recover their memory abilities is often boosted by environmental enrichment. For rodents, enrichment translates into having things to explore, climb, tunnel into, and chew. Children, you might suppose, would never be raised in environmentally deprived conditions. But sadly, this is not always true.

The Berlin Wall came down in 1989. Shortly after that, the regime in Romania ended with the joint executions of Nicolae and Elena Ceaușescu. Their deaths revealed to the rest of the world the scandal of the Romanian orphanages. In these institutions, many thousands of babies and infants suffered chronic deprivation. These children typically received exceptionally poor care, horrific levels of neglect, and were starved of social contact. After the scandal was exposed, some of these children were adopted oversees. Follow-up studies of adoptees in Canada showed that they often suffered a reduced I.Q., despite being raised in stimulating environments after adoption. Cognitive deficits were most evident in those children who had spent the longest time in an orphanage, while those children who had been confined for less than four months were, thankfully, less impacted.

Hints at the long-term effects of their time in a Romanian orphanage were revealed by the finding that over six years after adoption, levels of the stress hormone cortisol were often elevated. This finding is concerning as cortisol can adversely affect the hippocampus. Even more alarming was that more than 20 years after adoption the Romanian adoptees often showed smaller than normal brain volumes (Mackes et al., 2020). The longer the child had been in an orphanage, the greater the degree of brain shrinkage. The sad conclusion is that severe maltreatment in the first years of life can alter adult brain structure, even though the children were subsequently raised in enriched, stimulating environments.

The impact of the environment on brain health can also be 'transgenerational'. This term describes how parental experiences can be passed on to their offspring, independent of how they are subsequently raised. Put simply, the quality of your memory circuits can be influenced by the quality of the environment in which your parents lived during their youth. To reach this extraordinary conclusion, animal experiments have shown that the type of environment used to rear a female mouse can later impact on their offspring's synaptic plasticity and memory. For example, having a mother reared in a complex, enriched environment is associated with superior memory in that mouse's offspring, independent of the environment given to the offspring. This beneficial effect cannot be directly due to the mother's genes, as they are fixed. Instead, it seems to reflect how the expression of some genes is affected by the mother's environment. (The study of this phenomenon is called 'epigenetics'.) Some of these epigenetic changes in the mother can then be transmitted to her offspring, affecting their development.

3   Adulthood, aging, and superaging

With age comes wisdom, but sometimes age comes alone.

Oscar Wilde

It is natural to want to know when our memory capabilities reach their peak. At the same time, we are concerned that our powers of learning and memory will decline with age. Rather reassuringly, a self-belief of impending memory loss is often a poor predictor of what is going to happen. Feelings of struggling with memory often stem from our mood and stereotypes about aging rather than genuine insights into our declining memory.

Nevertheless, across the adult life span (20 years to 90 years), approximately 10% of all cortical neurons are lost. The average loss is around 85,000 neurons each day or about 1 every second. The weight of our brain peaks in our 20s and 30s, and then gradually declines. During this time, there is a decade-on-decade loss of the brain's white matter, which is made up of the fibres that transmit information between neurons. These changes point to the almost inevitable decline of cognition, including memory. This cognitive decline is of increasing concern as the percentage of the World's population aged over 60 years is projected to double by 2050 according to the World Health Organisation. But before we scare ourselves, it might be a good idea to look at the evidence.

How not to determine when aging affects memory: An obvious way to measure the impact of aging is to directly compare the memory test scores of different aged groups. If you do this, you will be shocked to discover that episodic memory peaks in our 20s and, thereafter, declines, decade after decade (Nyberg et al., 2012). There is better news for other types of memory. Priming, a form of implicit memory, may be unaffected by aging, while short-term memory only declines slightly in later decades. Meanwhile, semantic memory (general knowledge and vocabulary) may appear to peak in our 50s, before declining.

These conclusions come from 'cross-sectional' studies. As the name implies, in a cross-sectional study you pick one moment in time to ask the same question of different aged groups. Unfortunately, this is a poor way to find the answer. The principal problem stems from generation effects. Put simply, generation effects occur if upbringing, education, or environmental factors change across the generations, which they undoubtedly have. Indeed, we celebrate these changes in labels such as Baby Boomers, Generation X, Millennials, Generation Z, and Generation Alpha. For example, Generation Alpha is the first to grow up in an almost entirely digital world.

Try and guess the public health catastrophe labelled as 'The Mistake of the 20th Century'. Lots of possibilities spring to mind, but I doubt you will think of the villain – leaded petrol. Almost everyone born in the U.K. before 2000 was repeatedly exposed to fumes from

DOI: 10.4324/9781003537649-3

leaded petrol, even though it had been known for centuries that lead is highly toxic to the brain. During the previous century, about 50% of lead emissions originated from petrol. The long overdue U.K. ban in 2000 followed overwhelming evidence that car fumes cause brain damage, with children being especially vulnerable. (Unleaded petrol was only introduced to the U.K. in 1986.)

A recent estimate is that by 2015 leaded petrol had caused a national loss of over 824 million I.Q. points in the U.S. (McFarland et al., 2022). This corresponds to 2.6 I.Q. points per person, but with a much greater I.Q. loss for those individuals exposed to higher levels of car fumes. For much of my life I have been exposed to lead in this way (lead fumes are readily absorbed by the lungs) while thankfully my grandchildren are not. Apparently, trace levels of lead in the famous wine Chateauneuf du Pape parallel the rise and fall in exposure from leaded petrol. Exposure to lead is just one of many reasons why cross-sectional snapshots across the ages are flawed.

How to determine when aging affects memory: The best way to combat generation effects is to run a 'longitudinal study'. For this, you repeatedly test the same people at different intervals. This approach is not, however, without its own drawbacks. One problem is that repeated practice on a memory test might affect performance. There is, however, a far greater practical problem – the need to repeatedly measure the cognitive skills of the same person across their entire lifetime. To do this, you would need to have begun collecting data around 80 years ago and then repeatedly tested the same individuals over the following decades. There are various cohorts around the world in which children born at a certain time are now being followed over their lives. We will, however, have to wait many years to find out what happens to their memory when they reach their 70s and 80s.

Fortunately, there are clever mathematical tricks that make it possible to combine cross-sectional and partial longitudinal data. Using this approach, we can say that semantic memory, which is knowledge-based, can continue to improve with age, often peaking in our 60s (Nyberg et al., 2012). After that, semantic memory does eventually deteriorate, but this often only becomes apparent for those in their 70s. There are also subtle changes to auto-biographical memory with aging. There is, for example, a tendency for personal memories to become more generic, losing specific details.

These same hybrid longitudinal studies consistently show that episodic memory declines with age, though thankfully the degree of loss is far smaller than that seen in cross-sectional surveys (Frankenberg et al., 2022). Longitudinal data reveal a decline in episodic memory, typically starting in our 60s, which accelerates thereafter. (If you remember, cross-sectional studies indicated that this decline began from our 20s!) This decline in episodic memory is still appreciably earlier and steeper than that for semantic memory. Sadly, the subgroup of individuals showing the steepest decline in episodic memory are those most likely to go on to develop dementia.

The brief memory store known as working memory is also sensitive to aging, with one estimate based on visuospatial reasoning pointing to a decline starting around 55 years of age (Nyberg et al., 2012). This relatively early age probably reflects how working memory involves multiple processes that together manipulate cognitive resources (sometimes called executive processing or control processing). This cognitive control helps you to juggle and allocate the contents of working memory. A familiar executive task is to follow the television while also reading your smart phone. This same multiplicity of cognitive processes means that working memory is only as good as the worst component.

Executive control processes rely on the prefrontal cortex. The prefrontal cortex is not only one of the last brain areas to mature, but it is also one of the first to change with aging.

This time pattern helps to explain why aging effects are minimal for simple verbal span tasks such as digit span (short-term memory) but become more pronounced for working memory tasks, which require updating and switching, as well as inhibiting attention. A further challenge is that the elderly have more difficulty in supressing irrelevant items, another function related to prefrontal cortex.

In contrast, aspects of implicit memory, such as visual priming, appear to be far more resistant to the effects of normal aging, showing very little decline from the ages of 30 to 80. Even after considering differences in both levels of education and fluid intelligence, it becomes clear that some memory problems, such as associating items together in an episodic task, are far more affected by aging than other forms of memory, such as priming.

Explanations for the effects of aging on brain systems for memory fall into two categories. One category reflects the impact of widescale, non-specific brain changes. The second category reflects the idea that memory-related brain structures are particularly vulnerable to aging. As will become evident, both general and local aging effects take place in the brain, with the combination accentuating memory loss.

Non-specific brain changes and reaction times: The leading non-specific candidate for declining memory is a slowing down of processing speed within the brain. Processing speed is often seen as a core component of central nervous system fitness. To assess processing speed, people are typically timed on tasks such as decision-making, searching for a visual target, or reacting to the appearance of a signal. Of these three, I will focus on the reaction time taken to respond to the sudden appearance or change in a signal as this remains the most studied measure. One of the most dramatic examples of reaction time is at the start of a sprint race, as competitors react as quickly as possible to the sound of the gun. Incidentally, the quickest reaction times are set at 100ms, anything quicker is automatically regarded as a false start (Figure 3.1).

Reaction times, which slow with age, correlate with performance on complex cognitive tasks. This association was seen in a longitudinal study in which people were repeatedly asked to press a specific button on seeing a signal. The reaction times for this simple

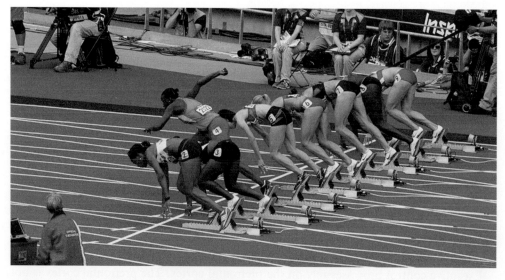

Figure 3.1 Test of reaction time (with a false start).

response task started to slow by the age of 45, while slowing on a more complex response task began a decade earlier in the mid-30s (Deary & Der, 2005). Those with faster reaction times performed better overall on a demanding cognitive task that together taxed attention, concentration, and memory, reflecting the multiple contributions from speed of processing.

Assuming processing speed is relevant, we can predict that aging will disproportionately affect those classes of memory where speed is most critical. The obvious candidate is working memory, as the ability to hold some forms of information in working memory is tied to the speed in which that information can be re-cycled. Evidence that working memory is often one of the first forms of memory to show an age-related decline fits this prediction. In people aged over 50, processing speed can also become a leading predictor of age-related changes in episodic memory. In contrast, processing speed does not predict semantic (factual) memory, as measured by tests of general knowledge, synonyms, or analogies. Instead, semantic knowledge often only begins to dip after 70 years of age. The preservation of semantic memory is consistent with how its demands are more self-paced and, hence, less dependent on processing speed.

You may have noticed that the age-related slowing of reaction times (starting after 30 years) typically happens before memory declines. The explanation for this apparent discrepancy is that we continue to enhance our skills in using memory as we age. With increasing knowledge, we are able to process experiences more efficiently, being able to encode and retrieve information more strategically, while also finding cognitive short-cuts. As will become evident in later sections, greater semantic understanding often results in superior learning, and semantic memory continues to improve into our 50s and 60s (well past the initial decreases in reaction times). The growing sophistication in our memory capabilities creates what has been called 'cognitive reserve', which is then able to combat detrimental effects on memory, including a fall in processing speed. So, just as children's learning accelerates as they acquire more knowledge, adults continue to benefit as they go through life.

Explanations for why processing speed declines with age concentrate on how messages are passed around the brain. Neurons often have axons; these are elongated processes that convey signals to other neurons. Many axons are wrapped in a fatty substance called myelin, which increases the speed of information flow within the brain. Together, axons and their surrounding myelin form the brain's 'white matter'.

The assumption is that with aging, there is a deterioration in the integrity of our white matter, disrupting information transmission. This idea gained considerable support from the discovery that the total length of the nerve axons in our brains decreases by about 10% every decade, resulting in as much as a 45% decrease from the ages of 20 to 80. This explanation also helps to explain why such a simplistic measure, like reaction time, can help predict changes in complex aspects of cognition, as both reflect common causes. Another shared feature of both reaction times and memory is that, with advancing age, performance becomes increasingly variable between different people. This variability only increases with added years.

It is interesting to briefly consider reaction times in sport. As I write this, the average age of a driver on the current Formula 1 grid is around 27 years. It is hard to imagine a sport that puts a bigger premium on rapid processing and fast reactions. Unsurprisingly, this mean age (27) is within the period when a person's reaction times are at their quickest. At 39 years, Lewis Hamilton is something of an age outlier. (The age record goes to Luigi Fagioli who was 55 when he won the French Grand Prix in 1951.) The internet credits Lewis Hamilton with a reaction time of less than 200ms, which is similar to other grand prix drivers but substantially quicker than the general population.

The loss of memory structures: The second category of explanations for the loss of memory with advancing years assumes that aging brings disproportionate changes to those brain structures vital for memory. Particular attention has been given to those brain sites supporting episodic memory, given its susceptibility to aging and importance for quality of life. A loss of episodic memory brings difficulties in remembering conversations, stories in books, programmes, or series on the television, as well an increased risk of becoming lost.

An obvious measure of brain health is brain volume. As you might guess, decreases in overall brain volume predict age-related cognitive decline. One focus has been on the cerebral cortex, the outer layer of neurons that cover much of the brain (Figure 3.2). Both episodic memory and working memory rely on the integrity of our cerebral cortex, as does the storage of semantic knowledge.

For those over 50 years-old, cortical volume decreases by about 0.5% a year. In many cortical areas this rate of tissue loss remains stable, but this loss is not equal across the brain's surface. One brain area that typically shows more rapid shrinkage is the temporal lobe. The temporal lobe contains the hippocampus and related parahippocampal cortical tissue, areas that are essential for episodic memory (see *Anterograde amnesia*).

Both the hippocampus (Figure 3.2) and the immediately adjacent cortices show faster than normal tissue loss over the age of 60. As might be expected, decreases in the size of the hippocampus can predict memory loss in the elderly. More surprising is that this relationship between episodic memory and hippocampal volume can be quite weak. One reason may be that, in addition to the hippocampus, a number of other cortical and subcortical sites are also vital for episodic memory and also appear sensitive to aging. Only from taking a more comprehensive approach will we understand the relationship between hippocampal volume, age, and episodic memory.

There is a useful rule-of-thumb that those brain areas taking the longest to mature are the most vulnerable to age-related changes, a pattern often referred to as 'last in, first out'. These late maturing areas tend to have a more complex cortical structure. Prefrontal cortex

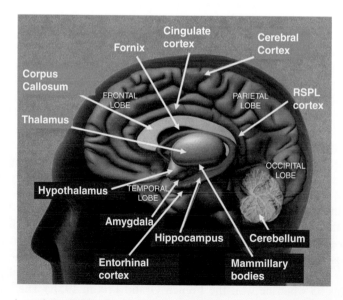

Figure 3.2 Side view of the human brain showing some major brain structures. The hippocampus and its major tract, the fornix, are shown connected. RSPL, retrosplenial cortex.

probably best fits this description, as it takes decades to mature but then shows relatively rapid tissue loss and shrinkage in later life. This combination of slow maturation and early degeneration is especially likely to affect working memory. This is because prefrontal cortex is important for many aspects of working memory. As might be anticipated, a smaller frontal cortex is related to poorer working memory performance in 70-year-olds.

Another component of brain health is the status of our white matter, which consists of the bundles of nerve axons that transmit information (see *W for White matter learning*). As mentioned above, a slowing of reaction times with aging is thought to represent a reduced efficiency in axonal transmission. Advances in brain imaging have now helped to confirm this belief. Declines in white matter integrity typically begin between our third and fifth decades, matching the reduction in reaction time performance. Following on from this, a study of people aged from 55-87 found that the loss of white matter integrity helped to explain the associated slowing of cognitive processing (Kerchner et al., 2012).

As white matter changes associated with aging are found in multiple brain pathways, there is the potential for widescale effects on cognition. However, the rate of white matter deterioration is not uniform across the brain, with tracts linking the prefrontal cortex often being particularly vulnerable. These tracts include the fornix (Figure 3.2). This pathway is of particular interest as it links the hippocampus with various brain sites also vital for episodic memory. More so than other brain pathways, age-related changes to the fornix reliably predict declines in episodic memory. Clearly, healthy white matter is good for memory, with some tracts being especially important.

Another way to study brain health is to compare neural activity across different sites. Functional neuroimaging makes this possible. Aging leads to decreased activity in a cluster of brain sites (hippocampus, retrosplenial cortex, parahippocampal gyrus, medial parietal cortex) that are all important for episodic memory and spatial processing. Of these sites, the retrosplenial cortex seems especially vulnerable to the effects of aging. Age-related changes in neural activity are also seen in the prefrontal cortex, with the potential to impact on working memory.

The overall picture is one of both grey and white matter loss that starts to become apparent beyond our mid-50s. In addition to the many widespread brain changes, there are brain sites critical for explicit memory that appear to be especially sensitive to the impacts of aging. This picture is exaggerated in those who will later go on to develop dementias (see *Losing memory: Alzheimer's disease and other dementias*).

Brain reserve and cognitive reserve: At the age of 93, Lorna Page published her first book to considerable acclaim, it was a thriller called 'A Dangerous Weakness'. Clearly, some individuals are more resilient than others to the effects of aging on cognition. There are two major components to this resilience: enhanced brain reserve and cognitive reserve.

'Brain reserve' is seen in those aged people who show a relative lack of age-related brain pathology. This preservation is not only seen in cortical and subcortical brain sites, but also in the brain's white-matter pathways, with resulting consequences for processing speed and cognition. When it comes to memory, researchers have understandably focussed on those brain structures most strongly implicated in learning, with the hippocampus at the top of the list.

Genetic factors play a part in hippocampal preservation. It is known, for example, that the ε4 variant of a gene called *APOE* is associated with a faster decline in hippocampal volume. (Much more will be said about *APOE* when discussing dementias.) In addition to not having 'bad' genes, there are a variety of life factors associated with improved brain reserve. Examples include good underlying health (such as lower heart rate), better blood circulation, emotional balance (for example, fewer depressive symptoms), higher educational levels, sufficient sleep, the availability of effective health care, reduced environmental pollutants, and positive lifestyle factors such as social living and exercise.

The hippocampus is vulnerable on many fronts. High blood pressure is associated with damage to hippocampal capillaries, which in turn, detrimentally affects hippocampal neurons. At the same time, hippocampal blood flow decreases with age, a decrease that matches a decline in spatial memory. Steroid hormones such as cortisol, which are released in times of stress, also affect the hippocampus. Adverse, uncontrollable stress disrupts hippocampal plasticity and reduces synapse numbers. However, it is not all doom and gloom. Exercise can have an important role as it helps to combat high blood pressure, improves circulation, and stimulates neurogenesis in the hippocampus. In addition, a diet that is high in fruit, vegetables, and grilled fish is associated with preserved hippocampal volume. Likewise, drinking little or no alcohol is also associated with good hippocampal status. Consequently, there is an array of life choices that should protect your memory in advancing years.

Just as it is important to preserve your hippocampus, so you should look after your white matter. Brain imaging studies indicate clear links between the decline in white matter integrity and factors that include high blood pressure, obesity, diabetes, and smoking. Other conditions related to white matter changes include hearing loss, social isolation, depression, and poor sleep patterns. On the other hand, physical activity, cognitive exercise, and a healthy diet may protect white matter during aging.

Cognitive reserve refers to how cognitive tasks are approached and solved. Individuals with higher cognitive reserve apply more efficient strategies to compensate for the effects of aging. Evidence for cognitive reserve emerges when you compare individuals that appear to have a comparable brain structural status yet show different rates of cognitive decline with age.

Factors related to superior cognitive reserve include levels of intelligence, years of education, and status of occupation. As none of these factors is readily altered in later life, the focus has moved to the potential benefits of additional activities. One pastime that has received considerable interest is engaging with cognitively stimulating problems such as sudoko or crosswords. The good news is that maintaining such cognitive stimulation can benefit cognitive reserve, and these benefits are additional to those provided by educational level and occupational status.

Other lifestyle activities appear to impact on both brain health and cognitive reserve. One of the more significant is having a rich social life. The impact is not just on cognition, but also on better health and improved death rates. The extent of one's social life has been measured by items such as internet friends, church attendance, shared leisure activities, and marital status. One positive example concerns the apparent cognitive benefits of singing in a choir. In contrast, widowhood is associated with cognitive decline, alongside other measures of poorer health. Intriguingly, having at least one living sibling may help to ward off the cognitive decline associated with being a widow. The loss of social interactions associated with deafness may also contribute to the reasons why hearing loss is linked with more rapid cognitive decline in aging.

A large piece of serendipity lies behind one of the most remarkable studies of cognitive aging. From that study we now know that some protective factors in old age are laid down in early life. For example, the I.Q. scores of 11-year-olds were found to predict working memory and episodic recall performance when the same people were aged 90 (Deary et al., 2013). This longitudinal study is truly astonishing because it required an 80-year follow-up.

In 1932 the Scottish Mental Survey tested 87,498 eleven-year-olds. That survey was followed by a second, large survey of Scottish children in 1947. Unfortunately, all of these test scores seemed lost. But in 1990, the results were rediscovered in the Moray House School of Education at the University of Edinburgh. The surviving participants were then contacted, making possible a truly unique, longitudinal study that still continues.

I.Q. is not the only long-term predictor of memory in much later life. One large category of people often less able to deal with the effects of aging are those millions who experienced adverse early-life effects, both medical and psychological. These adverse effects are closely linked to poverty.

Super-aging: There is enormous individual variation in how aging affects cognition. Terms such as 'successful' aging or 'super-aging' are used when referring to the subset of older individuals who maintain good levels of memory performance with advancing age. Examples include Lorna Page who started writing novels in her 90s. One definition of successful aging is being in the top third of your age category. A much more stringent definition is that the term applies to older adults who perform at or above the average level for younger adults and maintain this level over time.

Applying this more stringent definition, a 2007 study in Sweden initially identified about 8.0% of those over 70 as performing at or above the level for much younger adults. However, only a third of these same individuals maintained this level when tested five years later (now aged 75-90), meaning that true super-agers may comprise only about 3% of the population. This super-aging subgroup had more years of education and better health. They were also more likely to have no false teeth, a curious fact we will come across again much later when considering nuns and the risk of dementia.

While longer education may initially point to more 'cognitive reserve', and better health point to 'brain reserve', these two factors are not independent. For example, experiencing more years in education is associated with better health in later life. After factoring out these potential contributing causes it is still the case that superior episodic memory in super-agers is related to better preserved brain structure, in other words brain reserve. At the same time, cognitive reserve undoubtedly plays its part.

Studies of the brains of super-agers point to the relative preservation of sites such as the anterior cingulate cortex, the adjacent medial prefrontal cortex, and the hippocampus. Other features of super-agers include a reduced number of neurofibrillary tangles, which are twisted protein threads that contribute to Alzheimer's disease. The status of the entorhinal cortex is of much interest as it is both the information doorway to the hippocampus and one of the first sites to display Alzheimer's disease pathology. It is, therefore, fascinating that super-agers may have unusually large entorhinal cortex neurons and contain far fewer neurofibrillary tangles (Gefen et al., 2021). In contrast, their levels of amyloid plaques, another marker for Alzheimer's disease, can appear similar to those who age normally, as well as those showing early signs of dementia. Such information has galvanised research into how neurofibrillary tangles might promote Alzheimer's disease (see *Alzheimer's disease*).

I have left the very aged to last. June Spencer, who played a main character (Peggy Woolley) in the British radio soap opera 'The Archers' for over 70 years, was still performing when over 100 years old. Nicholas Parsons hosted the BBC's 'Just a Minute', for over 50 years, only stopping when he was 95 years old. Meanwhile, David Attenborough at 98 remains involved in ground-breaking television documentaries (Figure 3.3). Hopefully, these examples help to counteract stereotypes concerning extreme aging and cognition.

Terminal decline: A rather different time-course of cognitive decline is seen if cognition, including memory, is tracked back from the time of death. The 'terminal decline' model describes the acceleration of cognitive loss as we approach death. Some studies suggest that this acceleration begins three or four years before death, others suggest an onset beginning

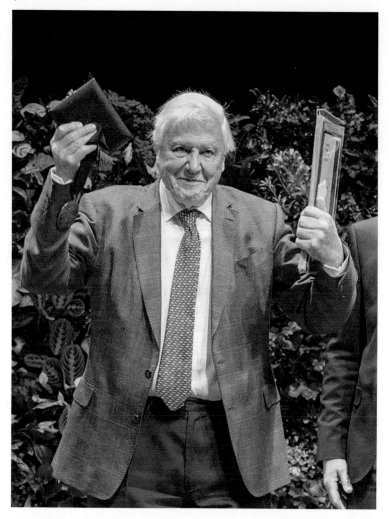

Figure 3.3 David Attenborough, still working on radio and television well into his 90s.

as much as seven or eight years before death. Increasing age further accelerates this terminal cognitive decline. One piece of good news is that the onset time and extent of decline varies for different cognitive abilities. While episodic memory and verbal speed display evident terminal decline, measures of semantic memory, such as extent of vocabulary, seem more resilient.

One cause of terminal decline is the accumulation of neurological dysfunctions, which can have snowball effects. While these dysfunctions may include those caused by the various dementias, there remains a large range of other, unexplained factors responsible for the accelerating loss of cognition. For your reassurance it is perhaps worth emphasising that not every person shows terminal decline, it is a population effect with many individual exceptions.

4 How accurate and durable are our adult memories?

Miss Prism: *Memory, my dear Cecily, is the diary that we all carry about us.*
Cecily: *Yes, but it usually chronicles the things that have never happened and couldn't possibly have happened.*

The Importance of Being Earnest, Oscar Wilde (1895)

This witty exchange captures the essence of what has, at times, been a highly acrimonious debate. The controversy centres around two related questions: whether our memories are permanent and whether they can remain accurate.

The idea that memories are permanent has a long history. In 1777, the German philosopher Johann Nicolas Tetens wrote: *"Each idea does not only leave a trace or a consequent of that trace somewhere in the body, but each of them can be stimulated – even if it is not possible to demonstrate this in a given situation"*. This sense of hidden but permanent memories is reflected in popular analogies with diaries and video recorders, which are favoured by over 60% of the public (Simons & Chabris, 2011).

The opposing view emphasises the fragility of our memories. Again, there were past champions. Here is what the polymath Francis Galton wrote in 1879 about his lost memories. *"The instances, according to my personal experience, are very rare, and even those are not very satisfactory, in which some event recalls a memory that had lain absolutely dormant for many years"*. The controversy is, however, not just about losing memories, it is also about whether we can unwittingly change past memories. If memories can be replaced, how can we distinguish what did or did not happen.

Some forms of memory are undoubtedly very long-lasting. Semantic memory is one of the two major classes of explicit long-term memory. This class of memory contains shared, factual knowledge about the world, including language and concepts. Long ago, as a child, I learnt the word and concept of a 'zoo-keeper', the very first career I wanted. By its very nature, semantic memory it is unlikely to suffer interference from conflicting information. It is also likely to be reinforced by repeated exposure to the same shared fact. I assume I will always know what a zoo-keeper does. Paris remains the capital of France, a fact that I have often heard or read, and one I trust I will never forget.

Likewise, some implicit memories appear very durable. Once acquired, perceptual-motor skills are unusually long lasting. The motor skills involved in riding a bike seems near-permanent, partly because we rarely experience competing information. Such learning typically follows many repeated learning experiences, adding to its durability.

In contrast, other implicit memories are less stable. A classically conditioned response (for example, blinking to the sound of a tone) will extinguish when the association between

DOI: 10.4324/9781003537649-4

the conditioned stimulus (the tone) and an unconditioned stimulus (a puff of air to the eye) ceases. This extinction may reflect the unlearning of the previous association or reflect overwriting by a new set of learnt contingencies, reflecting that the tone is now *not* associated with the air puff.

Habituation, the diminished reaction to a repeated stimulus, also shows forgetting. After a delay, 'dishabituation', the recovered reaction to the original stimulus, can be seen. Surprisingly, priming, the enhanced availability of a memory after a previous exposure, can sometimes be long-lasting. People can still show faster picture naming (priming) for images previously seen almost a year earlier. Even so, priming, a form of implicit memory, is not thought to be permanent.

In practice, the debate over memory permanence centres on episodic memory, our memory for the individual events in our life. Unlike skill learning and semantic knowledge, which benefit from multiple learning opportunities, episodic memory, by its very definition, arises from a single experience. In a heroic study from 1986, the Dutch psychologist Willem Wagenaar systematically recorded 1605 personal events in his diary over a four-year period (Figure 4.1). His diary entries not only included what happened, but also where and when it happened, and who was also present. Wagenaar then showed displayed amazing patience by waiting for another year before testing his memory for these events.

As might be expected, his memory was slightly poorer for those events furthest back in time. Of particular relevance was his ability to compare the effectiveness of different retrieval cues, namely what, where, when, and with whom. Could these cues help him to retrieve some or even all lost memories? Giving 'what' information was the most effective for recalling past memories, while 'when' information was the least effective. Combining the various cue types further increased the likelihood of recalling all four elements of an event, but levels of recall were never perfect. The number of irretrievable events rose to 20% for the longest retention period (five years), despite having multiple retrieval cues. Even after considerable prompting, these episodic memories simply appeared to be lost. Nevertheless, the surviving 80% keep alive the possibility of very long-lasting episodic memories.

The case for permanent episodic memories

> When I was younger I could remember anything.
>
> Mark Twain (1907)

Miss Prism's view – that memories for personal events are 'written down' in a permanent form, even if we cannot always retrieve them – has at various times proved highly popular. As explained, there are two elements to this view; that memories are permanent and that memories remain unchanged.

Memory engrams: Now might be a good time to introduce the word 'engram'. This word, coined by Richard Semon in 1904, refers to the brain's memory trace. More specifically, an engram is an assembly of neurons whose state creates a representation of a past experience so that it might be stored and later retrieved. As will soon become clear, the study of engrams has been revolutionised by recent research involving mice and laser lights.

It is worth pausing to say a little about the tragic life of Richard Semon. His academic career at Jena in Germany was irreversibly changed after a scandalous affair with the wife (Maria Krehl) of one of the professors. Richard and Maria moved to Munich and while there he developed his ideas about memory traces, though they made little impact at

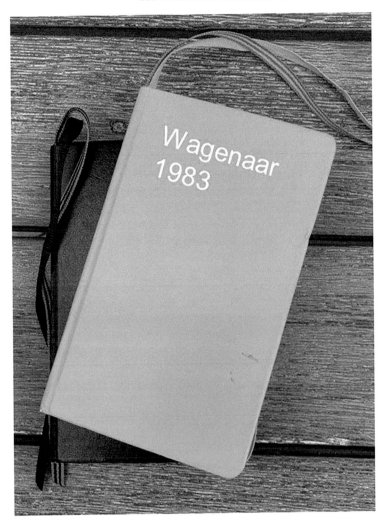

Figure 4.1 Willem Wagenaar recorded daily events in a series of diaries, then tested his recall 1–5
years later.

Source: Wagenaar, 1986.

the time. In 1918, Maria died of cancer. Later that same year, at the age of 59, Richard
Semon shot himself through the heart, while lying on Maria's bed covered in a German flag.

Semon's ideas helped to promote the search for the engram. One famous searcher, Karl
Lashley, asked whether destroying a restricted part of the rat brain might remove a specific
memory, based on the premise that it contained the relevant engram. After over 30 years of
research, starting in 1917, he concluded that the size of the tissue removed, not its location,
predicted the extent of any memory loss.

Despite Lashley's fruitless search, memory engrams suddenly looked far more plausible
following startling observations made by the neurosurgeon Wilder Penfield (Figure 4.2).
Beginning from the 1940s, Penfield would sometimes electrically stimulate the brains of
conscious patients during surgeries to alleviate epilepsy. Occasionally the patient would
describe scenes or spoken words evoked by the brain stimulation. Some descriptions seemed

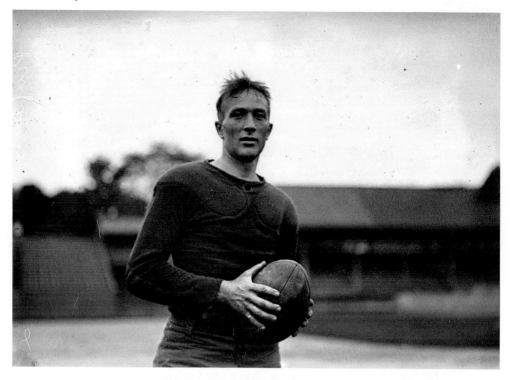

Figure 4.2 Wilder Penfield at Princeton long before his famous brain stimulation studies.

like genuine memories, with visual and auditory experiences akin to real-life sensations. These responses were called 'experiential'. Here are some examples of the experiential episodes recorded by Penfield (1968).

A young secretary MM reported the following *"Oh, I had a very, very familiar memory, in an office somewhere. I could see the desks. I was there and someone was calling to me, a man leaning on a desk with a pencil in his hand"*.

Patient JT *"Yes, Doctor, yes, Doctor! Now I hear people laughing - my friends in South Africa ... Yes, they are my two cousins, Bessie and Ann Wheliaw"*.

Another patient described *"a guy coming through the fence at the baseball game, I see the whole thing"*. A little later he explained: *"I just happened to watch those two teams play when the fellow came through the fence ..."*.

From these descriptions, Penfield became convinced of the existence of engrams. It is worth quoting what he said.

> *"It is clear that the neuronal action that accompanies each succeeding state of consciousness leaves its permanent imprint on the brain. The imprint, or record, is a trail of facilitation of neuronal connections that can be followed again by an electric current many years later with no loss of detail, as though a tape recorder had been receiving it all"*.

(Penfield, 1969)

Clearly Penfield believed he was releasing memory traces that had lain dormant for many years – switching on the brain's tape recorder. Penfield was not alone. Later neurosurgeons have confirmed that brain stimulation can sometimes produce 'experiential' responses in conscious patients (Curot et al., 2017).

Engrams updated: Penfield thought he had discovered the engram, though it remained a theoretical construct. The goal for many neuroscientists became the quest to track down and isolate the engram, should it exist. That goal has now been achieved, in both rodents and fish. The procedure is surely the stuff of science fiction, as it involves shining a light into a particular brain structure to seemingly release a memory.

The first step was to label just those neurons activated by a specific learning experience. There is a class of genes called 'immediate-early genes'. (They are 'immediate' because they are more directly stimulated into action than other genes.) Immediate-early genes, such as one called c-*fos*, are switched on in active neurons. In a typical study, a mouse learns that a certain location is associated with a mild foot shock. That same learning experience activates an array of neurons that turn on their c-*fos* genes. The trick is to engineer the c-*fos* gene so that when it is turned on during this experience it produces an additional chemical compound within that neuron. For 'optogenetics', that compound is both sensitive to light and alters the reactivity of the neuron. For example, when illuminated, the chemical excites the neuron.

The next step involves shining a laser light onto part of the brain. This helps to re-activate the c-*fos* positive neurons, as they are now light responsive. Their activation re-creates key elements of the initial learning event. For example, switching on the light causes the mouse to freeze. In other words, the mouse behaves as if it were suddenly back in the fear-inducing location, where it would remain motionless.

While the initial optogenetic studies focussed on hippocampal engrams, subsequent studies have found 'engrams' in other brain sites. Additional studies show how engrams are modified during consolidation. Engrams also show properties such as extinction and forgetting, adding to their resemblance of natural memories.

While animal engrams provide a unique platform from which to study the structure of a memory, there are many cautions. One concern is that these animal engram studies do not involve episodic memory. Rather, the tasks often rely on classical conditioning, limiting their generalisability. Another concern is that the techniques used to activate engrams often target restricted brain sites, such as the hippocampus. As is now evident, most memory representations reflect a wide array of subcortical-cortical interactions, alongside cortical-cortical interactions. While the ability to target and manipulate 'memories' raises many exciting possibilities, it also creates new ethical issues.

It is now time to return to the question of memory permanence. While the study of animal engrams is revolutionising neuroscience, it is yet to resolve the question of memory permanence. We know that engrams are modified during consolidation and are dynamic in nature, but these elements do not disprove their durability. One problem, already mentioned, is that animal studies cannot directly test episodic memory, having to rely on other categories of learning such as classical conditioning. A further, practical problem is the challenge of re-activating the same engram after an extended delay of months, or even longer, to test for permanence. So far, this has not been achieved. For these reasons, engram research in animals has yet to resolve the permanence debate.

The retrieval of 'lost' memories: Belief in memory permanence is helped by the familiar experience of a seemingly lost memory suddenly resurfacing. The most famous literary example is that of Marcel Proust (1913), who on smelling a madeleine biscuit dipped in tea was taken back to the Sunday mornings in childhood spent with his aunt. The strong impression is that the 'lost' memory was waiting for the right cue. A similar experience happens when re-visiting a holiday resort, the place brings back seemingly-forgotten memories from past holidays (*see 'Context-Dependent Memory'*). Likewise, Wagenaar, with his diary, showed how providing partial cues (who, what, where, when) helped the retrieval of many of this memories.

Other potential routes to lost memories include verbal-free association – saying the first word that comes into your mind when given a target word, which then leads to further associations. If I say candle, you might say 'church', which might you take you to a specific memory. (In my case it was Christmas carols in Winchester Cathedral). This method has been used by therapists to help uncover links to memories that may not normally seem available. There is no doubt that memory retrieval is aided by a variety of cues associated with the target memory. This effect was clearly demonstrated by Wagenaar's diary study. This same concept is embedded in influential ideas such as the 'encoding specificity hypothesis', which proposes that we automatically encode items with their surrounding cues. Those same cues subsequently promote recall of the linked memory. It is, therefore, entirely plausible that cues generated by free association could help bring old memories to the surface. But the difficulty is in knowing whether, with the right cue, *all* old memories could be retrieved.

The power of hypnosis: About 55% of the U.S. general public think that hypnosis is useful in helping witnesses accurately recall details of crimes (Simons & Chabris, 2011). This view stems from the common belief that seemingly forgotten aspects of a memory can be retrieved under hypnosis. In 1976, in Chowchilla, Californian, the bus driver Ed Ray was abducted, along with 26 students, and imprisoned in an underground trailer (Figure 4.3). According to Time Magazine, under hypnosis Ed Ray was later able to recall all but one

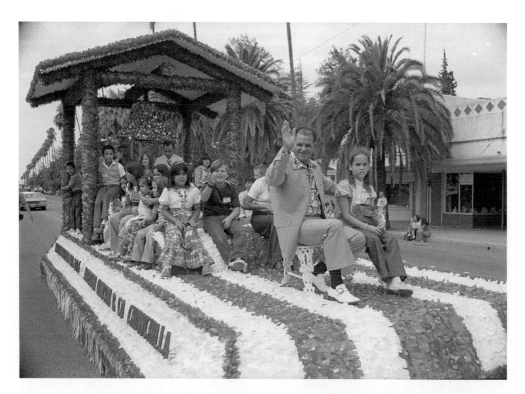

Figure 4.3 Parade for the Chowchilla kidnapping victims, with Ed Ray at the front from 1976.

digit from the licence plate of his abductors. This impressive feat implies that hypnosis might help in many criminal cases. While this one-off example may seem compelling, it is far from proof. Controlled scientific studies are needed to determine if hypnosis can indeed retrieve lost memories.

One influential experiment required participants to watch police training films that showed simulated violent crimes (Geiselman et al., 1985). Two days later they tried to recall the films. Recall when hypnotised gave an average of nine additional correct details, but no increase in the amount of false information reported. Explanations for this improvement include the possibility that hypnosis encouraged participants to mentally picture the location of the crime as well as re-instating the experience of watching the film. By mentally re-creating the experience and its context, recall should improve. Other studies have also reported that hypnosis can improve recall. Reflecting the potential gains from hypnosis, 13 U.S. States currently allow hypnotically induced testimony in legal cases. Furthermore, the U.S. Supreme Court holds that information and testimony from hypnotised witnesses cannot automatically be excluded if the hypnosis occurred under approved guidelines. (For more information see *H is for Hypnosis, memory, and the law*.)

Together, the combined evidence from brain stimulation, hypnosis, and the recall of old memories prompted by relevant cues, seems to show that some episodic memories are permanent, lying dormant and awaiting resurrection. A further source of evidence comes from those rare individuals with seemingly super-normal memory (see *'Exceptional memory'*).

The case against permanent episodic memories

> When I was younger I could remember anything, whether it happened or not.
>
> Mark Twain (1907)

As you may recall, Cecily (from *The Importance of Being Earnest*) felt that our memories chronicled things that have never happened and could not have happened. When asked in 2021, a panel of memory experts strongly agreed that 'memories are re-constructed', in other words, they are subject to later change (Patihis et al., 2021). The experts clearly sided with Cecily, and we will next see why.

Penfield's engrams re-visited: Let us begin with the memories released by Penfield's brain stimulation. The most obvious concern is that the experiences might not be real memories. Of the 40 patients Penfield reported as having experiential responses, only 12 described scenes with sounds, properties consistent with a real memory rather than an evoked image. The issue is whether the electrical stimulation had released a past memory or, instead, had encouraged the synthesis of different impressions. In other words, the experiences were re-constructed rather than re-lived. Of the described experiences, some portrayed plausible memories, but not all. One woman reported visiting a timber yard following brain stimulation, but later added that in real life she had never visited such a place. (There is the dilemma of whether she had never visited a timber yard or whether she had forgotten her visit.)

Following Penfield, other neurosurgeons have described how direct brain stimulation in conscious patients can evoke different sensations. Frequent reports include perceptual images and feelings of familiarity. Sometimes these perceptual sensations are drawn from semantic memory, such as 'seeing' a 'Bugs Bunny' cartoon or 'hearing' famous songs like 'Wish You Were Here' by Pink Floyd or the 'Star Wars' theme (Curot et al., 2017). Patients may describe a scene apparently drawn from memory, but that scene is often devoid of any specific memory. These static experiences do not move forward in time, with the exception of the hallucination of hearing music. Consequently, scenes do not progress as would happen in a story or a re-lived experience. For this reason, the patient remains passive and does not seem to actively participate in the hallucinated scene.

A thorough review of 80 years of experiential phenomena concluded that brain stimulation, especially of the temporal lobes, can elicit memory-like experiences but they are most frequently of a general autobiographical nature and do not chronicle specific events (Curot et al., 2017). Consequently, the large majority of these experiences lack the depth and detail of information consistent with episodic memory. Only around 14% of induced reminisces could be thought of as episodic-like, but many of these still lacked detail and were fragmentary. Only a small proportion of all evoked reminisces were described as strongly episodic (4%).

This still leaves an intriguing 4% of memories, suggesting that electrical stimulation might, just sometimes, release old episodic memories. If so, it is important to know how old those memories might be, given the question of memory permanence. As far as could be determined, this small set of episodic memories reflected events from between one day to several years ago (Curot et al., 2017). The furthest back in time, 14 years, concerned a picnic in Brewer Park, Ontario, when the person was eight years old.

Concerns about hypnosis: One of the reasons to believe in memory permanence came from the potential power of hypnosis to access lost memories. On the plus side, hypnosis might help people concentrate and mentally re-create past contexts to aid memory recall. While occasional studies do find improved levels of recall, such studies are more the exception. To complicate matters, there is the ever-present concern as to whether any 'lost' memories retrieved under hypnosis are real or whether they are unintentionally fabricated.

A recent survey from 2021 highlights the gulf between memory experts, who disagreed with the statement that 'Hypnosis accurately retrieves memories', while the general public agreed with the statement (Patihis et al., 2021). A frequent problem is that, under hypnosis, people show an increased willingness to provide an answer, even if they do not have the appropriate memory. Consequently, they will fill in missing parts of their memory with fabrications. This tendency is called confabulation. Although more correct details might be reported, more incorrect details are also supplied.

Hypnosis can also increase the belief in misleading information, creating a misplaced confidence in erroneous memories. One likely cause is the desire to fulfil the perceived wishes of the experimenter (so called 'demand characteristics'). To make matters worse, hypnosis increases susceptibility to leading questions. As we have seen with age-regression under hypnosis, it is possible to report events that could never have happened. A similar heightened suggestibility is seen when, under hypnosis, people inaccurately behave as if they have a specific clinical condition, such as amnesia or are suffering from delusions. Hypnosis is not a reliable way to enhance recall, and so its value in determining the permanence or accuracy of our memories remains highly questionable.

Implanting false memories: A major part of the debate over memory accuracy revolves around the creation of false memories. Please read the following list of 15 words:

hot, snow, warm, winter, ice, wet, frigid, chilly, heat, weather, freeze, air, shiver, arctic, frost.

We will return to these words just a little later.

If hypnosis is not the way to release lost memories, what of 'truth-serums'. As far back as the first century AD, Pliny the Elder referred to the proverb *"in vino veritas"* – in wine there is truth. By the 20th century alcohol was replaced by a wide variety of other drugs claimed to ensure truthful recollections. Alas, just as hypnosis can increase the readiness to supply answers, be they correct or incorrect, the same problem applies to so-called truth-serums (see *T is for Truth-serums*). At present, there are no pharmacological methods to target lost memories, unless they involve re-activating someone's physiological condition at the time of the original experience, which is called state-dependent learning (see *Context and memory*).

Now, without looking, try and recall that list of 15 words you read earlier.

Many people will recall the word 'cold', even though it was not present (Roediger & McDermott, 1995). People still make this error even if warned not to guess. The same trick also works for pictures of items that are closely related in meaning. This class of false memory task is referred to as the Deese-Roediger-McDermott paradigm (DRM for short), in honour of its various originators.

One remarkable aspect of this false-word effect is that people claim they can actually remember the non-presented word, re-experiencing the contextual, physical, and temporal details associated with its (non) presentation. By many measures, the false memory is often behaviourally and experientially indistinguishable from a true memory. Roediger & McDermott presumed that the never-present word (e.g., cold) is activated and then recalled because of its repeated associations with the list words. They thought that each word on the list promotes other associations, and the strength of the repeated associations with the word 'cold' often leads to the false memory. A related explanation is that each word creates a fuzzy trace, so that the 'gist' of the word is remembered. On retrieval, a strong associate such as 'cold' will be confused with a genuine target word. These false memories do not, by themselves, show that episodic memories cannot be permanent. Rather they show the enormous potential to be misled in what we recall. The false memory also shows that something that looks and feels like a real memory, need not be a real memory.

Equally damning would be the demonstration that memories can be changed ('re-constructed') after their initial encoding and storage. I have a friend who when introducing me in social settings will often recount anecdotes about our shared experiences. One example involves chasing someone riding a motorbike over sports pitches who turned out to have a knife. Over time I feel that his version of this story has repeatedly mutated, making it more and more dramatic. I am sure that my friend is completely confident that the latest version of these dramatic events is correct (just as I am sure of my own version). Indeed Marcel Proust, whose experience of a madeleine biscuit is often used to support the idea of surviving 'lost' memories, also went on to say that the remembrance of things past is not necessarily the remembrance of things as they were.

Countless experiments show that information given after a to-be-remembered event can alter your responses when questioned about the original event, as if a new memory had been implanted. The content of false memories includes non-existent tape recorders, stop signs, moustaches, hammers, car colours, and barns (Loftus & Pickrell, 1995). Methods used to generate such mistakes include 'false feedback', in which participants see or hear false information implying a change in the event that they experienced. In 'memory implantation' the suggested occurrence of the non-existent event is supported by false testimony from an individual's family members or doctored photographs. Finally, in 'imagination inflation' participants are instructed to repeatedly imagine events that have not occurred. As we will see, false responses do not necessarily prove the establishment of a new false memory, but they increase the likelihood that this can and does occur.

Many of the original experiments arose from concerns over the accuracy of eye-witness testimony. The significance of this research is underlined by claims that the single, leading cause of wrongful conviction in the U.S. is the false identification of an innocent suspect by an eye-witness. This same claim is supported by how DNA evidence has overturned several hundred cases highlighted by the Innocence Project. Famously, Elizabeth Loftus showed that later visual information, such as changing the traffic signals associated with a traffic accident (e.g., replacing a yield sign with a stop sign) could then alter the memory of the original film that showed the car accident. Even the wording of the questions used to subsequently assess someone's memory can seemingly affect recollection. Take the two questions: 'how fast were the cars going when they smashed into each other? and 'how fast were the cars going when they hit each other? The word 'smashed' not only gave higher speed estimates but also encouraged those participants to agree that they had seen (non-existent) broken glass.

On the 6th May 2002, the Dutch politician Pim Fortuyn (Figure 4.4) was shot and killed by an animal rights activist. Despite considerable media coverage, there was no video footage of the actual shooting (there was video footage of the dead body). A survey of peoples' memory for the murder included the question 'Did you see the amateur film of the Fortuyn shooting?' (Smeets et al., 2009). Follow-up questions asked whether those who had seen the (non-existent) film could provide more details. Here, interest focussed on those (false) details

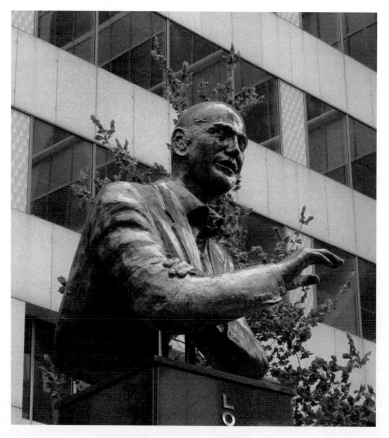

Figure 4.4 Statue in honour of Pim Fortuyn, Dutch politician.

that could only be seen from a video of the actual assassination, e.g., smoke from the gun and Pim Fortuyn collapsing. The confidence of any such false memories was also assessed.

Remarkably, two thirds of the participants claimed to have seen the non-existent video of the assassination, of these, 10% described imaginary details. Similarly, as many as a third of those who falsely reported seeing a video of the explosion of the No. 30 bus in Tavistock Square in London on 7th July 2005, added imaginary details. Finally, about 50% of participants in a study falsely reported seeing video footage of Princess Diana's fatal crash in 1997, though there was none.

Before concluding that these false memory errors are common, we need to pause. The misinformation findings are not without controversy. There is, for example, evidence that while the never experienced 'memory' may be given preferentially, if you test for the presence of the seemingly 'lost' correct information it can sometimes still be found. A related concern is that subjects might understandably trust the experimenter's memory more than their own, causing them to switch their response. Similarly, participants may be eager to please the researcher who provided the misinformation ('demand characteristics').

A further difficulty is how to best define a false memory. Does it require adding false details to the suggested event or is it sufficient to merely believe that the false version was experienced. A particular issue highlighted by the Pim Fortuyn study was that after careful debriefing, the large majority of participants who reported seeing the non-existent assassination video claimed they had misunderstood the critical question ('Did you see the amateur film of the Fortuyn shooting?'). They said that they thought that the question also referred to images of the aftermath of the shooting. Clearly, any ambiguity in the critical test question can have a big impact. That does, however, still leave us with the small but fascinating 10% who still reported details of the imaginary video even after being fully debriefed (Smeets et al., 2009). That subset may indeed have false memories.

For very good reasons, there is considerable interest in whether you can trust your childhood memories. In a famous study, adults were given four stories from their childhood and asked to write down as much as they could remember about these events (Loftus & Pickrell, 1995). Three stories referred to true events, the fourth story never happened according to their parents. One such false story was about being lost in a shopping mall as a child. Over successive interviews, a quarter of the participants repeatedly claimed to remember some details of being lost in a shopping mall.

In a related study using similar methods, about a quarter of the participants falsely remembered being at a wedding reception and spilling a punch bowl over the parents of the bride. Other events used in these memory implantation studies include putting Slime in a teacher's desk. In some studies, confidence in these false childhood memories is raised by asking participants to imagine a list of such events. These findings clearly strengthen the idea that people can develop false childhood memories, but they are not definitive given the issues of demand characteristics and the potential problem of placing your faith in the experimenter's memory.

For these reasons it is important to know if false memories differ in any way from true ones, and so might be distinguished. It is agreed that most false memories are less vivid and have less sensory detail. (Yet, statistical analyses of the recent TV show 'Traitors' reveals that participants are no better than at chance when trying to identify those who are lying.) False memories often come with lower confidence than real memories. Here, a major factor is plausibility. Our confidence is raised when implanted memories concern events that are highly feasible. This feasibility often stems from having genuine memories that overlap with aspects of the false memory, such as visiting shopping malls.

One solution might be to see if brain activity, measured with fMRI, is different for true or false memories. Increases in cortical activity are seen when people are encouraged to lie. Some of these differences, especially in prefrontal cortex, probably reflect the greater cognitive effort involved in deliberate deception, though this load may reduce if the lie is well rehearsed. To further reduce this load, we should look at false memories that are held to be genuine.

The false recall DRM task (described above) should be particularly informative as false memories, such as recalling the word 'cold', are unintentional and not unusually effortful. Comparisons using this method have found similar patterns of brain activity for true recall and false recall (McDermott et al., 2017), though there can sometimes be subtle differences in parts of the prefrontal cortex. Even so, brain activity is almost indistinguishable between a truth and an unintentional lie, and any differences are not reliable enough to serve as a practical lie detector. Given that U.S. courts have been asked to admit the results of fMRI-based lie detection scans as evidence during trials, there is cause for considerable unease.

We have yet to solve the question of whether false memories disprove the idea of memory permanence. For this we should consider why a false memory happens. Explanations include that the original experience was never encoded, that the false memory co-exists with the original memory (the false memory being preferred because of demand characteristics, its greater memory strength, or source misattribution), or that the new information blends or substitutes for the original, creating a revised memory trace (so the true original is lost).

To test the co-existence explanation, participants are offered a second guess to help find the correct information. This method often fails to reveal the correct memory. Likewise, offering monetary incentives rarely improves the recall of seemingly lost (correct) information. Similarly, warning people in advance of recall that they have may been exposed to misleading information often makes little difference, presumably because the misleading information has already been incorporated. However, none of these methods is definitive and there are probably multiple causes of the misinformation effect.

Memory construction, re-consolidation, and neurogenesis: There are further reasons not to trust our memories. Our experiences are not written down on a blank sheet. Rather they are interpreted (constructed) and retrieved (re-constructed) based on our prior knowledge and expectations. People with opposing views about a controversial topic, be it the legality of abortion, U.S. military action in the Persian Gulf, or U.K. Brexit, show a memory bias for information that supports their position. Interestingly, this bias is lessened in those with high prior knowledge about the topic. Such findings, which are explored at greater length in the next section, highlight the many biases that pervasively affect our memories and their subsequent recall.

Related conclusions come from the startling phenomenon known as 're-consolidation'. 'Consolidation' implies that once a memory is stored it remains fixed for the lifetime of that memory. But, what if memories become susceptible to alteration as soon as they become active again, such as during the recall of that same memory. Changes made to the memory at that later stage are called 're-consolidation' (Figure 4.5).

In one of the first experimental demonstrations of re-consolidation, rats learnt to associate a tone with a foot-shock (Nader et al., 2000). Days later, the acquired fear memory was re-activated by playing that same tone. As the tone was played, protein synthesis was blocked in a brain structure called the amygdala (known to be vital for fear-conditioning). Remarkably, this procedure caused amnesia for the fear learning, even though that same learning had been successfully acquired days before. Re-activation of the fear memory put it into a vulnerable state that could now be pharmacologically manipulated, in this case

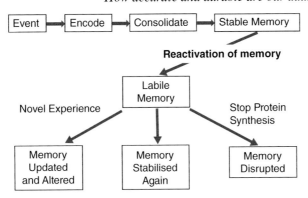

Figure 4.5 Memory re-consolidation: Re-activation of a memory with potential outcomes.

removed (Figure 4.5). Subsequent studies have demonstrated similar effects in animals for a wide variety of learning tasks and a variety of drugs.

In normal life, re-consolidation helps us to maintain and update memories. The process may also encourage new links between related events, thereby refining knowledge and building schemas. But re-consolidation may also lead to the loss and alteration of memories, creating errors. The latter property raises the spectre that the mere act of retrieving a personal memory puts that same memory at risk (as with my friend and his anecdotes).

At a clinical level, there is growing interest in the use of re-consolidation methods to help target and remove those traumatic memories that lie at the heart of the Post-Traumatic Stress Disorder (PTSD). The hope is to re-activate the traumatic experience while giving a drug that should interfere with that same memory, which is now in a vulnerable state. While the results of recent clinical trials have often been mixed, this approach holds considerable interest and potential promise. A more established treatment for PSTD known as 'Eye Movement Desensitisation and Reprocessing (EMDR) is thought by many to partly rely on re-consolidation processes.

The final piece of evidence in this debate comes from a most unlikely source – the Atom bomb tests in the 1950s and 1960s. The resulting clouds of radiation globally increased exposure to certain isotopes. By measuring levels of ^{14}C in post-mortem brain tissue it is possible to date the age of that person's neurons. These measures helped to confirm that a region of the hippocampus (called the dentate gyrus) produces new neurons throughout life. But, in addition to neurons being replaced, there is the loss of neurons over time that exceeds the numbers of new neurons. Both effects will impact on the permanence of our episodic memories if it is assumed, as many do, that the hippocampus remains vital for their consolidation and retrieval. Consequently, critical elements of a memory will be lost or replaced over time. Either way, key properties of the original memory will change, so it cannot remain as an exact copy.

We should now be in a position to appreciate the insights held by the attendees at the 2010 Psychonomic Society meeting. Almost 100% of these 'experts' disagreed with the idea that 'once you have experienced an event and formed a memory of it, that memory does not change' (Simons & Chabris, 2011).

5   Comprehension, encoding, and recall

You see, but you do not observe.

Sherlock Holmes to John Watson.
A Scandal in Bohemia, Arthur Conan Doyle (1891)

As Sherlock Holmes astutely pointed out, we may see the same thing but extract very different information. What we subsequently remember is shaped by our prior knowledge and attitude. Indulge me with the following football score from 2020, *Manchester United 1 Tottenham Hotspur 6*. If you have no interest in football this score may mean next to nothing. If you are a neutral, you would probably be very surprised. If, like me, you endure the ups and downs of supporting Spurs (the only Football League team named after a Shakespearean character), you will never forget the result. If you support Manchester United, you will try and forget this aberration. (I will discuss *Directed/Motivated Forgetting* later.)

Clearly the same piece of information, a football score in this case, means very different things to different people and is remembered differently. In fact, we best remember the scores of those football teams we most like and most dislike. Unsurprisingly, opposing fans perceive and recall the same match in very different ways. We do not walk around with a blank tape on which to record our memories, rather our prior knowledge and expectations dramatically affect what we encode and remember. In this way, past memories guide our new memories.

Meaning, memory, and schemas: Please read the following, rather ambiguous, passage. It comes from a landmark experiment that is both elegant and simple. (Apologies if you have read this before.)

> The procedure is actually quite simple. First arrange things into different bundles depending on make-up. Don't do too much at once. In the short run this may not seem important, however, complications easily arise. A mistake can be costly. Next, find facilities. Some people must go elsewhere for them. Manipulation of appropriate mechanisms should be self-explanatory. Remember to include all other necessary supplies. Initially the routine will overwhelm you, but soon it will become just another facet of life. Finally, rearrange everything into original groups. Return these to their usual places. Eventually they will be used again. Then the whole cycle will have to be repeated.
>
> (Bransford & Johnson, 1972)

Your task is to remember as much of the passage as possible. But the experiment has a clever twist. Half of the participants were told the subject matter of the passage *before* hearing the

DOI: 10.4324/9781003537649-5

text. The other half were told the subject matter immediately *after* hearing the passage. You might want to guess the subject matter of the passage. You also might want to predict the result. Those who were told that the upcoming passage was about washing clothes recalled twice as many details as those given the title after hearing the passage. Having a title for this ambiguous text made a huge difference as the participants could far better understand and assimilate its contents. We now know that this is a highly reliable effect. One consequence is that subheadings can help considerably when reading technical text.

Consider the next passage.

> The voyage was long and the crew was full of anticipation. No one really knew what lay beyond the new land that they were heading for. There were, of course, specula-tions concerning the nature of the new place, but this small group of men would be the only ones who would know the real truth. These men were participating in an event that would change the face of history.
>
> (Hasher & Griffin, 1978)

In a clever variant, people were given another ambiguous paragraph but this time it had one of two titles ('Columbus Discovers a New World', or 'First Trip to the Moon'). Depending on the title, people remembered different elements of the passage. Again, what you recall is shaped by your expectations and prior knowledge. Similarly, when people read the same house description but from the perspective of either a potential house buyer or a burglar, different house details were recalled.

During our life we learn what to expect in different situations. We amass generic infor-mation about a host of distinct events. These events concern almost every aspect of life, from having breakfast to cleaning our teeth, heading to work, buying a coffee, watching television, or going to a birthday party. Each separate cluster of knowledge is called a 'schema'. Each *schema* creates a cognitive framework that helps us to interpret and organ-ise relevant information. Most of us will have a schema for washing clothes. That schema helps you to understand the ambiguous text above and, as we shall see, understanding is a short-cut to richer encoding and remembering. That understanding includes deciding how the clothes washing description matches your expectations. The title also helps you to add appropriate imagery to the description, which further aids memory.

We are surprised when events or information violate existing schemas. Unexpected events usually receive more attention, for example, a tractor in a supermarket. One of the most memorable opening lines in literature uses this same trick – "*As Gregor Samsa awoke one morning from uneasy dreams he found himself transformed in his bed into a gigantic insect*" (*The Metamorphosis* by Franz Kafka, 1915). This startling image challenges our preconceptions about sleep, dreams, and insects (Figure 5.1). (In fact, there is some debate about exactly what animal Gregor Samsa is transformed into as there are different transla-tions.) A personal favourite opening line is "*It was the day my grandmother exploded*" (*The Crow Road* by Iain Banks, 1992). By breaking our expectations about grandmothers, the sentence grabs our attention and demands additional processing (also see *S is for Surprise*).

When memory is tested by *recognition*, atypical information is often better remembered. For instance, after hearing a story about going to a restaurant, people were more likely to recognise the event of buying some mints after paying the bill (atypical) rather than order-ing dinner (typical), both of which occurred in the story. Comparing the *recall* of typical and atypical information is trickier as typical information is more likely to be arrived at by guessing, being more strongly associated with the relevant category, in this case, going to a

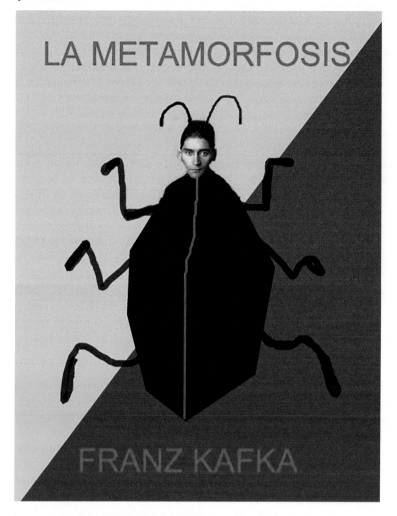

Figure 5.1 The Metamorphosis, Franz Kafka (1915).

restaurant. While the recall of atypical events may be superior at short retention intervals, over time, more typical events tend to dominate people's memory. This pattern is seen when people are asked to recall what they had eaten over preceding weeks.

While deeper understanding and engagement encourages learning, superficial process-ing can leave us embarrassingly ignorant. It is all too easy to demonstrate our readiness to process information at an alarmingly shallow level. The following is a series of memory challenges that should be incredibly easy, but in reality are surprisingly hard.

What is the precise layout of numbers, letters, and symbols on a phone keypad? Can you draw and colour the single letter logo for Google? Which letter occupies the centre of the nine letters in middle row on a standard keyboard? Can you draw the roadside sign (shape, colour, and content) for an upcoming zebra crossing? Can you draw from memory both sides of the Elizabeth 5p and 10p coins? (or whatever currency you might choose, be it euros or dollars).

These memory challenges are much harder than they should be. Most relate to informa-tion that almost every adult will have seen repeatedly, yet that information is surprisingly difficult to recall. In real life, there are numerous examples of how merely seeing or hearing something over and over again can fail to establish a stable memory. The relevance of this learning failure for education is self-apparent.

Part of the explanation for these examples of poor learning centres on how we normally use that information. We need to recognise different coins, but rarely more than that (Figure 5.2). We do not, for example, think about why they are designed the way they are. (If you put together the tail-sides of the Queen Elizabeth 1p, 2p, 5p, 20p, and 50p coins you make a single, joined-up image of the Royal Shield of Arms.) Car drivers have to engage with road signs but only at the level of identification, no deeper elaboration is required (Figure 5.3). If you want to remember some information, you should engage with it. One effective way is to explain that information to another person. In doing so, you are forced to understand the meaning of that information.

Levels-of-processing: The importance of understanding brings us to a topic often called 'levels-of-processing'. The simple, but powerful, idea is that the deeper you process information the better it is subsequently remembered. Imagine I give you a list of words. Rather than telling you to memorise them, I simply ask you to perform what is often called an 'orienting' task.

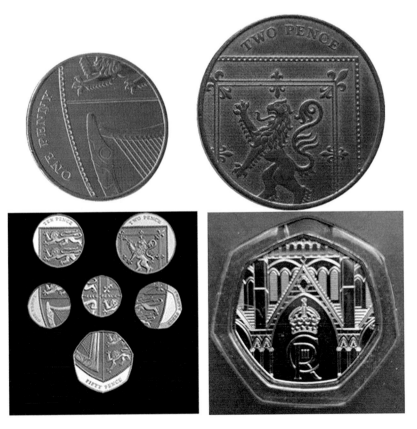

Figure 5.2 U.K. coins to recall. 1p and 2p tail sides (upper). Bottom left the shield made when the tails are combined. Bottom right, detail of new King Charles III 50 p tail.

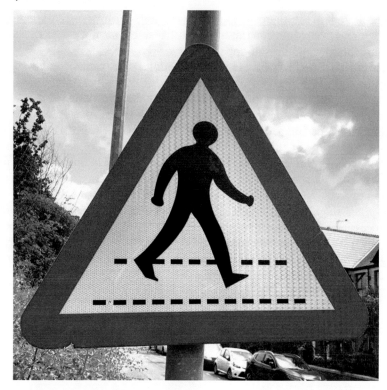

Figure 5.3 Road sign for an upcoming zebra crossing.

For some words you have to decide if they are in upper case or lower case, for example, 'TABLE?' – this is an example of a structural decision. For other words you have to focus on what they sound like by assessing a possible rhyme, for example, 'does crate rhyme with weight?' – this is a phonemic decision. For other words you are asked to make a semantic judgement, 'is a shark a kind of fish?' – this category decision forces you to examine the meaning of the words. After completing the orienting tasks there is an unexpected memory test for those same words in the list. Any learning is described as 'incidental' to the orienting task, as it is a secondary consequence of making the word judgements.

This type of incidental learning task consistently gives the same pattern of results – the poorest word recall happens for the 'structural' (upper/lower case) condition, while the best recall is for those words processed at a 'semantic' (meaning) level. These differences persist even when subjects know beforehand that they will be asked to remember the words. The favoured explanation is that analysing the appearance or sound of a word only requires 'shallow' encoding, resulting in poor incidental learning. Deciding the semantic quality of a word (is an ostrich a bird?) requires 'deeper' encoding that creates greater elaboration of the ostrich 'trace'. This elaboration involves related domains of knowledge. In this way, the memory for 'ostrich' is weaved into place with other items in memory. That same meaningful processing leaves the trace more resistant to loss and more distinctive for retrieval.

A further finding in many levels-of-processing studies is that intentional learning (being told that a memory test would follow) and 'deep' incidental learning (with no prior warning of a memory test) give similar memory scores. In other words, being told to learn a list of words can be no better than being asked to perform a deep (semantic) incidental task. Again, the implications for education are clear.

While the levels-of-processing model predicts the effects of prior knowledge on learning, as a complete account it is not without problems. The most pressing problem is how to independently define 'shallow' or 'deep' processing. Clearly, it is vital to avoid the circular definition that deep encoding produces better learning, while shallow processing produces poorer learning. Intuitively, 'deep' relates to semantic meaning while 'shallow' relates to superficial features such as surface form and colour but confirming that this is case can become circular. The search for an independent measure of depth has, however, proved challenging. One initial candidate, the time taken to process information, with the assumption that 'deeper' takes longer, has unfortunately proved to be unreliable.

An alternative approach has been to find out whether different brain activity patterns can distinguish levels of processing. It is often supposed that deeper processing recruits extra frontal lobe and temporal lobe activity, consistent with top-down processes that strategically guide encoding. (The term 'top-down' refers to processing that is affected by prior models and predictions). This explanation is supported by the repeated activation of a set of frontal, temporal, and parietal cortical brain sites during language tasks that stress word meaning. In this way, brain imaging techniques, such as fMRI, could help to distinguish deep from shallow processing.

Irrespective of whether we can find a precise brain signal that measures depth of processing, the key message is unchanged. Semantic elaboration is a tried and tested route to better learning and memory. To underline the point, I will finish with two personal stories. Both taught me that giving a talk to others about a novel topic forces you to understand the details and implications of that topic, leading to much better learning.

I was at a conference in Trieste, Italy. Very unexpectedly, the day before the main speaker was scheduled to give her talk, she discovered that for family reasons she urgently needed to leave. Before leaving she asked me for a favour – could I deliver her 45-minute talk on Developmental Amnesia? Not only did I have to give her talk but I found myself answering audience questions. Several years later, at a scientific meeting in Liverpool, I was asked at the very last minute to giving someone else's talk as the speaker was in a hurry to leave – she gave birth to her baby later that same day! Both times I realised that I had gained a much better knowledge of someone else's area of scientific endeavour by having to present their findings.

Expert knowledge: Anyone watching the BBC quiz 'Mastermind' will be struck by how some contestants know an astonishing amount about a specific topic yet have mediocre general knowledge. (Specialist topics have included famous British poisoners, Led Zeppelin, the wines of the Loire valley, and burial grounds of London.) We all have pet subjects where our memory shines. This phenomenon, known as 'expert knowledge', highlights the value of deep encoding and rich schema. Mastery of a subject (expert knowledge) brings remarkable advantages when acquiring new information that falls within that same area of expertise. The benefits to memory of expert knowledge have been experimentally confirmed for bird-watchers, chess-players, football fans, baseball fans, physicists, your favourite soap opera, indeed almost any domain of interest.

When a topic is new to you, acquiring additional information is often challenging. But the more you understand a subject, the easier it becomes to add more information about that same subject. In truth, we are all experts at something, and may display impressive memory skills for that particular subject, be it the TV series 'Stranger Things' or 'Friends', Bruce Springstein, the Marvel Comic universe, or cooking recipes.

Expert knowledge is often highly specific. In a famous study, chess players looked at a chess board with 24 pieces in place for five seconds. They then reproduced the position of each piece from memory. Experts remembered four times as many chess positions as novices (Chase & Simon, 1973). Incredibly, this advantage completely disappeared when the chess pieces were placed in random positions on the board, positions that could never occur in a game. The superior performance of the experts for real game positions came from their ability to perceptually group sets of pieces by characteristics such as colour (black versus white), mutual defence between pieces, their proximity, and their ability to attack over small distances. At its extreme level, this expert knowledge translates into the ability of chess grandmasters to play multiple games simultaneously (as seen in 'The Queen's Gambit'). If that is not enough, in 2017 the world record for blindfold chess was claimed by Timur Gareyev, a 28-year-old U.S. grandmaster. He played 48 games simultaneously (losing only six) while wearing a blindfold. He also covered the equivalent of 50 miles on an exercise bike while playing these matches.

In a less dramatic fashion, football fans are better at remembering soccer scores than non-fans. Like chess masters, this benefit is lost when given made-up football scores. Real scores promote richer encoding because of their impact on league standings. My contribution to the study of expert knowledge involved regular listeners of the radio show 'The Archers'. Set in a fictional farming community, 'The Archers' is the world's longest running soap opera. Regular listeners showed a clear advantage over non-listeners when recalling a fabricated 'Archers' episode set in a cattle market. That advantage was lost when the fabricated episode was about a visit to a boat show, even though the two scripts were almost identical. The recall difference occurs because 'The Archers' never visit boat shows, so that particular story received little expert benefit, while cattle markets are a regular feature.

I feel honour bound to mention bird-watching. This is an ideal area for research into expert knowledge as there are so many bird-watchers, of whom I am one. (When my wife and I compare past holidays, she remembers what we ate, I remember the birds I saw.) As you might predict, bird-watchers show better memory for pictures of birds than novices, a difference that is greatest for families of birds with which the person is familiar. Consequently, expert European bird-watchers were better at remembering not only a familiar bird (Eurasian nuthatch) but also an unfamiliar one (Pygmy nuthatch), as the latter has features that identify it as a type of nuthatch, aiding memory (Figure 5.4). Reflecting this difference, experts process pictures of novel birds by grouping them within different bird families (taxonomy) while novices focus on superficial features, such as colour. This superior knowledge also helps experts to reduce interference between seemingly similar birds.

I have often wondered why some people have a store of jokes that they can happily deliver, while others (like me) can never remember a single joke. In 2014, the Australian comic Taylor Goodwin told 571 jokes within an hour at the Arkaba Hotel in Adelaide, breaking the previous official record of 449 jokes. There is a questionnaire called the Humor Perceptiveness Test (which includes 32 very dated gags) that assesses both our memory and comprehension of jokes. Not only can people be categorised as either 'good' or 'poor' comprehenders of jokes, but these two groups show different patterns of brain activity when told a joke. There is also a high correlation between being interested in humour, for instance knowing the names of funny films and comedians, with being able to remember jokes. This association reflects how a growing depth of knowledge (expertise) enhances the ability to remember and retrieve gags. Finally, as we find humorous material easier to remember than equivalent non-humorous material, the good comprehenders of jokes may benefit further, as they are the more amused.

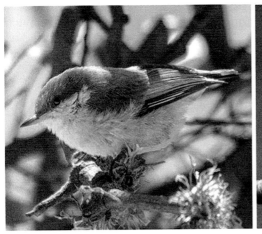 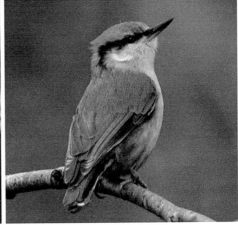

Pygmy nuthatch   Eurasian nuthatch

Figure 5.4 Expert bird-watchers are better at remembering both familiar and unfamiliar birds.

We are almost all experts at distinguishing faces. This ability is so important that we have a critical brain area for processing faces called the fusiform cortex, which is positioned at the base of the temporal lobe. (Fusiform means resembling a spindle, in other words, tapering at both ends.) Remarkably, when bird experts are shown bird images, that same human face area is activated, but this does not happen for pictures of cars (Gauthier et al., 2000). Conversely, when car experts are shown car images, their face area is activated, but this does not happen for pictures of birds. In other words, expertise can lead to marked changes in the way the brain processes information within that specific area of knowledge. For bird-watchers (and car enthusiasts) this processing change reflects how experts learn to distinguish birds (cars) in a holistic manner. When a bird-watcher identifies a distant bird from the briefest of glances, it is rarely by using one diagnostic feature, rather it is the simultaneous bringing together of many small elements. A similar process allows us to discriminate and identify the multitude of faces we encounter. We do not rely on one feature, instead we bring together an ensemble of features in order to identify faces. In this way, expert bird identification mirrors processes that we all use for face identification.

Another group of experts are London Taxi drivers. Famously, they are required to acquire 'The Knowledge'. This involves learning your way around about 26,000 London streets. It normally takes several years to master. Seizing on this natural experiment, in 2000 Eleanor Maguire looked at the brains of London Taxi drivers to see if their extraordinary spatial learning had altered their brains. She found that there was a difference in the proportions of the hippocampus, a brain structure required not only for memory but also for spatial maps. This structural change was not, however, seen in London Bus drivers, who provide a perfect comparison as they only drive set, defined routes. As this hippocampal change takes place as training progresses, we can assume it reflects how the gaining of expert knowledge can alter something as fundamental as brain structure (Woollett & Maguire, 2011). Related research focussing on the brain's white matter shows again how extended practice and expertise can alter brain structure (see *W is for White matter learning*).

Eleanor Maguire's initial taxi driver study was awarded an Ig Nobel in 2003. This dubious prize is usually given to frivolous or downright weird research, but in this case they accidentally gave it to a highly influential study that led the way in showing how our brains can react and respond to training at a structural level. (Other Ig Nobel winners in that same year included a study of homosexual necrophilia in the mallard duck and an analysis of the forces required to drag sheep over various surfaces.)

Perceptual learning: A further aspect of expert knowledge is a phenomenon called perceptual learning. This term describes how repeated experiences can refine our ability to discriminate sights, sounds, smells, tastes, and touch. Examples include trained musicians distinguishing pitch, poultry sorters sexing day-old chicks (surprisingly difficult and surprisingly important), separating cell types down a microscope, and yes, bird-watchers distinguishing subtle differences in plumage. Acquiring these perceptual skills is typically slow and can involve hundreds, even thousands, of practice hours. However, once acquired, the skill is resistant to forgetting.

I should add a footnote concerning 'sommeliers', people who through practice acquire expertise at distinguishing wines. The problem is that even self-styled experts are hugely influenced by prior information such as the cost, origin, and colour of the wine. In 'blind' tastings, when this information is removed, our ability to distinguish wines plummets. Incredibly, a study of 6000 blind tastings found that, on average, people enjoyed more expensive wines slightly *less* (Goldstein et al., 2008). Expert drinkers are sometimes the most prone to be deceived by the colour of wine, giving it expected rather than real qualities. Famously, when Frédéric Brochet gave students of wine science a white wine that had been dyed red, the students described the taste and smell of the dyed wine as if it were red. They gave quite different descriptions for the same wine when it was in its original white state. The visual clues had created a perceptual illusion.

Back to perceptual learning. While some examples may seem rather trite, others are life-changing. With extensive practice, radiologists learn to discern subtle changes in X-ray and MRI images while histologists learn to identify cancerous cells. Unsurprisingly, a considerable amount of perceptual learning takes place as we develop through childhood. Just one of the countless examples is the learnt ability to hear appropriate breaks in one's own language. (This is why foreign languages seem to be spoken rapidly, without breaks.) But, even as adults we can, with extensive training, refine something as fundamental as our ability to distinguish between lines drawn at similar, but slightly different, angles.

The conclusion is that expert performance is often a combination of a finely tuned cognitive skills alongside refined perceptual and motor abilities. These same refined skills leave a fingerprint in the brain. The vocal skills of trained opera singers are, for example, associated with increased activity in a cortical network for fine motor control and enhanced sensorimotor guidance. In particular there is additional sensory cortical activation for those areas receiving feedback from the mouth, tongue, and larynx.

Stereotypes and bias: Up to now, prior knowledge has been seen as an aid to memory, but this is not always true. One concern is how our acquired stereotypes may distort memory. This effect is sometimes called a 'false prior'. It is very hard to avoid deploying stereotypes, which is why 'unconscious bias' can be so difficult to combat. I am sure there are stereotypes about bird-watchers (male, middle-aged, green waistcoats with pockets – to which an American survey added 'creepy', oh dear).

While we often find it easier to remember information that is consistent with our stereotypes, these same stereotypes can unwittingly distort our perception and memory. For example, when people were given lists of stereotypical female roles (including secretary and nurse) they falsely remembered additional, related roles (such as dancer) and traits (for instance, caring) that were not on the list, but consistent with female stereotypes. Conversely, when given lists of stereotypical male roles (including lawyer and soldier), false memories typically matched male stereotypes (Lenton et al., 2001).

Our biases affect our selection of information. Some people immediately turn to the sport's section of any news service, others to politics. But our biases can have more insidious effects. One frequent example is the confirmation bias. This term is given to the way in which we seek and retain information that supports our prejudices. This behaviour is quite natural, as it feels uncomfortable to expose ourselves to information that clashes with our worldview. Consequently, we may go to considerable lengths to avoid this upsetting experience, instead we seek information consistent with our existing expectations. If you asked a Conservative voter and a Labour voter to read both 'The Guardian' and 'The Mail' newspapers, I have no doubt they would show predictable differences in what information they target, how it is judged, and how it is retained. (For the U.S. it might be the 'New York Times' and the 'Wall Street Journal'). In the current world, selection bias is increasingly prevalent. Unseen filters act on social media platforms helping to ensure that we only see content with which we agree, while excluding opposing information. In this way, the hidden algorithms amplify our confirmation biases.

The debate on many important world issues is marred by confirmation bias. One example is the way in which information concerning climate change is sought and retained. There is a greater sense of empathy and message effectiveness when encountering text consistent with one's pre-existing position on climate change. Confirmation bias is also rife when it comes to the use of vaccines, including those for COVID-19. Without mechanisms to combat confirmation bias it is hard to see how public health messages can reach their desired goals. This task is made all the more difficult as we live in an era of self-selected news gathering.

Unsurprisingly, confirmation bias is one of the main props for conspiracy theorists, making it all the more difficult to change to a rational viewpoint. Once a belief is formed, the person seeks out confirmatory information, creating a positive feedback loop. Indeed, belief reversals in areas such as politics and religion as so rare that they become truly noteworthy. In living memory (for some), surely the most significant political U-turn was that of Mikhail Gorbachev, who ended the Cold War and allowed the separation of countries from the Soviet Union. (More will be said about confirmation bias and other biases in the next section, which looks at why we forget.)

The effects of acquired stereotypes and bias have long been studied in the field of criminality. We are all prone to create ill-informed stereotypes, including those concerning gender, race, religion, sexuality, age, height, weight, and even dialect (a pervasive issue in the U.K.). These conscious and unconscious effects have the power to alter our current memories. One famous set of studies by Gordon Allport in the 1940s provided a wake-up call when considering the credibility of eye-witness testimony. In these studies, a subject describes the content of a picture to a second person who could not see the picture. That second-hand description was then passed on to a third person, who had just entered the room and also could not see the original picture. This chain of conversations continued until the passed-on description reached the sixth or seventh subject.

The best-known example from these studies concerned the drawing of a white man holding a razor knife who is apparently confronting a black man in a subway carriage. In over half of the tests, at some stage in the series of reports, the black man (rather than the white man) was said to hold the razor in his hand. Some second-hand descriptions of the original experiment have since implied that the weapon jump occurred even more readily than reported in the original study. This is ironic given that the original study was about memory distortions, such as those seen in second-hand reporting.

As an aside, in Britain the children's game of passing whispered messages from one to another is often called 'Chinese whispers' (Figure 5.5). The U.S. equivalent is often called the 'telephone game'. It is not clear why the British whispers are 'Chinese'; one suggestion is that people imagined that the language was deliberately unintelligible to foreigners. Prior to that, the game was sometimes called 'Russian Scandal' or 'Russian Gossip'. It is easy to see how stereotypes emerge and become reinforced.

There is an understandable belief that aging comes with poorer memory. A fascinating consequence is that when seniors are first given negative stereotypes about old age they then tend to perform poorer on subsequent memory tests than those seniors who were given positive stereotypes. An even more remarkable effect was seen when people were first asked about their belief in age-related stereotypes using sample statements such as 'Old people are absent minded'. The greater the belief in such stereotypes, the poorer was their subsequent performance on memory tasks when aged 60 or over (Levy et al., 2012). The exceptional thing about this study was that the measures of age-related stereotypes were taken *decades* before the memory tests, suggesting long-term effects of such beliefs.

Sadly, it is no surprise to discover that our stereotypes mean that we are biased to think that someone from an ethnic group other than our own is more culpable in a simulated crime. Reflecting this misbelief, we are more likely to wrongly identify someone of different ethnicity as the guilty party. Some of our racial stereotypes can have unforeseen consequences. There is a widespread belief that Asians are shorter than Caucasians. This same belief led to the height estimates of an Asian man in a staged robbery being reduced. Adding to these problems are how we are poorer at distinguishing faces from ethnic groups with which we have less experience. This poor performance largely reflects a lack of perceptual learning.

Bias effects can occur at almost every stage of the criminal and legal process. They can even begin at the earliest stages of information processing. White perceivers often direct more attention to black faces rather than white faces, an effect partly reflecting threatening stereotypes and less prior interaction. Likewise, anxious participants who were exposed to terrorism-related words showed a visual bias toward Middle Eastern faces. Our prior beliefs and expectations also affect how we process what we hear. When the same eye-witness testimony is repeatedly delivered by the same witness, it is rated as less favourable when given

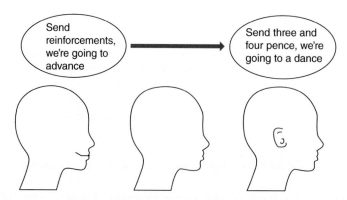

Figure 5.5 How information can become distorted and changed (Chinese whispers).

with a foreign accent. Similarly, identical court testimony given by aged witnesses and by children is interpreted differently than that given by middle-aged witnesses.

We suffer from what are called 'halo' and 'devil' effects. The 'halo' effect describes our tendency to believe that because one aspect of a person is pleasing, so their other characteristics must also be positive. Physical attractiveness can have a strong halo effects. Male markers give higher scores to essays they think were written by more attractive female students. Similarly, I.Q. estimates for men are higher when their faces seem more attractive. As you can imagine, marketing plays on the halo effect, just think of almost every advert you have seen.

The 'devil' effect refers to the opposite bias. In this case, one disliked aspect of a person spills over to make us believe that they are bad in other ways. It is no surprise that villains are often portrayed as being physically unattractive as it makes it easier to believe that they might be evil in other ways. Examples range from Quilp ('The Old Curiosity Shop') to The Joker ('Batman'). Thankfully, there has been a recent backlash against the portrayal of those with physical abnormalities as villains, as it feeds this unfortunate prejudice.

Should you ever find yourself in court, it may matter what you wear. Unsurprisingly, the best advice is to dress conservatively, given the importance of first impressions and resulting halo effects. GOV.UK advises you to dress smartly if you can. High on the list are dark suits for men and a modest dress or business suit for women. What not to wear might include sleeveless shirts, exercise outfits, revealing clothes, T-shirts, flip-flop shoes, or sports shoes. Other suggestions are to cover up tattoos, wear little or no jewellery, and make sure your hair is well groomed. We are all prone to making snap judgements about others that are difficult to undo. (In U.K. courts the only rule about clothing is that you cannot wear anything on your head unless it is for religious reasons.)

Expectations, change blindness, and inattentional blindness: Up to now I have been discussing how our prior learning can affect what we take in and remember, for better or for worse. Our expectations can alter short-term as well as long-term memory. When people are briefly shown sets of letters that include mirror-images, such as Ɔ instead of C, after just a couple of seconds the Ɔ is likely to be recalled as a C. Such illusions of short-term memory highlight again how many obstacles we have to overcome in order to recall events accurately. These instances often arise from the predictive nature of both our sensory and memory processes.

If we misperceive what is in front of us, we will end up with faulty memories (Figure 5.6). The accompanying photo of the author having a drink is rather an extreme example of how our perceptual processes can be fooled. (I will leave you to work it out, but the photo is a true reflection of what the camera saw.)

Sometimes, however, we fail to record what is right in front of our eyes, again creating faulty memories. Imagine you are asked to look at five different objects on the same computer screen. The screen briefly goes blank then comes back on again. Observers often failed to report that the objects have switched places, or that one object has been replaced by a new object. This failure is called 'change blindness'.

If what I have just described sounds underwhelming I would strongly recommend that you take a minute to look on the internet at the 'Changing Rooms Illusion' by Michael Cohen. This visual illusion came second in The Best Illusion of the Year competition for 2021. (Yes, there really is an annual competition). You will be utterly astonished at how poor we are at processing the world in front of us. Other remarkable examples of change blindness include how people failed to observe a switch in check-in personnel at a hotel when the person behind the desk briefly disappeared from view and was replaced.

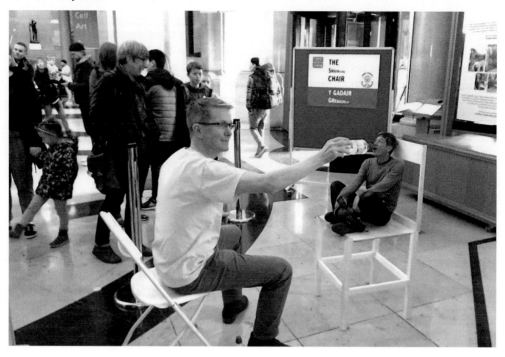

Figure 5.6 Things are not always as they seem. (The author having a drink.)

A far less dramatic example of change blindness is our constant failure to notice continuity errors in films. These errors occur when there is a sudden change, such as in clothing, hair styles, or the weather, within a supposedly continuous scene. Almost all films have continuity errors that largely go unnoticed. There are even websites devoted to highlighting these mistakes. These sites will tell you that 'Apocalypse Now' may top the list with 456 continuity errors, followed by 'The Birds' (450) and 'The Wizard of Oz' (301). Apparently, when Dorothy first encounters the Scarecrow her pigtails change repeatedly between short and curly to long and straight. There is even a brief moment in 'The Wizard of Oz' when Dorothy's famous red shoes become black. Clearly, these mistakes do not stop us from enjoying these classic films, partly because so many continuity errors go unnoticed.

While change blindness can occur for stimuli in front of our eyes, it is most prevalent for items at the periphery of our vision. Unsurprisingly, this has worrying implications when driving, where a sudden change may reflect a potential hazard. Change blindness also has social consequences. One example is how we frequently overestimate the ability of others to notice our actions – we think our behaviour is in the spotlight when, in reality, it is not. Appreciating that another individual has changed their sweater during a memory test often goes unnoticed, yet for the person who removed their sweater it seems all too obvious as they hold the false belief that they are in a spotlight. Instead, because of change blindness, this action (changing a sweater) will often go unnoticed by others.

A related phenomenon, inattentional blindness, reveals how an unexpected event can be completely overlooked if we are attending to something else. Ulric Neisser asked people to attend closely to the details of a basketball game on a video. Remarkably, the observers often failed to notice a woman with an open umbrella who strolled through the game. That study was the springboard for the famous 'invisible gorilla' experiment.

There are few more dramatic experiments in Psychology. It has a bit of everything, being both theatrical and astonishing in its findings. It shows that when you attend to a particular aspect of the world in front of you, quite extraordinary events can be missed, even though they occupy centre stage. For the invisible gorilla experiment (it is well worth seeing the video on the internet), you are asked to watch a video of a group of people playing basketball (Simons & Chabris, 1999). Your task is to count the number of passes made by those players with white tops. After a short while, a woman in a gorilla suit walks into the middle of the players, beats her chest, and then leaves. Despite being visible for 5s, half of the observers failed to report seeing the gorilla. Some subjects asked for the video to be replayed as they could not believe that there was a gorilla. Yet, if you are not asked to track the basketball players you will undoubtedly see the gorilla. (The study, which revels in the glorious title 'Gorilla in our midst', received an Ig Nobel in 2004).

Change blindness and inattentional blindness have fascinating implications for what we do and do not encode, and then subsequently remember. These phenomena lie at the junction of perception and memory. We now believe that instead of passively receiving external sensory information, we continually construct predictive models of the world around us. These expectations, based on past learning, will include top-down information about what is most likely to occur in a given situation. In this way, schemas help us to both interpret and anticipate events around us. For much of the time this anticipatory approach is highly efficient as most objects are stable or only change slowly, but as we have seen, this mechanism can sometimes be fooled.

6   Why do we forget?

If we could recall everything, we would be as incapacitated as if we could not recall at all; a condition to remember is that we must forget.

William James (1890)

We forget things all the time. This is not always a bad thing. Indeed, it is hard to conceive of memory without also having forgetting. Apparently, every animal studied that shows learning also shows forgetting. As the great psychologist William James observed in 'The Principles of Psychology' from 1890, learning and forgetting go hand-in-hand.

Some of our memory lapses are relatively trivial, such as forgetting where I put my glasses, but some are catastrophic. An unwitting consequence of urging parents to use baby seats in the back, rather than the front of the car was a rise in instances of accidentally forgetting that your baby was in the car. This lapse is bad enough, but tragically it may have caused between 15 and 24 deaths a year in hot cars in the U.S.

It is natural to think of forgetting as just being the gradual fading away of a memory trace. In reality, there is rarely one reason why something is forgotten. Sometimes the memory trace is degraded, losing its original information. Sometimes a memory is replaced so that the original is overwritten or disappears. One form of replacement already described is 'reconsolidation'. At other times the memory remains but, for a variety of reasons, it becomes inaccessible. For practical purposes, all of these examples constitute 'forgetting' as the final result is the same, even though they may be caused by errors in encoding, consolidation, or retrieval. Consequently, there are multiple culprits.

One helpful framework is Daniel Schacter's 'seven sins of memory'. The seven sins are absent mindedness, blocking, transience, misattribution, suggestibility, bias, and persistence. To this list, Schacter later added directed forgetting (Schacter, 2022). This final term refers to our ability to deliberately forget targeted information when urged to do so. It does seem incredible that we can consciously summon up the appropriate brain mechanisms to lose a particular memory, but the evidence shows that we can. This same ability also highlights why the term 'sin of memory' may be a misnomer. Rather, these errors and changes are often the by-product of an otherwise effective memory system. Consequently, memory is increasing seen as a dynamic constructive process, in which errors and distortions are a relatively small price to pay. Furthermore, some forgetting can be beneficial, such as those concerning distressing events.

Absent-mindedness, as horrifically demonstrated by those parents who forgot that their babies were in the back of the car, is largely a result of poor initial learning. In these tragic cases, contributing factors included being distracted, mind wandering, and a lack of sleep.

DOI: 10.4324/9781003537649-6

The loss of a reminder cue normally provided by a baby in the adjacent passenger seat, then added to the problem.

A frequent memory challenge is remembering whether you have locked the front door, something I repeatedly struggle to recall. So yes, I am that person who sets off on a journey and agonises over whether I locked the house, often having to turn around just to be sure or even telephoning a neighbour (Figure 6.1). This type of absent-mindedness typically arises when we fail to attend to the task, so we do not mentally tag the critical event. This failure is most common for frequently executed routines that are largely the same, day after day. Aspects of such routines may become implicit, e.g., how to turn the key to ensure it locks, while the explicit episodic memory of the event will seem very similar to the many previous occasions when you locked the door. Consequently, these explicit components are shallowly processed and easily forgotten, while what remains is readily confused with similar, previous experiences. One solution is to have a deliberate thought or image tied to locking the door, and then later recalling that thought or image to confirm your action. (But do not use the same image every time.)

Mind-wandering is another cause of absent mindedness. In other words, thinking about other events and not attending to the matter in hand. Again, this is very likely to happen

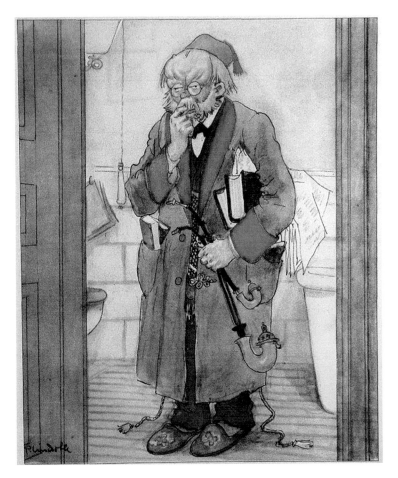

Figure 6.1 The stereotype of the absent-minded professor has a long history.

Source: Per Lindroth (1878–1933).

when leaving the house as you start to mentally anticipate your interactions for the upcoming day. Mind-wandering is especially common when performing a regular action, as the ease of that action releases you to think about other things. Another common cause of mind-wandering is not being engaged by the information in front of you. Unsurprisingly, mind-wandering bedevils student learning. Just to be really sure, this was put to the test and yes, experiments confirm that student mind-wandering leads to poorer retention of taught material.

There is a strong link between absent-mindedness and levels-of-processing. As detailed in the previous chapter, the way in which we engage with information makes an enormous difference in its memorability. Absent-mindedness is often accompanied by superficial processing caused by mind-wandering, distractions, or the fact that the action to be remembered is routine.

Blocking is the curse of crossword solvers. The term refers to how retrieving the wrong information can leave the desired information harder to find. The wrong answer repeatedly comes to mind, getting in the way of the solution and making the task of finding the right answer so much harder. This phenomenon has also been called retrieval-induced forgetting, in which the favoured memory (be it right or wrong) helps to inhibit the retrieval of similar traces.

We experience blocking when trying to retrieve information that we know but cannot quite reach. Try naming all seven dwarves in Snow White or all of Santa's nine reindeer. You may find this task simple, or you may struggle to name them all. If you struggle you might experience 'tip-of-the tongue', where you have a 'feeling-of-knowing' that is often accompanied by fragments of information. A closely related phenomenon is 'presque vu', (almost seen) where you feel you are just on the brink of recollecting something, but it will not materialise.

Tip-of-the tongue is found across all languages and cultures. This includes American Sign Language, for which it is appropriately called 'tip-of-the finger'. When tip-of-the tongue occurs, something blocks or interferes with the retrieval of the target information. The target information has been sufficiently activated to produce the feeling-of-knowing but there is insufficient activation to trigger recall. A feature of blocking is that some of the retrieval cues for the desired memory are shared with the undesired memory. For this reason, tip-of-the tongue generates words with meaning or attributes similar to those of the target word.

Tip-of-the tongue occurs for both episodic memory (that last item on the shopping list) and for searches of semantic memory (for example, in which town in Pennsylvania is set the film 'Groundhog Day' or what is the full name of 'Doc' in the 'Back to the Future' films). Diary reports indicate that younger people experience tip-of-the tongue once or twice a week, increasing to once a day for older adults, though these are probably underestimates. In about half of our tip-of-the tongue experiences we know that the 'answer' that comes to mind is incorrect and is blocking retrieval of the correct answer. This blocking action increases with aging. Whenever my grandmother tried to remember my name she would have to first go through the names of six or more other grandchildren before alighting on mine.

A fascinating feature of tip-of-the tongue is how the fragments of information we can access are not random. In over half of our tip-of-the tongue episodes we can correctly guess the first letter of the word that we wish to recall, while in about a third of cases the initial sound (phoneme) of the word is correctly guessed (Figure 6.2). The final letters can also be generated, less well than the first letters but better than those in the middle of the word. We can also often correctly guess the number of syllables in the word we cannot recall.

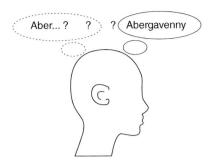

Figure 6.2 My most recent tip-of-the-tongue was for the place name 'Abergavenny'. All I could recall was Aber.

After experiencing tip-of-the tongue, the large majority of sought words are retrieved over the following few days. A natural question is how often do the target words spontaneously pop-up? This question is difficult to answer but estimates suggest that spontaneous pop-ups represent about a third of retrievals. Once tip-of-the tongue is overcome, subsequent retrieval of that lost word is slightly enhanced, probably reflecting the heightened attention and effort initially given to that word, along with contributions from priming. (The town of Punxsutawney, Doc Emmett Brown)

A final example of blocking is when a well-trained motor action overrides the less frequent, but appropriate, action for the situation. This error is more likely to occur when our attention is distracted. On the rare occasions I drive an automatic car, I sometimes find my left hand searching for the non-existent gear stick when slowing down or accelerating. I hasten to add that this has not affected my ability to drive safely.

Transience and interference: Over time, memories seem to decay. When Wagenaar was recalling the entries to his diary in 1986, he found that the oldest memories were the least complete. When people repeatedly used the same Cambridge car park, their memory for the spaces they had used also declined over time. The clear implication is that the passage of time causes forgetting.

Famously, in the 1880s Hermann Ebbinghaus systematically looked at forgetting from long-term memory. He deliberately stripped the problem to its essentials (Ebbinghaus, 1885). To remove the effects of prior knowledge he created non-word syllables that could be pronounced but had no meaning, e.g., POQ, WIB, and so on. He then systematically varied factors such as the time spent learning and the length of the retention interval before subsequently retesting his memory. In this way, he compared his ability to recall information after minutes, days, or weeks. It has been estimated that for one set of studies (on varying the numbers of learning trials and its effect on forgetting) he learnt and re-learnt 420 series of 16 syllables. Together, the learning and re-learning required slightly over 15,000 recitations. This was a Herculean effort.

Ebbinghaus found that for his lists of syllables there was an initial rapid rate of forgetting, followed by a gradually decreasing rate of forgetting (Figure 6.3). As a consequence, forgetting for Ebbinghaus followed a gradually decelerating curve, making it logarithmic rather than a straight line. A corollary of this finding is Jost's Law (1897), which states that when two memory traces are equally strong, the older of the two memories will, thereafter, be forgotten more slowly, as its rate of decay is flatter. Many subsequent studies have converged on Ebbinghaus' conclusion that the rate of forgetting is initially rapid but slows down as time progresses. This process is only arrested if memories are retrieved and rehearsed.

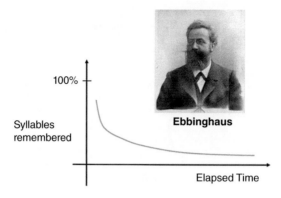

100%

Syllables
remembered

Ebbinghaus

Elapsed Time

Figure 6.3 Memory decay function across time found by Ebbinghaus.

Although Ebbinghaus has been criticised for being reliant on one subject (himself) and for using artificial learning tasks, his forgetting curves (rapid at first, but then slowing down) are seen again and again for other material. Many of us learnt a language many years ago at school but have barely used it since. Using that past learning, Harry Bahrick compared adults' knowledge of Spanish when it had been studied up to 50 years previously. As you might guess, while the decline in Spanish was rapid over the first few years, it thereafter declined at a much slower rate. A similar pattern of forgetting, rapid at first, then slowing down, has been demonstrated for past news items from one day to two years ago and for our ability to recall the names of class-mates from two weeks to 57 years ago.

There is little doubt that time typically increases overall forgetting. The mechanism is often called 'trace decay'. Put simply, memory representations are presumed to degrade, a process that continues over time. The rapid initial forgetting is seen to occur as there is more of a complete representation to suffer some kind of break-down, while the more resilient aspects survive longest.

The principal criticism of 'trace decay' is that time itself cannot cause forgetting, there has to be an action that continues across time to degrade the memory. The favoured action is called 'interference'. This explanation assumes that there is inadvertent competition between different memory traces. The greater the similarity between the memory traces, the greater the interference, creating more forgetting as the original memory is increasingly corrupted.

'Proactive interference' is the term for the competition that is generated by information previously learnt, i.e., *before* the target information. 'Retroactive interference' describes competition from information learnt *after* the target information. It is called retroactive because it works back in time, while proactive interference works forward in time. In the Cambridge car parking study, there was remarkably little location forgetting over time if the participant only used the facility once. But when the car park was used repeatedly, older parking locations were most likely to be forgotten, an example of retroactive interference.

Another example of interference may arise when recalling your car registration (Figure 6.4). When remembering the plate on your current car you might suffer interference from the registration numbers on your previous car (*proactive interference*). If, however, you should try to remember the registration plate of your previous car you might struggle as the numbers and letters on your current car get in the way (*retroactive interference*).

Interference contributes to several of the sins of memory, including *blocking* and *misattribution*. Cue-competition at retrieval ('blocking') has already been mentioned. Cue-competition typically increases as the similarity grows between the item-to-be-recalled

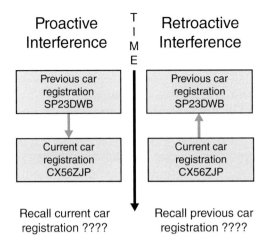

Figure 6.4 The different temporal actions of proactive and retroactive interference.

and its competitors. The problem further increases when more memories are attached to the same cues, creating greater interference. Remembering your daily commute exemplifies how the same retrieval cues are linked to a host of different memories from similar, but separate, days. While yesterday's commute may only suffer proactive interference from previous commutes, last week's commute will suffer both proactive and retroactive interference, making it all the more difficult to isolate and remember details from any given day.

To test interference in the laboratory many studies have examined how learning one list of words affects the recall of a second list. Classic studies by Benton Underwood confirmed that making the words increasingly similar in meaning increases interference and impairs memory. Likewise, the more times you learn the competing list (the one not recalled at test), the greater the interference from that list. This means that unique, unusual experiences can be better remembered, as they suffer low levels interference. Given this finding, Underwood wondered why students in some experiments showed steep forgetting curves for nonsense syllables, as hopefully they are not part of the education syllabus and should be unfamiliar. The explanation was that these same students had already participated in multiple psychology experiments involving nonsense syllables. In contrast, naïve students showed much better retention when first asked to learn nonsense syllables.

To understand the true nature of interference it would make sense to look at the level of the neuron. Here, we might find out what happens to a memory trace (engram) over time and identify time-dependent mechanisms that cause change and decay. It is reasonable to assume that forgetting involves a collection of process that create circuit changes, so that engrams transition from being accessible (where they can be reactivated by natural recall cues) to inaccessible. This change could occur in the engram, in the rest of the brain, or both.

Candidate neuronal actions underlying interference include changes in the availability of neurotransmitters at the critical synapses, alterations in the shape of the neuron including its dendritic spines, the loss of synapses, and alterations in the balance of excitatory and inhibitory inputs to the engram. Furthermore, similar information might be expected to occupy an increasing number of overlapping nodes with the target engram, creating instability or inhibition. Another factor, already mentioned, is the changing neuronal composition of the hippocampus with neurogenesis, so that access to past memories may become increasingly difficult. Any, or all, of these factors could accumulate over time, highlighting again how 'time' as a cause of forgetting is really a shorthand for one or more processes.

Misattribution refers to errors in distinguishing the source of information. Such errors can lead to misplaced recall and recognition. Misattribution can even help to create events that never existed. This last situation is exemplified by the Deese–Roediger–McDermott paradigm, the test in which people often remember the world 'cold', even though it had never appeared on the list of words to be learnt (see *The case against permanent episodic memories*). Explanations for this kind of misattribution centre on the idea that, in addition to the target, we activate representations for words or images that have similar meanings to the target. These activated associates, such as 'cold' can then feel as though they are a real memory. Older adults seem more susceptible to this kind of misattribution error.

Errors in source attribution more typically refer to correctly retrieving information but falsely believing where or when that information arose. Such source confusions also become increasingly common in the elderly. There are understandable concerns that this type of confusion may affect eye-witness testimony. In this way we might unwittingly transfer information from an innocuous context to a crime scene. Indeed, there are a number of famous examples where just this has happened. In 1988, the psychologist Donald Thomson described how he was accused of rape, based on his identification by the victim. By a twist of fate, Thomson was giving a live television interview on memory when the rape occurred, providing an airtight alibi. The misattribution arose because the victim had been watching that same TV interview just before being raped.

Another form of misattribution occurs when we believe that we have generated an original idea when in reality we are retrieving someone else's (so called 'cryptomnesia'). While this error may seem relatively harmless, it can take on nightmarish proportions. For the scientist there is the constant worry about whether I really had that great idea, or whether I simply forgot that I had previously read it. For this reason, plagiarism can be unwitting ('inadvertent plagiarism'), just as it can be deliberate. This distinction hits the headlines whenever a musician is taken to court over claims that they had copied an earlier piece of music. In a famous case in 2022 involving the singer Ed Sheeran, the judge, Mr Justice Zacaroli concluded that Sheeran 'neither deliberately nor subconsciously' copied a phrase from the song 'Oh Why'. The reference to 'nor subconsciously' specifically relates to inadvertent misattribution.

Suggestibility is closely akin to misattribution. Suggested information after the event is incorporated to create a false recollection that is placed in a real context. In contrast, misattribution can occur spontaneously, and so it does not need an overt suggestion.

There are two main reasons for wanting to understand how and when suggestibility might affect our memories. The first comes from studies into the accuracy of eye-witness testimony. The second concerns the extent to which childhood memories are robust or whether they can later be influenced to create false narratives. The importance of this second topic is underscored by the therapeutic and legal issues surrounding childhood abuse.

Examples of suggestibility already described include creating false memories of childhood events, such as being lost in a shopping mall or spilling drinks at a wedding reception (see *How accurate and durable are our adult memories?*). These studies show that suggestive or misleading questions about a past event can change reports of past childhood events. The likelihood of describing an event that never occurred does, however, depend on its plausibility. In one study, for example, while 20-30% of subjects falsely recalling a plausible childhood event, none recalled having a rectal enema as a child. While these suggestibility studies are not without criticism, there is agreement that false reports can develop without any intention to lie.

As implausible made-up events are less likely to be adopted you would believe that you could not get someone to falsely recall having committed a crime. You would be wrong. Students were asked to describe an event from their past. Those in the criminal condition were told that they had committed a crime between the ages of 11 and 14, resulting in police contact. They were encouraged to remember this mythical event over successive sessions. The students were prompted with specific (false) cues such as their age at the time and the season of the year. When a student could not 'recall' the false event, the experimenter encouraged them to try and remember details, including imagining the crime. After completing three interviews at one-week intervals, 70% of the students described false memories of being involved in a criminal event (Shaw & Porter, 2015). The crimes included assault and theft. These are startling numbers, leading to justifiable concerns about the contribution of social coercion during interrogations. Even after considering obedience to the researchers' wishes, around 25% of the students still recalled false memories of committing a crime.

While the previous study was constrained by ethics, real interrogations can be far more exhaustive and threatening. They also contain numerous opportunities to plant false information. Advances in DNA fingerprinting have helped to confirm that miscarriages of justice resulting from coercive confessions are all too common. The Innocence Project estimates that for overturned convictions in the U.S. involving murder or rape, a false confession was made in about 25% of the cases.

Confession, even if subsequently recanted, is probably the most powerful evidence when used in court (Figure 6.5). Experiments show that mock juries will still vote for conviction even when they know the confession was produced by coercion. An array of factors conspires to make us believe the original confession, come what may. We often show an alarming perseverance for past beliefs that are now clearly in error. Once we have made up our minds, we are very resistant to change.

Many factors can encourage someone to provide a false confession. These include youth, low I.Q., the attraction of a certain over an uncertain outcome, the preference for immediate resolution, and our social desire to be compliant with others (in this case, the interrogators). Our social compliancy was famously highlighted by Stanley Milgram's 1963 studies showing how, with varying degrees of coercion, subjects would 'administer' electric shocks of increasing intensity. Furthermore, when psychologists were subsequently questioned, there was an almost complete disbelief that any participant would show full obedience, yet many did. There are clear parallels with the disbelief that jurors show to the possibility of a suspect making a false confession, even under duress.

Duress can come in many forms. You may be relieved to know that torture was banned in the U.K. in 1709, though that has not stopped its use across the world. I should add that the use of torture to obtain a confession is both abhorrent and ineffective. Nevertheless, physical beatings as part of an interrogation were not banned in the U.S. until 1936. Over 100 countries, including the U.S. and U.K., now comply with the 'Miranda' rules, which include telling suspects that they have a right to remain silent and the right to a legal defence. (The name 'Miranda' originated from a 1966 case in Arizona.)

Interrogations in the U.K. are now covered by the Police and Criminal Evidence Act (PACE). PACE was introduced in 1984 following high profile miscarriages, including the Birmingham Six and the Guildford Four where confessions were coerced by physical and psychological abuse. It is because of PACE that U.K. police interviews are recorded, as we now see in countless TV cop shows. A further goal, to adopt more appropriate interview techniques, arose in the U.K. from a collaboration of police officers, psychologists, and

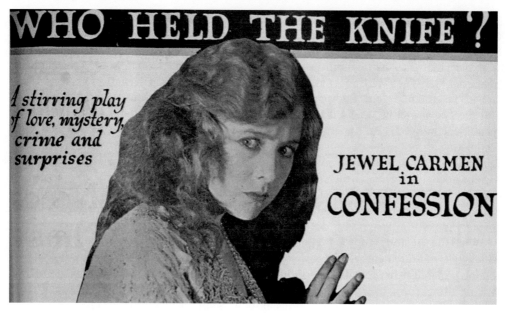

WHO HELD THE KNIFE ?

A stirring play of love, mystery, crime and surprises

JEWEL CARMEN
in
CONFESSION

Figure 6.5 Poster from the 1918 film *Confession* about a man wrongly convicted of murder.

lawyers. The resulting strategy, introduced in 1992, has the mnemonic PEACE, which captures its five main elements (Preparation and Planning, Engage and Explain, Account, Closure, and Evaluate).

Bias occurs both when encoding and recalling past memories. There are many forms of bias. Listings of different cognitive biases give more than 50 different types. Some of these biases have the potential to alter how we process or retrieve information, creating errors. One form of egocentric bias to which I am prone has been called the 'bias blind spot'. This is the belief that I am less biased than other people and more able to detect their cognitive biases. Another is the 'frequency illusion', which is the tendency to notice something more often after it first comes to your attention. You buy a pair of red shoes, and now you suddenly see red shoes everywhere. This illusion, which is a result of selective attention, can, for example, apply to ideas, objects, songs, and phrases.

One prevalent form of bias, already introduced, is confirmation bias. We seek, interpret, prefer, and remember information that accords with our prior beliefs. At the same time, we tend to ignore or superficially dismiss information that runs against our preconceptions. While not wishing to betray my political convictions, I have little doubt that my memories of a certain past U.K. Prime Minister, the former MP for Uxbridge and South Ruislip, are shaped and reinforced by my present beliefs about how he conducted himself in office. Of far more concern is the worry that a doctor may make an initial diagnosis, but then seek confirming evidence rather than look for evidence that may disprove that diagnosis. Likewise, jurors are likely to reach a decision about their verdict early in the court proceedings, leading them to pay particular attention and then recall the evidence that is consistent with their initial decision. First impressions really matter.

We can see how confirmation biases help to support the world of 'fake news'. Pro-life, anti-abortion supporters in Ireland were more likely to think that they 'remembered' a fabricated, negative story about supporters of abortion rights, and *vice versa*. It should be no surprise

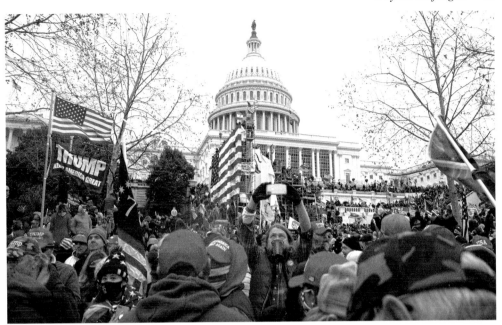

Figure 6.6 Storming of the U.S. Capitol in 2021.

that partisan bias has also been shown for peoples' memory of the events at the Capitol riots in the U.S. on 6th January 2021 (Figure 6.6). Put simply, Democrats and Republicans remember the events differently, recalling more events that favour their political party. Furthermore, the likelihood of holding false memories about the riots is associated with a belief in conspiracy theories. When bias and misinformation combine, alarming outcomes can arise. The problem is that confirmation biases can rarely be overcome, though they may be moderated by education, including training in critical thinking and evidence evaluation.

The three major constituents of confirmation bias are the unequal search for information, its biased interpretation, and the resulting memory distortions. The combination of these three factors helps to polarise attitudes, so that the same evidence can drive two opposing parties further apart. Just think of the climate change debate. To compound the problem, the seeking of confirmatory evidence encourages belief perseverance. This is a classic trap that scientists often fall into – the priority should be looking for evidence that disproves your ideas.

As one moves into the terrain of conspiracy theorists, there is growing tendency to falsely see correlations between events or situations that have no bearing on each other. Consider the fact that those countries with the highest chocolate consumption also have the highest number of Nobel prizes per capita. There is also a positive correlation between drownings in American swimming pools and the power generated by US nuclear power plants.

Rather wonderfully, in some European countries an increase in the number of storks is associated with an increase in the number of children. This spurious correlation should not be seen as evidence that storks deliver babies (Figure 6.7).

Those who believe in conspiracy theories, such as the moon landings being faked or that the AIDS virus was created in a laboratory, are more likely to see a causal link between real-life, but completely unrelated, correlations. The illusion of causality suggests that those holding conspiracy beliefs try to find order in events that would otherwise seem random or outside of one's control.

Time to consider another bias. The 'consistency bias' describes our tendency to retrofit our memories to help them better match our current knowledge, likes, and beliefs. This bias stems from the notion that our past and present attitudes are stable and, therefore, largely unchanged. This means that we tend to remember how we would wish to have behaved or think, given our current perspective. While I like olives and, therefore, feel that I remember liking them when young, this is probably false given their bitter taste. Such biases can be seen in romantic relationships. When relationships flourish, participants will exaggerate how positively they rated their partners at the start of the relationship. Conversely, when relationships break down, remembrance of partner ratings made at the start of the relationship become more negative than they had originally been.

Persistence involves memories one would like to forget, but persistently resurface. Such memories can block out others. In people suffering from depression there is a greater access to negative memories, creating a dangerous, self-perpetuating cycle. Unsurprisingly, excessive rumination over negative events can prolong depressive episodes. Traumatic events are high on the list of persistent memories. I have persistent, bittersweet memories of my late son, Hugh that I do not want to lose, even though they are troubling. For some people there are traumatic memories best forgotten as they can become disabling. This situation is common in Post-Traumatic Stress Disorder (PTSD).

The brain has a number of mechanisms that help to explain our ability to remember events associated with heightened arousal. One mechanisms begins with the release of adrenaline by the adrenal glands, which can bring about increased levels of a variety of neurotransmitters in the brain, including noradrenaline. Increased levels of noradrenaline in the amygdala make emotional memories stronger and longer lasting. It is thought that interactions between the amygdala and prefrontal cortex are then especially important for the persistence of traumatic memories. One piece of extraordinary evidence was the finding that veterans of the Vietnam War who had sustained injuries to either the amygdala or prefrontal cortex were *less* likely to develop PTSD.

Directed or motivated forgetting refers to the active removal of memories. Some memories are unwanted, raising the question of whether we can help to forget them. Many people have upsetting memories they would dearly love to forget. The notion of removing these memories is strongly linked to Freud's controversial idea of 'repression' – that we can block

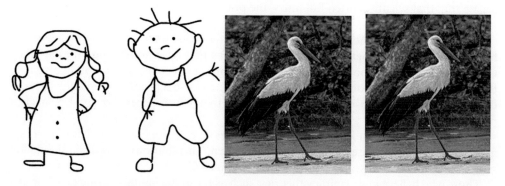

Figure 6.7 Correlation is not the same as causation.

traumatic memories, even though they may continue to affect us. Rather than discuss highly emotional memories, I will just consider whether we can wilfully forget everyday information. (Traumatic information is covered when discussing *Psychogenic Amnesia*.)

Imagine you are shown a list of single neutral words, but after each word comes the instruction to remember or forget. Subsequent memory tests show that to-be-forgotten words are less well remembered. This effect is all the more intriguing as the instruction to remember or forget follows the offset of each word, so than the initial encoding of these items is the same. This 'forgetting' is not done to just please the experimenter (so-called demand characteristics) as it seems impervious to being offered money to help retrieve actively forgotten items.

We appear to be able to moderate and suppress memories, both at encoding and retrieval. At encoding, directed forgetting of a specific item is aided by our ability to limit any active rehearsal of that item. However, other more active inhibitory processes contribute. It is thought that the instruction to forget increases prefrontal cortex and parietal cortex activity that helps to inhibit the encoding of the to-be-forgotten items. More specifically, top-down prefrontal processes are thought to help depress hippocampal activity at the time of initial learning, encouraging successful forgetting (Anderson & Hulbert, 2021).

Similarly, at retrieval, there is a suppression of unwanted memories. By not allowing a retrieval cue to give a learnt, but unwanted answer, subsequent memory for that association can diminish. This effect is called retrieval suppression. Forgetting increases each time an item is successfully suppressed. This suppression appears to involve cognitive control processes that are mediated by prefrontal cortex but then affect other areas, including the hippocampus. One aspect of this process has been called 'thought-substitution'. Here, active suppression helps to redirect your attention to a different cue target, taking you away from the to-be-forgotten item. Another component has been called 'context-inhibition'. The belief is that prefrontal cortex can inhibit the ability to bring to mind the context in which the to-be-forgotten memory occurred. One potential consequence of this suppression is that the directed forgetting spills over to affect innocent bystander memories, in other words, associated information. This spill-over creates what has been called an amnesic shadow.

Active forgetting may have many beneficial consequences. Evidence that active forgetting occurs in other animals, including fruit flies and rats, adds to this idea. The most obvious benefit for humans is the ability to suppress upsetting memories, but other benefits may include maintaining self-beliefs in the face of contradictory evidence, helping us to forgive others, maintaining false beliefs or deceptions, and helping to generalise across experiences. The clinical benefits of effective forgetting are probably most evident when we consider how unwanted, intrusive thoughts are a core feature of conditions such as anxiety and PTSD.

Other causes of forgetting include changes in our context. As will be discussed in the following Chapter (*Context and memory*), the context surrounding an event can provide a powerful retrieval cue. Consequently, a change in context will remove those cues, and so encourage forgetting. Contextual retrieval cues can be external, such as the location of the to-be-remembered event, but they can also be internal, for example your physiological or emotional state at the time of the to-be-remembered event. By re-instating these cues, such as by returning to your old school, a host of old memories, for better or for worse, are likely to resurface.

7 Context and memory

The past and present rose side by side, at that supreme moment.

The Moonstone, Wilkie Collins (1868)

A priceless diamond has been stolen, with blame falling on Franklin Blake. To solve the mystery and save his reputation, Franklin re-enacts the evening when the diamond was stolen with the others who were there. This re-construction causes old memories to resurface and helps to solve the mystery. These dramatic events occur in one of the earliest detective mysteries, 'The Moonstone' (1868). Wilkie Collins, the author, was clearly aware that recreating a past environment can trigger memories associated with that place and time. A more accessible example is when we return to the location of a previous holiday, many seemingly forgotten memories and emotions resurface from that earlier visit. Odours can also provide particularly strong cues to past memories. For some, the smell of cut grass evokes memories of summer. For me, the aroma of roasting malt takes me to Cardiff Central train station where, in the past, you could smell the Brains' Brewery.

These evoked memories are all examples of 'context-dependent memory'. Their retrieval occurs because we often simultaneously combine ongoing events with the context within which they occurred. Re-experiencing that same context then prompts retrieval of that particular event. The power of contextual cueing was apparent in the five-year diary study of Willem Wagenaar from 1986. He demonstrated how cues, such as the where and when an event occurred, enhanced later retrieval. Likewise, distinctive places bring back memories of previous visits, be they to a supermarket, the dentist, or a friend's house.

Just as re-visiting a context can enable recall, so a change in context can cause forgetting. When I am out cycling I often think that I have a great idea to put in this book, but then fail to remember it when back in my study as the context has completely changed. For the same reason, holidays can be especially relaxing as they remove many of the prompts that remind you of day-to-day cares.

Demonstrating context-dependent memory: Despite the apparent power of a place to prompt the retrieval of past memories associated with that place, demonstrating context-dependent memory in the laboratory has often proved surprisingly difficult. It is for this reason that the most cited experimental demonstration of this phenomenon used extreme changes of outdoor context, changes far beyond those normally possible in the laboratory.

The cognitive psychologist Alan Baddeley knew that professional scuba-divers reported a curious problem. If they did not record their observations underwater, they often forgot them after surfacing. He also knew that laboratory studies involving context changes often failed to affect memory or had to use bizarre manipulations that they bore no resemblance

DOI: 10.4324/9781003537649-7

to real life. One example was strapping people to a board which was then spun with participants either lying flat or upright. As he wryly observed, such experiments lack real-world validity.

For their classic study, Godden & Baddeley (1975) asked scuba-divers in the sea off Scotland to learn lists of words, which they later recalled. The experiment required four conditions:

learn underwater – recall underwater (same context)
learn underwater – recall dry-land (changed context)
learn dry land – recall underwater (changed context)
learn dry land – recall dry-land (same context)

If context matters, word recall should be best for the first and last conditions (when learning and recall are in the same context) but worst for the middle conditions (when learning and recall are in changed contexts). This was exactly the pattern of results they found.

A few years later they repeated their diving study, but now tested word recognition rather than word recall. For this task, divers heard lists of words and then later attempted to distinguish those same words from novel words. Once again there were four groups, with testing in either the same or changed contexts. In stark contrast to the recall experiment, there was no evidence that the context change (underwater – dry-land) disrupted recognition memory.

I was later able to repeat this pattern of results in Durham City swimming pool (Figure 7.1). Those who changed context (between being underwater or on dry-land) after learning a set of safety instructions were poor at recalling those same instructions. In contrast, the same context shift had no impact on either word or face recognition memory. Thus, while free recall can be sensitive to context changes between learning and recall, recognition memory is often unaffected.

Despite the challenge of demonstrating reliable context-dependent memory in the laboratory, psychologists have persisted. We now know that a wide variety of laboratory-based context shifts can occasionally affect recall, although the effects on memory are typically small and rarely robust. Effective context shifts have included the appearance and location of a room, background music, and background smells. Other contextual cues include the

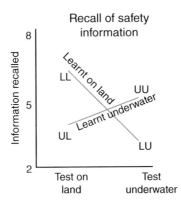

Figure 7.1 Superior recall when learning and recall were in the same context (either both on land – LL or both underwater – UU).

presence of the experimenter. For this reason, having the same experimenter at learning and test can reduce context-switch effects. Of growing interest will be how the context switch between officeworking and homeworking, initially driven by the COVID-19 pandemic, affects our ability to transfer between the two very different environments.

One explanation for the weak context effects seen in laboratory-based studies is the inadvertent use of procedures that draw attention away from the learning and test environments. As I write these words, a song by the (Dixie) Chicks is playing. The song instantly takes me back to a specific memory of driving along the M27 in Hampshire with my son Hugh when we first listened to this song together. The particular situation is relevant because when driving you cannot ignore the changing environment, creating conditions that should encourage context-dependent memories. Indeed, when driving along a road I have not been down for some time I very often experience strong context-dependent memories from the previous journey. I suddenly remember a conversation or what was on the radio at a particular point in the journey. I very much doubt I am alone in this.

Viking smells and memory: There is a widespread belief that smells are especially powerful at evoking past memories. Is there a way of experimentally testing this anecdotal effect in the real world? For this, you need a distinctive odour at a place where people experience the same set of events, so you can date-stamp and confirm any retrieved memories. I realised that the city of York is the perfect test location.

York is famous for many things, including the Jorvik Viking Centre. The Centre recreates York as it was over 1000 years ago. As you travel through the displays in a time capsule, you experience the sight and smells of Viking York. The smells, some of which are particularly pungent, include the Viking toilets, a favourite with children. We decided to find people who had visited Jorvik many years previously, and then allowed them to smell the various Jorvik odours. We then tested their memory of the exhibits. As predicted, the smells improved peoples' memory of their Jorvik experience. Even though the smell-exhibit association came from a single visit, the effect was long-lasting as the museum visit was an average of six years before the test.

In a similar way, distinctive smells from the past, such as shoe polish and the odour of coffee, have been used to help adults recall old memories, including those suffering from Alzheimer's disease. Sadly, the ability to recognise smells is very often affected in Alzheimer's disease. This is to be expected as the entorhinal cortex, part of our smell brain, is one of the first brain areas to show neuropathological changes in this disease. It is, therefore, fascinating how anecdotal reports suggest that smells can still prompt memories in people with Alzheimer's disease, even when the smell cannot be named.

The power of smells to evoke old memories may reflect properties of the olfactory system. The way that the nose identifies smells helps to segregate their individual signals, reducing competition between smell-linked memories. The route by which smells gain access to the brain is also very different to that used by sights and sounds. Olfactory signals have a more direct route to parts of the brain important for memory, such as the entorhinal cortex, ventral prefrontal cortex, and the amygdala. Consequently, odours may create stronger memory links than those usually found for other sensory modalities. As already mentioned, these same brain sites are also capable of boosting emotional memories. This property ties in with how emotional memories may be especially prone to odour-retrieval. Vietnam veterans with PTSD may react excessively to a smell (diesel) linked to their combat experience, showing how trauma-related smells can create strong emotional reminders. For more positive reasons, some people crave the smell of their dead loved-ones. Indeed, a company was set up to try and produce the right individual aroma for a price. (The smell of my son's clothes still causes an intense emotional rush.)

State-dependent learning – drugs and emotions: Up to now, the term 'context' has referred to the external world – its sights, sounds, tastes, and smells. However, one reason why the diving experiment (underwater versus dry-land) was so effective at demonstrating context-dependent memory is that the contextual changes not only involved the external visual and tactile sensations of being underwater, but also the internal physiological sensations caused by diving. The physiological aspect of the context switch is captured in the notion of 'state-dependent learning'. Here, the emphasis is on the internal bodily state and whether it changes between learning and recall. As you might predict, a change in your physiological state between learning and recall can reduce performance at retrieval.

State-dependent disruptions of recall can be induced by a variety of drugs that have marked physiological effects. This means that recalling memories when, for example drug-free, may be difficult if the events to be recalled happened when you were under the influence of a drug (Figure 7.2). Likewise, recalling memories when in a drugged state can be affected if that information was acquired when you were drug-free.

Unsurprisingly, one of the reasons why alcohol disrupts memory is that it causes state-dependent effects, meaning that when sober, people forget the alcohol-related events of the night before. Anecdotally, heavy drinkers who might hide alcohol or money when drunk, may need to resume drinking to remember where those items were hidden. Just to be certain, careful laboratory-based experiments have confirmed how alcohol has state-dependent effects on memory recall. It is also worth remembering that alcohol has many additional actions that disrupt learning and memory, which in extreme cases can lead to amnesic states (see *Alcoholic blackouts*).

Given its worldwide consumption, there is considerable interest in whether caffeine can have state-dependent effects. The short answer is yes. There is evidence that caffeine-caffeine and placebo-placebo conditions are better for memory recall than caffeine-placebo and placebo-caffeine, showing that state-dependent effects can sometimes occur. Nicotine is also known to have state-dependent effects, with obvious implications for

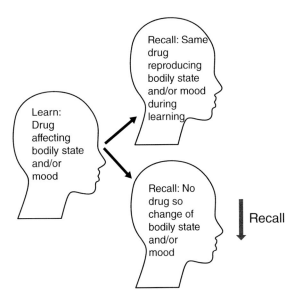

Figure 7.2 State-dependency. How a change in bodily (and/or emotional) state can impair recall.

cigarette smokers. You might predict that vaping would have especially strong context effects given the combination of nicotine and distinctive tastes and odours.

The internal states associated with 'state-dependency' also include our emotional feelings. Consequently, changing our emotional state between learning and recall can also disrupt memory. Psychologists have, for example, measured recall when people are happy at learning but then sad at recall (compared with; sad then happy, happy then happy, sad then sad). The best performance occurs when you are in the same emotional state at learning and recall. It is probably no coincidence that many recreational drugs that can cause state-dependent effects such as nicotine, alcohol, cannabis, and amphetamine, change both our physiological and emotional states.

A closely-related, clinically important effect is 'mood congruency'. Here, people find it easier to remember sad events when they are already sad (or happy events when they are happy). Mood congruency is medically important because it creates a situation in which a depressed person is biased to recall more unhappy memories, and so perpetuate their condition. Appreciating this unfortunate bias and how to escape its effects has obvious therapeutic implications.

Explaining context-dependent memory: The 'encoding specificity hypothesis' introduced by Endel Tulving and Donald Thomson helps to explain the effects of context on memory. The hypothesis assumes that as we encode a piece of information it is associated with other concurrent information, such as the place, the time, and our internal state. Subsequent remembering is then aided by matching features from the earlier encoding with those at retrieval. A part of the recollective process involves distinguishing the target information from competing memories. This task is aided by an increasing amount of appropriate contextual knowledge. Indeed, it may be that the ability of context to help us to discriminate the correct target from its competitors is a major component of context-dependent memory.

This same role in target discrimination may help to explain one of the oddities of context-dependent memory. As already mentioned, while memory *recall* can be sensitive to context shifts, *recognition* memory is often unaffected, even following extreme context shifts, such as going underwater. One explanation, the 'outshining hypothesis' follows directly from the idea discussed above – that context information helps us to discriminate a target from its competitors. For recognition memory (deciding which stimulus is novel and which is familiar) the familiar stimulus provides its own inherent cues that take precedent over other cues and so 'outshine' any associated contextual cues.

Using context-dependent memory: Context need not be physically present to aid recall, it can be imagined. If you start thinking about a past holiday by picturing the place and its surroundings, associated memories will come to the surface. A related, imagery-based process is employed when eye-witnesses are asked to recall the details of a crime. An effective strategy is to ask open-ended questions and encourage the person to describe the events leading up to and surrounding the crime, rather than just the crime itself. In doing so, contextual cues will emerge. Better still would be to go back to the actual crime scene to aid recall, but this raises both practical and ethical issues. Remember though that recognition memory is often immune from context effects, so re-instating the context of a crime need not help with recognising mug shots.

In recent years, virtual-reality has been used to construct different environments with which to test context-dependent memory. Not surprisingly, switching between being underwater and being on the planet Mars, or switching between a virtual-reality office and a real-world office can affect recall. These context-shift effects provide a caution when transferring virtual-reality based education to the real world. Others argue that virtual-reality context-shift effects are often inconsistent and small, and so of less concern. This is a rapidly emerging field and while we have yet to reach a consensus, it remains likely that switching to and from virtual-reality will impact on memory.

For students there is the obvious issue of context and the taking of exams. There are rumours that a university accidentally placed some exam students in the lecture theatre used for that course, while others from the same course sat in an unfamiliar exam hall. In theory, the former group should have been at an advantage. Whether this story is true or not, it should be possible reduce context effects by visualising where and when you first learnt the information to be recalled. Likewise, picturing the rest of the page or the relevant PowerPoint slide can help to cue seemingly forgotten information. At the same time, the stress of sitting an exam is likely to change your mood and physiology, potentially inducing state-dependent effects that may impair recall. For the same reasons, differences in caffeine or nicotine levels between revision and exam-taking may upset retrieval.

But perhaps it is best not to exaggerate the potential impact of some context changes. Many experiments have found that shifting a room between learning and recall has small or inconsistent effects. We might also be reassured by the finding that shifts between a clinical setting (bedside) and an educational setting (classroom) produced no discernible context shift effect on memory recall. Even when medical students were given lists of words to learn and later recall, shifting contexts between a surgical theatre (in gown and mask) and a tutorial room produced no apparent context effect (Coveney et al., 2013). The lack of any obvious effects serves to remind us how context-shifts create such erratic findings in formal studies, even though they seem to be ever-present in the real-world. One critical difference may be how real-world context effects are associated with both spatial and temporal sequences, as we move through space. This potentially important aspect is often absent in laboratory studies.

Up to now, I have described how re-visiting a context can aid memory recall. There are, however, occasions when maximising a context change is beneficial as it helps us to forget. One of the pleasures of being on holiday (a context shift) is that the day-to-day cares of life seem to disappear as they less readily come to mind. Exercising in the gym, using a sauna, swimming, surfing, walking in the countryside, and cycling are all activities where the context shift from work or home could scarcely be greater. Perhaps it is no surprise that people often find that these same activities reduce stress as they all involve switches in both internal and external states that can take you away from the memory of day-to-day pressures.

8   Superior memory in individuals

Mnemonists, memory champions, and savants

What are the 39 steps?

The 39 Steps (1935 Film)

This classic Hitchcock film opens in a London variety theatre with a performance by 'Mr Memory', whose act is to answer questions about almost anything. At the end of the film our hero, Richard Hannay, challenges Mr Memory to answer the question "*What are the 39 steps?*" I won't tell you what happens next in case you have never seen this classic movie. I begin with this film because it exemplifies the belief that there are rare individuals with amazing powers of recall. These people are sometimes called mnemonists. (I might add that Mr Memory was a dramatic device for the film and never appeared in the 1915 book by John Buchan.)

Mr Memory from the film of 'The 39 Steps' was based on a real act. James Maurice Bottle began performing from 1901 in British Music Halls as 'Datas, the Memory Man'. His act was to answer any question posed by the audience, just like Mr Memory. To do this, he had devised his own memory techniques. In case you think that memory acts no longer exist, you would be wrong. Paul Sinha recently hosted his version of a Pub Quiz on BBC radio. In one impressive section he answers unscripted general knowledge questions from the audience, just as in the opening of 'The 39 Steps'.

Before proceeding, we should remember that we all possess a degree of 'expert knowledge' for topics that hold a particular fascination. That fascination results in the superior retention of facts from that same topic, be it sports statistics, the TV series 'Buffy the Vampire Slayer', train locomotives, or the Kardashians. In 1937, Chess Master George Kotanowski set a world record by playing 34 games simultaneously while blindfolded, yet it was found that other aspects of his memory seemed normal. (As noted earlier, his record was beaten in 2017 by Timur Gareyev, who played 48 games simultaneously.)

In some instances, expert knowledge has been combined with rehearsed cognitive strategies to produce astonishing feats of memory (Ericsson et al., 2004). The undergraduate S.F. trained for more than 230 hours to increase his memory span. This measure is the number of digits you can repeat back in the correct order after just hearing them. (Think telephone numbers.) S.F.'s span was originally a typical seven, but eventually rose to a truly remarkable 79. This feat was made possible by transforming sets of digits into times (minutes and seconds), which were recoded as sequences of running times for various races. This achievement was only made possible by his expert knowledge of athletic events.

The idea that rare people exist with truly exceptional memory is reinforced by TV shows with characters such as Sheldon in 'The Big Bang Theory', Spock in 'Star Trek', Sherlock

DOI: 10.4324/9781003537649-8

in 'Sherlock', and Astrid, in 'Astrid in Paris'. The same device is also seen in films, most notably 'Rain Man'. These same shows also emphasise the common idea that exceptional memory is accompanied by difficulties in aspects of human interaction, such as those caused by autism. While this description is often true for one category of mnemonists, namely 'savants', it is not applicable to the many trained mnemonists.

Innate versus trained mnemonists: We need to distinguish between those rare individuals who seem to be blessed (or cursed) with remarkable memory abilities from childhood and those individuals who start with relatively normal memories but have deliberately trained with cognitive memory aids (mnemonics). An example of the latter is the journalist Joshua Foer who practised for a year until he could eventually break the U.S. record for playing card memorisation. The message is that we can all train to become mnemonists, should we have the time and tenacity.

A famous challenge is to memorise π (Pi), which closely approximates to 22 divided by seven. Pi starts as 3.141592.... but it is as an 'irrational number', which means that the digits after the decimal point are never-ending, a fact first proved by Johann Heinrich Lambert in 1761. After seven years of training, taking up to 13 hours a day, the Chinese businessman Chao Lu recited the first 67,890 digits of π. This was a new Guinness World Record. To achieve this feat, he converted pairs of numbers to images or words, then combined them into vivid stories and locations. Subsequent formal testing showed that his digit span was not out of the ordinary unless he was able to apply his mnemonic strategy.

The conclusion is that Chau Lu's memory record came from exhaustive training, and not from an exceptional, innate ability. This conclusion agrees with studies of another memory man by the name of Tomomori. Despite learning the first 40,000 digits of π, his memory span for visually presented digits was only eight. Again, he did not differ from other people on a range of other memory tests. Likewise, the civil servant TE had astonishing memory skills. At the age of 15 he responded to a newspaper advert promoting a book to develop a 'super-power memory'. He successfully mastered a variety of mnemonic methods, yet his basic memory abilities often seemed normal. These individuals further highlight the importance of distinguishing those with innate abilities from those with trained abilities.

Innate mnemonists: Let us first consider those very rare individuals with remarkable, innate abilities. My favourite mnemonist has always been 'S', who was described in detail by the Russian neurologist Alexander Luria in the book *The Mind of a Mnemonist: A Little Book about a Vast Memory* (1968). 'S' was Solomon Shereshevsky (1886–1958), a journalist. His colleagues noticed that Shereshevksy never seemed to take notes yet had a verbatim memory. At their first meeting, Luria thought that Shereshevksy was a rather disorganised and dull-witted person, but soon discovered that he had both an exceptional memory and an extraordinary mind.

Shereshevsky could recall any number of words and digits, as well as memorises whole pages from books on any topic. Furthermore, his memory did not seem to erode over time. To make this possible, he created intense images of the world around him, often employing a combination of senses. Shereshevksy had a particularly florid and wide-ranging form of synaesthesia, a condition in which stimuli in one sensory modality are also perceived in another sensory modality. Unusually, for Shereshevsky it affected all of his senses. He memorably described the Russian psychologist Vygotsky as having 'a yellow crumbly voice'. He reported not buying some ice cream because the vender's voice was as if 'a pile of coals and black cinders came bursting from her mouth'. These examples of synaesthesia involved the transfer of sound to colour and texture. Apparently he found it difficult to remember things while eating, because the tastes created vivid images across the senses.

With his intense imagery, Shereshevksy could retain complex mathematical formulas and letter arrays for years. He would endlessly create visual images so that abstract items were transformed into concrete images. Each number, for example, had a specific character. The number '6' was a man with a swollen foot, the number '7' (which for S would have been 7) was a man with a moustache, while '8' was a stout woman. The number 87 was seen as a woman next to a man twirling his moustache, while the square root sign √ is a tree with roots. He could also look at number matrices on a blackboard, close his eyes and then 'see' that same matrix on a table.

Like Mr Memory, Shereshevsky performed as a professional mnemonist, but disillusioned he later became a taxi driver in Moscow. Because his memory was so vivid he struggled with competing past memories and had great difficulty recognising faces as they often changed from how he had meticulously memorised them. To remove unwanted images, he could place them on a visualised blackboard and then mentally erase them. From Luria's book it becomes clear that being able to remember almost everything comes at a cost, and Shereshevksy had a difficult life.

The lines between an innate mnemonist and trained mnemonist can become very blurred. The mnemonist Rajan Mahadevan (1957–) has an exceptional memory for digits and words. In 1981 he memorised the first 31,811 decimals of the mathematical constant π. After years of testing, it was concluded that Rajan had vastly superior basic abilities, making him an innate mnemonist. His abilities were then supplemented by considerable skilled training. As evidence, when his digit span was first tested in the U.S. it was already around 15, far beyond the normal range of five to nine. When rapidly memorising lengthy lists of digits he would break the task down into long groups of around ten digits, integrating each group with previously learnt numerical information.

Nevertheless, there remains some debate over whether Rajan does possess innate, exceptional memory skills or whether his abilities can all be explained by relentless training – the 'skilled memory' theory (Ericsson et al., 2004). That three-part theory describes how remarkable memory feats can be acquired without the need for an exceptional basic capacity. The theory first assumes that to reach extraordinary levels of memory performance, the individual relies on prior knowledge and patterns to interrogate and group items in long-term memory (the 'encoding principle'). Next, the encoded information is linked with cues during study, cues that later enable retrieval from long-term memory (the 'retrieval structure principle'). Finally, with more and more practice, individuals become increasingly efficient so they can encode and store the same amount of presented information in less time (the 'speed-up principle').

In the debate over Rajan's abilities, key issues are whether his superior memory is restricted to those areas of additional training (digits and letters), as might be predicted by the 'skilled memory theory', or whether his ability to create and combine long groups of digits was largely innate. When tested with symbols, rather than digits, his initial performance was like that of normal controls, only surpassing them when he was able to substitute symbols into digits, a pattern consistent with the skilled memory theory. Other examples of apparently normal memory include Rajan's modest ability to remember the orientation and position of objects. Furthermore, prior to his first memory tests in the U.S., Rajan spent between 200 – 400 hours learning the first 10,000 decimals of π in order to receive a funded trip to that country, creating ample opportunity to refine his mnemonic techniques. Consequently, the idea that Rajan was an innate mnemonist remains in some doubt. Like some other famous mnemonists, he appears to be someone with a foot in both camps, possessing some superior aspects of cognition combined with endless practice.

Professor Alexander Aitken (1895–1967) may be a stronger contender for someone with exceptional innate skills. His powers of memory encompassed broad swathes of information, including mathematics, music, English literature, English and Latin verse, as well as having an unusual degree of precision for the names, dates, and locations of past events. His letter span was about ten, while his digit span approached 15, double that of most people. Aitken's breadth of achievements is unusual among mnemonists, but he did not have total recall. As far we know, Aitken did not use mnemonics in a deliberate manner. Instead, his learning abilities were centred around interest, meaning, and expert knowledge. While Shereshevsky operated in a world of perceptual maps, Aitken created rich conceptual maps, employing deep processing of unusual sophistication.

Another contender is the mnemonist V.P. As a five-year-old, V.P. is said to have memorised the street map of the Latvian city of Riga along with its rail and bus timetables. As an adult, V.P. could play up to seven simultaneous matches of chess when blindfolded, and at least 60 correspondence games of chess with no notes. He could recall long lists of nonsense syllables and vast sequences of numbers. He memorised a lengthy, complex First Nation's tale called 'The War of the Ghosts' producing it nearly verbatim after two readings, and again a year later. V.P. used a variety of verbal recoding methods, based around his exceptional linguistic knowledge. He could seemingly associate any three-letter string with a word, while number matrices could be recoded, for example, as dates. As V.P. is thought to have spent considerable time practising memorising and recoding, aspects of his ability can be explained by skilled memory theory. At the same time, his precocious talent points to a combination of innate and acquired skills.

One way to distinguish innate mnemonists from trained mnemonists might be to compare their brains. Put simply, are the brains of innate mnemonists unusual? Unfortunately, we lack sufficient information because of their rarity and their individuality. Consequently, the best information concerns trained memory athletes. Here, the short answer is that the brains of trained mnemonists are remarkable for being so unremarkable.

Eleanor Maguire and her colleagues used brain imaging (MRI) to examine ten people noted for their superior memory (eight had been very successful at the World Memory Championship). Unlike their performance on memory tests, their scores on general cognitive tests, including measures of I.Q., were not exceptional, being in the high to average range. All relied on extensively practised mnemonics. Despite their superior memory abilities, no structural brain differences were detected. Interestingly, when performing memory tasks, they showed heightened activity in brain areas associated with space and navigation, including the retrosplenial cortex and the right hippocampus. This activation pattern most likely reflects the visual and spatial imagery deployed in the mnemonics that they almost all practised.

Subsequent MRI studies of Memory Champions have also found no clear evidence of altered brain structure but there may be changes to the patterns of brain activity across visual, spatial, and memory-related areas when performing memory tasks. These patterns are again consistent with the deliberate deployment of visual and spatial imagery. In a clever twist, a group of naïve people undertook six weeks of intensive mnemonic practice (Dresler et al., 2017). After this training, their patterns of brain activity during memory tasks became increasingly similar to those of the memory athletes. The message again is that many mnemonists do not have exceptional brains, or even exceptional cognitive skills. Areas closely associated with memory do not appear to be enlarged. Rather, with persistence and diligence these memory athletes have perfected the art of using mnemonics to optimise how the brain links and remembers specific types of information.

Highly Superior Autobiographical Memory: A small number of individuals, less than 100 so far, have been labelled as having Highly Superior Autobiographical Memory (HSAM). This very rare condition, also called hyperthymesia, concerns the ability to remember past personal events with exceptional precision and very little forgetting. The first recorded case, A.J., contacted the eminent neuroscientist Jim McGaugh with an email that included the following statement

> Some people call me the human calendar while others run out of the room in com-plete fear but the one reaction I get from everyone who eventually finds out about this "gift" is total amazement. Then they start throwing dates at me to try to stump me.... I haven't been stumped yet. Most have called it a gift but I call it a burden. I run my entire life through my head every day and it drives me crazy!!!....
>
> To Jim McGaugh's astonishment, A.J.'s claims proved correct (Parker et al., 2006)

People with HSAM show a remarkable ability to recount their past experiences without deliberately using mnemonic techniques. These rare individuals often first become aware of their unusual memory skills at around 10 years of age. Some HSAM adults claim to remem-ber almost every day of their lives, starting from their teens. When given a date they can often provide the corresponding memory. Apparently, if you give the actor Marilu Henner a random date in the past, she can recall it with unusual clarity (Figure 8.1). On being given the date April 30, 1980, she recalled. *"It was a Wednesday"*, *"I was in Cancún, Mexico, with my boyfriend at the time, who was soon to be my first husband"*. *"I drank tequila for the first time, and then never again for 25 years!" "The weather was beautiful that night, but it poured rain the next day,.."*.

This ability is not the same as calendar calculating. That skill is displayed by some indi-viduals with autism, who name the days of the week from their dates, rather than what personal events happened on specific dates. Furthermore, unlike Shereshevsky, who could seemingly remember anything, people with HSAM show a narrow ability, focussed on their autobiographic experiences and memory for public events, especially those that impinge on their lives. The performance of HSAM individuals on other tests of memory is often normal.

Surprisingly, a study of 27 HSAM individuals concluded that their initial encoding of autobiographical events is largely normal because their memory for recent events did not differ from controls in the first week. But, thereafter, forgetting by the HSAM individuals was far slower (LePort et al., 2016). Over time, the control subjects increasingly relied on gist, while the HSAM participants retained detailed individual memories. This enhanced retention of personal events could be seen for episodes stretching back at least ten years.

So why is their autobiographical memory so good? Individuals with HSAM appear to benefit from superior consolidation and retrieval skills. Many HSAM individuals organise their memories by date and location. Their memory skills often appear to be aided by an almost compulsive rehearsal of past autobiographical events, sometimes as a way of lulling themselves to sleep or as a form or relaxation. A five-year diary study by Marigold Linton in 1975 (who did not have HSAM) established that the repeated, spaced retrieval of past autobiographic events substantially improved their retention. In HSAM that effect is con-siderably magnified. That said, given the extent of their autobiographical knowledge, the amount of time needed for explicit rumination would soon become prohibitive. Consequently, deliberate rehearsal cannot be a sufficient explanation for HSAM. Instead, this repetitive rehearsal of past events probably employs incidental or automatic, processes of which HSAM individuals are unaware.

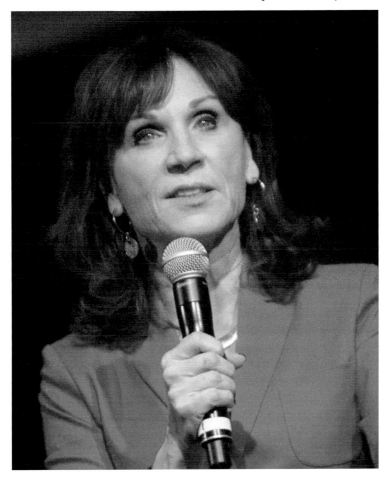

Figure 8.1 Marilu Henner, who has HSAM.

Source: Gage Skidmore, https://creativecommons.org/licenses/by-sa/2.0

Again, we would like to know if the brains of HSAM individual are unusual in some way. Unfortunately, single case studies are notoriously difficult to interpret (Einstein's brain is discussed at the end of this Section). One of the very few group studies involved 11 HSAM people who received brain scans (LePort et al., 2012). Nine brain regions showed evidence of differences, with a mixture of increases and decreases in brain indices. It was suggested that changes to the temporal lobe cortex might be linked to superior autobiographic memory, while increased grey matter in two subcortical areas (the right putamen and caudate nucleus) might reflect the obsessive nature of these individuals. Even with this impressive numbers of participants for such a rare condition, these conclusions remain very tentative.

Super-recognisers: Another group with superior memory skills are called 'super-recognisers'. Our individual ability to discriminate between familiar and unfamiliar faces is very variable. The top 2% have been given the title super-recognisers. Such individuals only recently hit the spotlight. In 2009, four individuals came forward who claimed to have exceptional memories for faces, but only for faces. They reported frequently recognising others who did not, in return, recognise them. This mismatch meant that they sometimes pretended not to recognise others in order to avoid confusion and embarrassment. They had the subjective feeling that they almost never forgot a face. Formal testing confirmed that these four individuals were superior at naming the faces of people before they were famous, as well as being superior at distinguishing a novel face from a familiar face shown earlier in the experimental session.

In eye-catching news, some super-recognisers have been used by police forces to create special task forces to pick out suspects. The Metropolitan Police (London) is said to have 200 super-recognisers at its disposal, although advances in AI will almost inevitably replace humans. Before getting carried away, we should examine just how much better they are than the general public and whether this has real, practical benefits. One estimate is that being in the top 2% of people recognisers only translates into a real-world gain of about 12% in performance, which is not a lot, though the size of this lift has been disputed. For example, it has also been suggested that super-recognisers are as far above the norm as those with prosopagnosia are below the norm. (Prosopagnosia is a clinical condition characterised by an inability to identify familiar individuals from their faces.) Unfortunately, as yet we know very little about brain activity in super-recognisers and whether these people have special neurological attributes.

Savants and eidetic memory: The most frequently portrayed group of people displaying spectacular feats of memory are known as 'savants'. The word comes from the French for learned or wise. The term savant is usually reserved for people with developmental challenges who are neurodiverse, but nevertheless display an island of genius. The historic term 'idiot savant' was first introduced by John Down in 1887, a physician more famous for his work on Down's syndrome. His unfortunate label, now discarded, arose because some savants do have a low I.Q., as measured by standard tests.

While many neurodiverse savants are diagnosed as autistic, only a small minority (about 10%) of people with autism show some savant skills. As there is an increased prevalence of synaesthesia in autism, this link may partially explain some individual instances of enhanced memory among autistic savants.

Far rarer are 'prodigious savants', whose particular abilities can tower above the rest of the population. Areas of prodigious savant achievement include music, art, calendar calculating, mathematics ('lightening calculators'), and visuospatial skills. A frequent feature of these savant abilities is their exceptional depth of knowledge and learning within a narrow domain.

Calendar calculating, the ability to name the day of the week from any given date, is one of the abilities more often seen in savants. There is an algorithm to solve this problem but that is probably not how savants tackle this challenge. Likewise, it is probably not through an unusually large working memory (that might speed calculations) or an encyclopaedic knowledge of all individual past and future dates. Instead, some savants take advantage of how the calendar repeats every 28 years, alongside known specific anchor dates, while other savants may benefit from visualising calendars. The impression is that a variety of methods are used by different individuals. Nevertheless, a common theme is a heightened interest in the dates of specific events, helping to create a calendar-related knowledge-base.

Different methods for calendar calculating are even seen in twin savants. The twins George and Charlie were both calendar counters. Even though they would struggle with simple mathematic problems, they could correctly give the day of the week for past dates. That said, they did they not account for the switch of 13 days with the change from the Julian to the Gregorian calendar, so adjustments had to be made for dates before 1752.

(Russia did not adopt the Gregorian calendar until 1918, causing their shooters to miss the London 1908 Olympics as they arrived days too late). George, the more accomplished of the twins, consistently gave correct days of the week from A.C.E. 100 in the past to the year 40400 in the future. George appeared to have learnt a 400-year cycle of calendar dates, along with subpatterns within that cycle. Charlie, on the other hand, appeared to have rote learnt the past 200 years, and so was unable to determine the days of future dates.

The most famous fictional portrayal of a savant was by Dustin Hoffman in the 1988 film 'Rain Man'. The inspiration for that character was the prodigious savant Kim Peek (1951–2009), nicknamed the 'Kimputer' (Figure 8.2). He was not autistic but suffered developmental damage from birth. He is described as having an encyclopaedic knowledge of 15 different areas of expertise, including American history, sport, music, the bible, and Shakespeare plays, which he learnt word for word. He knew all the U.S. area codes and major city zip codes, along with how to get from one U.S. city to another, and then how to successfully navigate that city street by street. He is said to have read over 12,000 books and then recite details decades later. Kim Peek was described as the 'Mount Everest of Memory' by a world expert on savants, and it is hard to disagree.

Despite these utterly incredible achievements (and many more), Kim Peek suffered extensive central nervous system (CNS) damage from the time of his birth. One consequence was that he had considerable difficulties with fine motor skills, for example, buttoning his shirt. As an adult he had an unusually large head, while brain imaging revealed a malformed cerebellum and an absent corpus callosum, the white-matter tract that links the two cerebral hemispheres. He also lacked the anterior and posterior commissures, further isolating his two hemispheres. The absence of these major tracts does rather raise questions

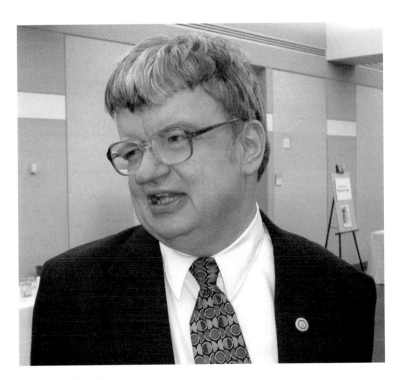

Figure 8.2 Kim Peek – the 'Kimputer'.

about the value of these pathways for cognition. His brain also showed abnormalities in the left hemisphere, and it has been noted how damage to the left hemisphere is linked with some reported cases of 'acquired savant' syndrome, when older children and adults suddenly develop savant skills. Despite these various abnormalities we simply cannot pinpoint what gave him his astonishing memory skills.

A very different savant is Stephen Wiltshire who draws incredibly complex cityscapes from memory. Stephen was diagnosed with autism at the age of three. As a child he became famous for his detailed sketches of London landscapes, which were drawn from memory and without prior training. Since then, he has reproduced cityscapes all over the world. Not only are his drawings remarkable for their accuracy, such as the number of windows or columns on individual buildings, but he also requires an astonishingly short time to memorise a vast, complex scene. After a single helicopter ride, he is able to draw cities from memory. Following a 45-minute helicopter ride over Rome, he completed over three days, a startlingly accurate drawing of the city. The drawing, on a five and half yard canvas, detailed the city, street by street, building by building, in great precision and accuracy. Likewise, his drawing of Mexico City, which took four days, began the day after a 30-minute helicopter ride over the city (Figure 8.3).

The obvious question is how do savants do it? To which the answer is, we really don't know. One possibility is that they might be more reliant on less conscious, habit-based learning. Current explanations are often based on the idea that their neurodevelopmental disruptions caused an area to shut down, thereby releasing the brake on another brain region that then galvanises the savant's special ability. This idea gains support from the subgroup of 'acquired savants'. (This is the term given to those who acquire savant skills in adulthood after a brain insult.) Narinder Kapur reviewed such instances of paradoxical facilitation following brain injury, including examples from animal studies. The cases highlight how direct or indirect neural damage can sometimes facilitate a range of psychological domains, including memory, language, sensory, and perceptual functions.

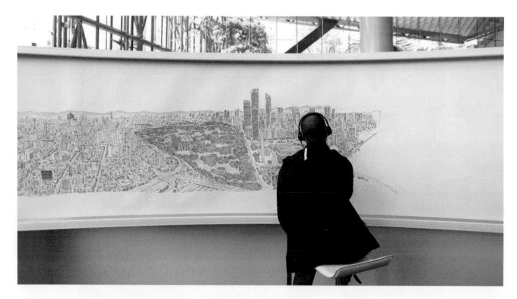

Figure 8.3 Stephen Wiltshire drawing Mexico City from memory, based on a 30-minute helicopter ride the previous day.

Nevertheless, just to be clear, brain pathology typically impairs brain function, any facilitation is highly unusual.

This uncertain picture helped to fuel studies into whether the brain activity of savants is unusual during memory tasks. Some studies of memory savants point to increased activity in right visual areas, possibly reflecting an enhanced used of pictorial representations. However, other studies emphasise just how variable any brain changes are between individual savants. While structural changes and altered connectional activity are repeatedly seen, it is extremely difficult to discern a general pattern given the small number of cases and their apparent uniqueness.

Nevertheless, one repeated suggestion is that left hemispheric dysfunction 'releases' the right hemisphere and, thereby, facilitates the use of imagery. Support for this idea includes evidence that disrupting the left hemisphere in neurotypical brains (by a magnetic process called TMS) can release savant-like tendencies within the domains of drawing, numerosity (the ability to guess how many objects in a large array), and proof-reading. The intriguing implication is that we all have latent savant skills, but with normal development these remain hidden.

A final category of superior memory skills concerns what is called 'eidetic memory'. This term, which is not the same as 'photographic memory', captures the sense that some people, children in particular, are able to retain vivid visual images long after looking away from a scene. Unlike a photograph, this mental image is not static and can be voluntarily manipulated.

Traditionally, individuals were given a picture to inspect, the picture was then removed, and the person described it from memory. This method led to estimates that between 0 and 11% of children have eidetic imagery. One speculation was that eidetic memory reflects the more concrete representations that we form as children, but which gradually become more abstract in later years, hence, the loss of this potential ability. This explanation has, however, been challenged by evidence that eidetic abilities remain stable over early school years and that there is no obvious correlation between levels of eidetic imagery, abstract thinking, or reading.

It is probably fair to say that interest in eidetic memory has waned over recent decades with the growing uncertainty as to whether normal imagery and eidetic imagery are qualitatively different. Adding to this uncertainty is the growing realisation that within the normal population there is enormous individual variation in the spontaneous use of imagery, from those who seemingly lack imagery (see *A is for Aphantasia*) to those with exceptional rich imagery ('hyperphantasia'). It is, however, important to remember that hyperphantasia is not equivalent a 'photographic memory'. The former is about creating images, the latter is about maintaining highly accurate visual information. Stephen Wiltshire, the drawer of cityscapes, is a rare example of the latter.

Einstein's brain: To conclude this section, we might come back to the question of whether the brains of individuals with exceptional cognitive abilities are also exceptional. We know that the brains of mnemonists who rely on trained memory drills look essentially normal. But we also know that the brains of savants are often not typical, suggesting that some neurological features promote the syndrome. The difficulty in identifying those special neurological features is highlighted by the case of Albert Einstein's brain. Surely, if we can make a detailed study of the brain of a great genius like Albert Einstein, we must be able to uncover what made that person so special?

Although Albert Einstein's brain has been examined, the lessons to be learnt may not be what you might anticipate. The fate of his brain is a labyrinthine story, so weird that you could not make it up. When Einstein died in 1955 it is thought that he requested for his entire body to be cremated. But the temptation to save the great man's brain proved too great. The pathologist Thomas Harvey, who conducted Einstein's autopsy, removed his brain, which weighed 1230g, a fairly normal weight for a man of his age (76 years). Harvey photographed the brain and then sectioned it into 240 blocks. He later took the blocks from Princeton to Philadelphia, where they were stored in his basement, before moving to the Midwest. Bizarrely, Einstein's eyes were removed and remain in private 'hands'.

Einstein's brain was finally rediscovered by the journalist Steven Levy in Wichita in 1978. The brain was still in Harvey's possession. The precious brain sections had been preserved for decades in alcohol in two jars within a Costa cider box under a beer cooler. Eventually, in 1985, the first details of his brain were published. In this initial paper it was claimed that Einstein's brain had an unusually high ratio of glial cells to neurons, but this claim has been much criticised. Likewise, earlier claims that the overall appearance of his cortex was seemingly abnormal, have been disputed.

In 2010, the estate of Thomas Harvey released 14 previously-unseen photographs of Einstein's brain, helping to revise previous opinions. The photographs help to confirm the presence of an enlarged left primary motor cortex and an enlarged left primary somatosensory cortex. The significance of these features with respect to his genius has, however, been much disputed, not least because I doubt that anyone in advance would have predicted that these particular areas might have anything to do with his genius. Indeed, if you had asked an expert to list those sites most likely to be altered, these cortical areas would probably have been close to the bottom of the list. To make matters worse, interpreting any apparent brain difference as contributing to his genius is hopelessly compromised by *post hoc* reasoning. The temptation to attribute apparent brain changes to his genius can be too hard to resist, even if such changes (if real) might arise for other reasons, such as from his being bilingual or from his early music training. A further problem is the likely reluctance to publish any findings that seem to show that his brain was normal.

The reality is that the structure of Einstein's brain may have contributed to his genius but linking that genius to any particular brain feature has become a game of inconclusive speculations. The lesson is that interpreting a single case, no matter how special, is fraught with numerous problems. A further lesson is the need to respect an individual's wishes.

9 Superior memory for all

Mnemonics, imagery, and skilled performance

If I hear it, I forget.
If I see it, I remember.
If I do it, I know.
  Old Chinese Adage

Mnemonics

Competitors at the World Memory Championships, which is administered by the World Memory Sports Council, compete in ten memory disciplines (Abstract Images, Binary Numbers, Random Numbers, Names and Faces, Speed Numbers, Historic/Future Dates, Random Cards, Random Words, Spoken Numbers, and Speed Cards). These competitors rely heavily on mnemonics that centre around the use of imagery. Records from the World Memory Championships include learning 4620 random digits in one hour, 335 random words in 15 minutes, linking 224 names with 224 faces in 15 minutes, and memorising a deck of 52 playing cards in an astonishing 12.74 seconds (one card every 0.245 seconds). It is worth pausing for a moment to appreciate these mind-boggling records.

Just as amazing as these feats of memory is the evidence that the brains of such mnemonists are not unusual. Their prodigious learning feats are largely the result of exhaustive training. The goal is to perfect a variety of processing tricks to establish stronger memories – these memory enhancing devices are called mnemonics. Most mnemonics involve conscious, effortful processing. Many also incorporate visual imagery. Anyone who has watched the highly successful BBC series 'Sherlock' may remember how he uses his 'mind palace' to visualise and arrange his memories and thoughts. (I should add that the original Sherlock Holmes never mentioned any use of mnemonic techniques, despite having a razor-sharp memory.)

To appreciate how mnemonics work it is helpful to describe a number of techniques. Variants of the first technique to be described (The Method of Loci) are popular with competitors in the World Memory Championships. These competitors include Joshua Foer who, as you may remember, trained for a year before beating the American record for playing card memorisation.

The Method of Loci: This is one of the oldest mnemonic techniques. The Method of Loci is attributed to the Greek poet Simonides of Ceos (556–468 BC). The story has it that Simonides was invited to a banquet by Scopus, a nobleman from Thessaly. During the feasting, Simonides was called away by some visitors. (In some versions he was interrupted by the twins Castor and Pollux.) This interruption proved most fortunate for Simonides,

DOI: 10.4324/9781003537649-9

but no one else, as the banquet hall collapsed killing his fellow diners, including Scopus. The devastation was so complete that the bodies of his fellow diners were unrecognisable.

Simonides was subsequently asked to identify the victims so that they could be buried. Simonides could picture the seating and who sat where, thereby, naming the unfortunate victims. He then realised that he could use his visual memory to help recall other material. For this, he visualised a complex room (his 'mind palace') in which he carefully placed images of items in different locations. To recall them, he simply re-imagined the room and looked for the items in their correct places or 'loci'. His mnemonic strategy, which was adopted by Roman orators such as Cicero, has remained popular ever since. (It is worth adding that the story of Simonides and the ill-fated banquet creates vivid images, making the origin story highly memorable.)

To experience the Method of Loci, practise visualising the same, repeated walk through some of the rooms in your house or visualise a familiar walk starting from your house. Along the way, pause at ten locations. Leaving your house, you might start with the porch (location 1), followed by the front gate (location 2). You might next turn right at the gate and look at the pavement (location 3), before crossing the road to enter the park and look at the nearest bench (location 4), and, so on, for another six locations. Next, you practise visualising these same ten consecutive loci. It should become easy as one location takes you to the next.

Imagine you now have a shopping list of ten items: milk, baked beans, apples, red wine, yoghurt, butter, tomatoes, broccoli, honey, and pizza. To memorise the list, you simply follow your 'walk' and place an image of each item in each of the ten locations – starting with a carton of milk on the porch, a tin of baked beans resting on the gate, apples dropped on the pavement, and bottle of red wine on the park bench, and so on. To recall the list, you simply retrace your steps and 'see' each item in its place. To help you remember it was red wine and not white wine, you could picture a spill of red wine rather than a bottle.

With practice you can generate much longer lists of loci, as well as multiple sets of routes or locations for different memory tasks. Skilled mnemonists learn to re-use the same routes, though the closer together the re-use, the greater the risk of interference. Abstract items pose more of a challenge as they may not readily translate into images. One solution is to create concrete associates, so that for 'peace' you might picture a white dove, for 'love' a heart, and for 'courage' a lion.

Related mnemonics employing imagery: I have described the Method of Loci at length partly because it is so popular and partly because it highlights some of the core features found in many other mnemonics, namely: a pre-learnt set of retrieval cues (in this case your route), elaborative ('deep') encoding (you have to think about the nature of each item), and the use of imagery.

One of the simplest mnemonics is the link system, which again uses the power of interactive imagery. This method involves making consecutive images of the to-be-remembered items, linking them in a chain of events to create a narrative. These interactions not only add to the imagery but create additional semantic processing and promote their associations. The mnemonist Shereshevski used this method when converting a complex mathematics equation into a highly visual story in which each symbol became an item that interacted with the next to form a linked story.

For the link system to work each image needs to interact with the next, rather than merely be placed alongside (Figure 9.1). As long as you can recall the first word and its image, the chain of events should help you to recall the series, e.g., a *dog*, jumps onto a *table*, tipping it over to break a *window* which falls onto a *swan*, which puts on a *hat* .....

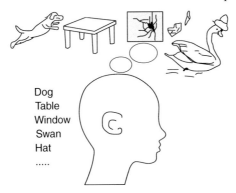

Figure 9.1 Depiction of the link system used to help remember word list. The images need to interact.

(Not that I can imagine when you might ever want to remember this list of words.) You might suppose that the more bizarre the imagery, the better the later recall, but this relationship is often not found. What does matter is that the images interact with each other.

Peg-word mnemonics use a pre-learnt set of items that are then linked to the information to be learnt. In this sense they operate like the Method of Loci, but instead of using places, they employ names to create the pegs. In one class of peg systems, numbers are used to generate sequences.

To begin, you might learn a series of rhymes, such as 'one is bun, two is a shoe, three is a tree, four is a door,' and so on, creating a unique image for each number. That image is then linked with an image of the to-be-remembered item. One advantage is that you can go directly to a specific item. The eighth item, for example, is the image interacting in some way with a gate (eight is for gate). This saves you from having to go through seven previous items as you would need to do with a link system.

A much-promoted system developed by Tony Buzan is known as 'memory-mapping' or 'mind-maps'. Here, the core idea within a body of knowledge is placed in the middle of a sheet of paper. The student then draws radiating links to the categories of information that feed into that core concept. These major links may be distinguished by colour. Further branches can then radiate off these major categories (Figure 9.2). These links can be both named and represented in drawings.

This method can be used as an alternative to note-taking but also as a revision device. Because mind-mapping combines elaborative sematic processing, visual imagery, and self-generation, it has many advocates in education. Key attractions include how the learner works to create their map, rather than simply reproducing something already made. This effortful, self-generation aspect is thought to encourage critical thinking (see *G – The generation effect*). Subsequent sharing and discussion should promote further analysis.

Mind-mapping has, for example, been introduced in a variety of medical settings, although quantitative tests of mind-mapping have given mixed results, with some studies finding clear benefits while others see no advantage. Furthermore, any map is only as good as its initial construction, so that unwitting errors might be introduced and retained.

What is special about imagery? The power of imagery is not restricted to mnemonics. Imagery provides an effective boost for a wide range of memory processes. For example, picture recognition is superior to word recognition. Likewise, the recall of concrete words is superior to the recall of abstract words. In both instances, pictures and concrete items encourage imagery, helping to explain their superior recall. This explanation is

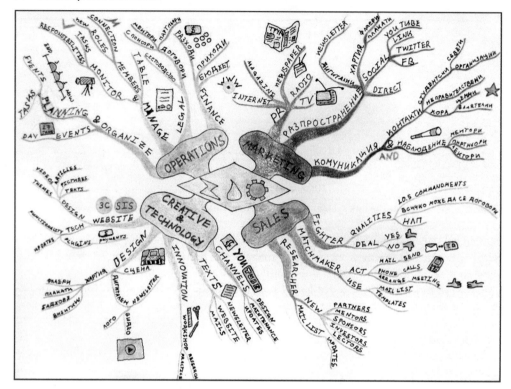

Figure 9.2 Mind-map for the topic of economic operations and strategy.

encapsulated in the dual-code theory, proposed in 1971 by the Canadian psychologist Allan Paivio (Figure 9.3).

Put simply, Paivio's dual-code theory presumes that verbal information and imagery are processed separately in distinct channels, creating parallel sets of representations. Consequently, both new verbal information and new pictorial information can generate independent, additional imagery and verbal codes. At recall, both classes of information are potentially available. This additive property leads to better retention as you have more access points for retrieval.

In addition, imagery is thought to be especially durable as it initially requires greater cognitive effort – what does a white dove actually look like? Furthermore, the task of manipulating images as part of a mnemonic adds to the need to consider the nature of the item, again promoting deeper encoding. Also, an individual image, such as a white dove, is likely to be more distinctive and, for that reason, suffer less interference than its verbal counterpart, adding to its durability. (Allan Paivio, who championed the dual-code theory, was a dedicated body builder, winning the title of Mr Canada in 1948. There is a photograph of Allan Paivio in the book 'Universal Hunks', published in 2013.)

The dual-code theory is not without its critics. One criticism is that it seems to limit cognition to words and images. Another is the argument that rather than have parallel constructs, an image is a mental description. This idea is central to 'propositional theory', which regards representations as stored mental propositions rather than words and images. These propositions provide the underlying concept of an idea without the need for images

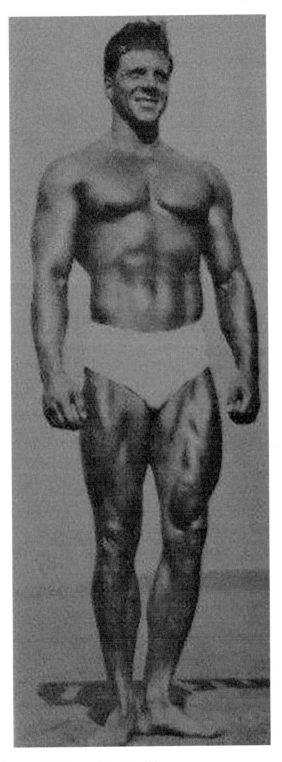

Figure 9.3 Allan Paivio, psychologist and body builder.

or verbal information. Consequently, images are derived from these more basic processes. Despite these potential alternatives, the dual-code theory remains highly influential, not least because it provides an intuitive explanation for why information that can readily be converted to images is often so much better remembered.

Other mnemonics

Not all mnemonics rely on imagery. The phrase 'Spring forward: Fall back' is invaluable for changing the clocks. Rhymes feature in many mnemonics, probably most famously for remembering the number of days in each month of the year. 'Thirty days have September ....' The rhyming element is powerful as it precludes some wrong options (as they don't rhyme), it guides you to potential answers, and gives a rhythm to the mnemonic that acts as a further cue. I should add that I could never spell the word 'rhythm' until my niece explained that 'rhythm has your two hips moving'.

Other useful rhymes include 'I before E, except after C', but beware, there are quite a few exceptions (including 'science', 'seize, 'vein', 'their', and 'species'). Other well-known mnemonics include 'In fourteen hundred ninety-two, Columbus sailed the ocean blue'. There are also long, rhyming mnemonics that name all of the Kings and Queens of England since 1066. Recent suggestions of how to update this list include 'After Liz, who will it be? The next in line is Charlie Three'.

One of the most used mnemonics is ROYGBIV – the colours of the rainbow. Many mnemonics simply take the first letter of a series of words to be remembered and then convert each first letter into a different word to make a sentence. In this case ROYGBIV often becomes Richard Of York Gave Battles In Vain. An arbitrary sequence of colours is converted into a sentence that is not only high in imagery, but the constraints of the English language restrict the order of the words. Furthermore, Richard Of York becomes a single entity, while the entire sentence has a coherent meaning. To apply the mnemonic, Richard becomes R - red, Of becomes O - orange, York becomes Y- yellow, and so on.

This famous mnemonic is an example of an 'acrostic', the name for a puzzle in which the first letters provide the key. Acrostics are especially effective for arranging familiar names into their correct order. A glance at the internet will provide an 'acrostic' for just about everything that a student might wish to remember. One well-known example concerns the notes on the treble clef lines (e.g., **E**very **G**ood **B**oy **D**eserves **F**ruit),

Other acrostics give the order of the planets and the twelve cranial nerves of the brain. My Very Educated Mother Just Sent Us Nine Pizzas gives you the nine planets in order from the Sun – Mercury, Venus, Earth, etc. (I have included the dwarf planet Pluto.) Meanwhile, a popular medical acrostic for the numerical order of the 12 cranial nerves is – On Old Olympus's Towering Top, A Finn And German Viewed Some Hops. The first letters signal the Olfactory nerve, Optic nerve, Oculomotor nerve, Trochlear nerve, Trigeminal nerve, Abducens nerve, Facial nerve, Auditory nerve, Glossopharyngeal nerve, Vagus nerve, Sensory (accessory) nerve, and Hypoglossal nerve. Sometimes the first letters form a word, making the task all the more efficient. For example, HOMES give you the first letter of each of the Great Lakes in America.

Up to now, the memory challenges I have mentioned may seem artificial, divorced from real world experience. So let us consider the real problem of remembering someone's name. As a teacher I find this a perennial challenge. There are a number of reasons why remembering a person's name can be so problematic. On introduction we often focus on the person and largely ignore the name. This is why it is fine to immediately ask again for the name – delaying the request becomes more and more socially awkward.

A major difficulty is that names are arbitrary. My first name is John but, as far as I know, there is nothing inherently John-like in my face. A related problem is that my full name, John P. Aggleton, is not naturally imageable. (Incidentally, if you ever meet an Aggleton anywhere in the world, they will be a relation, so do pass on my best regards.)

The arbitrariness of names is highlighted by how we are far better at remember face-occupation pairings than face-surname pairings. Intriguingly, this difference persists even when the same word, such as baker, can be used as a surname or an occupation. In other words, it is harder to remember that this person's surname is Baker than remembering that this person is a baker. It may be that face-occupation pairing gives you the opportunity to process the face alongside your prior knowledge about that occupation, for example, mentally visualising and testing how appropriate the pairing looks. This process is rarely possible for face-name pairings as names are typically arbitrary. When people are allowed to generate and assign names to faces, based on what they think is an appropriate name, recall is considerably improved.

There are mnemonics that will help with name recall. If you are introduced to 'Duncan' you may try and link that person with another Duncan you already know. The first Duncan that comes to my mind is a very keen surfer, so I could 'place' a surfboard on a distinctive feature of the person I am meeting. Another option is to tweak the name 'Duncan' to give an image and then, again, link that image to some distinctive feature of the person. Duncan could become a dustbin (not many other names start Du..) and that person might be standing in a dustbin.

Many years ago, I taught a student called Kirsty. She had a very distinctive nose piercing, and so I imagined water pouring out of her piercing and linked that to 'thirsty' (as it rhymes with Kirsty). While the mnemonic proved incredibly effective and difficult to forget (I still remember it), it created the awkward situation of looking at her nose to find her name. When tested in the quiet of a laboratory there is good evidence that such complex methods markedly improve the recall of names from faces.

More important is what happens in a realistic, social setting. Peter Morris and colleagues invited university students to a party having told them that they should learn the names of other party-goers. Some of the students were trained using an imagery mnemonic, similar to those described above, others were asked to try and retrieve the names at increasing intervals after first hearing them. For this second method, students were told that shortly after hearing each name they should test themselves by attempting to recall it. Then, after a longer interval they should try once again to remember the name. Now and then afterwards, they should look round the room and try to recall the names of the people that they had met earlier. A third group did not receive any memory improvement instructions. The results were clear. Repeated-retrieval was considerably better than the other two methods, with the imagery mnemonic group doing somewhat worse than the control group. Clearly, complex mnemonics need to be tailored to the practicalities of the situation and they are not a panacea for all memory problems.

It is worth finishing this section by revisiting the 'skilled memory' theory (Ericsson et al., 2004). This model captures the many elements of mnemonics and highlights their potential. To enhance memory, you should use prior knowledge and patterns to deeply analyse and group items (encoding principle). Next, by establishing links with retrieval cues during study, those same cues can then be used to promote recall (retrieval structure principle). Imagery is often a key element in these first two steps. Finally, with practice, you become increasingly efficient so that the same amount of information can be stored in less time (speed-up principle).

Imagery and skilled performance

Does imagery help in sport? Next time you watch a top footballer take a penalty or an elite athlete just about to tackle the high jump, consider their mental preparation. They are in deep concentration, often visualising their upcoming actions. There are very good reasons for this preparation. Experiments have shown that imagery training can improve penalty taking by professional footballers. Likewise, high-jumpers trained to use internal motor imagery achieve higher bar clearances. It is thought that most elite athletes (70-90%) use motor imagery to improve performance, with professional sportsmen and women using imagery more than amateurs. An example is the great golfer, Jack Nicklaus, who wrote that *"I never hit a shot, not even in practice, without having a very sharp in-focus picture of it in my head."*

Imagery can benefit motor performance across a wide range of situations. Performance improvements have been described for both laboratory tested actions and for real sporting skills. The many sports in which imagery benefits have been described include swimming, football, running, jumping, gymnastics, and volleyball. One popular way to assess the effects of imagery has been to compare performance on the 'free throw' in basketball. Here, the player stands on a specific spot and tries to throw the ball through the hoop. Studies from all over the world have shown how visualisation training can improve the percentage of successful shots. It might be added that while not every study finds improvements associated with imagery, competitive sport is all about marginal gains.

It is possible that the many basketball experiments involving imagery were partly inspired by a much earlier study of free throw accuracy. Rather curiously, the internet repeatedly describes a 1996/1950s study (it cannot make up its mind on the year) on basketball free-throws by a Dr. Biasiotto/Blaslotto from the University of Chicago showing how the improvement following 30 days of visual imagery was almost as good as physically practising shots for an hour a day. A remarkable result. Not only are there internet inconsistencies in spelling the supposed author but it is, in fact, the wrong author. The study was actually described by the Australian psychologist Alan Richardson in 1967. One reason for mentioning this misrepresentation is that it highlights how internet users can generate and then perpetuate errors – so beware.

Imagery offers multiple benefits. In addition to promoting skill learning and performance, imagery can be used to help build confidence and motivation, control arousal and anxiety, complement rehabilitation after injury, and make 'training' possible when facilities are inaccessible.

Reflecting these different benefits there are different forms of imagery. Perhaps the most obvious distinction is between external and internal (motor) imagery. The former is principally visual. This can involve seeing yourself externally as others would or seeing the challenge through your own eyes, thereby incorporated kinaesthetic aspects. For example, seeing yourself run the hurdles from your own perspective. The second form of imagery, internal, involves mentally recreating the desired sequence of motor actions and their kinaesthetic attributes. Many programmes emphasise motor imagery. However, for reasons that will become clearer, the ability to use internal motor imagery effectively depends on already having the basic skill. This means that imagining I am Patrick Mahomes, Simone Biles, or Harry Kane will not assist my sporting prowess.

Imagery protocols have been tailored to match the cognitive demands that relate to a specific challenge, such as penalty taking, or are designed for more general benefits, such as planning and strategy. Likewise, imagery has been used to assist with different aspects of motivation, such as staying focussed, regulating emotions, and appreciating the long-term steps to a goal.

Reflecting the complexities of performance, the influential motor imagery model (PETTLEP) was devised. The letters form an acronym standing for the Physical response to the imagined sporting situation, the Environment, the imagined Task, its Timing and pace, the Learning or memory component of imagery, the Emotions elicited, and its Perspective, which refers to the type of imagery, for example external or internal. A review of the effectiveness of PETTLEP found evidence for improvements in volleyball, golf bunker shots, and bicep curls, along with aspects of rhythmic gymnastics, football (soccer), ice hockey, and field hockey (Morone et al., 2022). In most of these studies the imagery training protocol lasted up to six weeks. Before concluding that imagery has seemingly magical properties it is worth reminding that in some studies the benefits of imagery appear minimal, and sometimes are simply not evident at all.

Those with better imagery skills seem to receive better training effects. In practice, this means engaging as many senses as possible to create the image, i.e., the sight, sound, and feel of the action. To help, trainers have developed different imagery scripts ('guided imagery') for different sports. This approach is attractive as it offers a complementary regime that minimises risk of injury and fatigue, and which is not affected by bad weather or lack of access to equipment.

Those who regularly use imagery include dancers and musicians, as well as athletes. Their anticipatory images can help the planning and execution of future movements, thereby, increasing efficiency, temporal precision, and economy of movement. Consequently, both auditory and motor imagery skills help in the learning of new pieces. Musicians might benefit from how imagery can help to counter music performance anxiety. Imagery can also be used for training in less obvious domains. For example, guided imagery was successfully used to help student nurses perform their first injections. Mental imagery has also moved into patient rehabilitation, including retraining after a stroke, recovering muscular strength, and aiding pain management.

Why might imagery work? We now know that visual imagery activates a network of brain regions from frontal to sensory cortical areas, creating a weak version of the real thing. Likewise, imagining a motor action sets up activity in motor cortex that can be augmented by training. It is this ability to internally mimic real events that helps to explain why imagery can be effective.

The Functional Equivalence theory builds on the discovery that when someone engages in imagery, they activate areas of the brain similar to those that would become active if the individual actually executed the task. If you imagine yourself kicking a football, then areas of the brain which normally become active when you kick a football should become active. Consequently, imagined actions share brain activity sites with those associated with real movements, though the activity patterns are not identical.

Starting from this premise, the Functional Equivalence theory promotes several factors thought to contribute to more effective imagery. These factors include trying to match the durations of the executed and the imagined tasks, giving appropriate time for more complex movements, and trying to equate the force required for the motor task execution with the mental effort during its imagination. One speculative reason why this can be effective is that motor imagery may increase brain plasticity in those key sites required for the motor-skill learning. Other possible explanations include the idea that motor imagery creates faint activity in relevant peripheral muscle groups. A more cognitive explanation is that motor imagery aids the coding and rehearsal of key elements of the desired action.

Finding exactly how motor imagery aids performance will inevitably lead to better training protocols.

Up to now, the focus has been on imagery, but the mere observation of well executed actions can also benefit training. Like imagery, observing actions can induce relevant brain activity. Just watching someone kick a ball will increase activity in pre-motor brain areas. However, observation and imagery are not equivalent, despite many overlaps. Imagery is thought to be top-down, driven by our knowledge of the desired actions. In contrast, observation of a skilled-action is more bottom-up in that it involves the passive interpretation of that information.

Part of the explanation for why passive observation influences the brain in this way comes from the discovery by Giacomo Rizzolatti of 'mirror neurons'. Mirror neurons fire *both* when the individual makes a specific action, e.g., reaching out their hand, *and* when observing another making that same action. Although first discovered in the brains of monkeys (Figure 9.4), it is assumed that humans also possess mirror neurons. Consequently, making an action, observing an action, and imagining making that same action, can all activate overlapping populations of mirror neurons. In this way, better connections can be made when observing or imagining faultless performance. A further feature of mirror neurons is that they are more active the more practised an individual is in making the observed action, a feature that is clearly relevant when considering training regimes. This same feature helps to explain why imagery may not help the learning of a novel movement or action as any mirror neuron activity will be low.

The complementary conclusion is that imagery will be more effective in those who can already execute the skilled actions. A comparison of active and naïve high-jumpers showed brain activity differences when asked to imagine jumping. Practised athletes activated motor areas while novices activated visual areas. In another study, practised players of volleyball and basketball showed more restricted brain activation patterns, contrasting with more diffuse activation in novices. The clear implication is that you should establish precise motor representations of the desired skill before you can mentally translate that into a helpful internal representation. Consequently, if you cannot perform an action physically, you will not be able to imagine it in a way that delivers a high level of functional equivalence. This is probably why I will never be a great golfer.

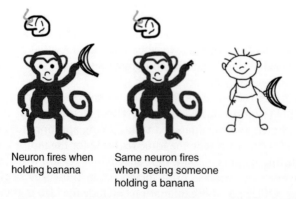

Neuron fires when
holding banana

Same neuron fires
when seeing someone
holding a banana

Figure 9.4 Mirror neurons fire (jagged arrow) when performing an action and when observing the same action.

A concern is that mirror neurons might 'force' an observer to mimic the actions of those they are watching. Consider for a moment sitting next to a trained musician at an orchestral performance – thankfully their arm actions to do not reflect what they are seeing. In reality, overt motor mimicry does not typically happen, even though some mirror neurons seem to be directly linked to motor output relays. Thankfully, the same system has suppression mechanisms that stop the automatic mimicry of other peoples' actions. (However, when I watch a sport, such as rugby, my body will often twitch and move, reflecting what I am watching. My family wish that my suppression neurons could do a better job.)

10 'Smart drugs', supplements, and self-brain stimulation

Never be the smartest person in the room.

Attributed to Confucius

The quest for cognitive enhancers

The dream of finding a drug that will increase your cognitive powers is irresistible. The 2011 film 'Limitless' plays on this very dream, with the creation of a pill that liberates the (supposed) inaccessible 80% of your brain. This belief is fueled by the very rare individuals who have cognitive skills that are truly exceptional, often for reasons that we do not fully understand (Chapter 8). The belief also feeds into the persistent notion that we have untapped reservoirs of cognitive powers that, for some unknown reason, we persist in not using (see Chapter 19). For students there is the allure of taking the right pill before an exam and reaping the rewards (Figure 10.1).

Potential cognitive enhancing drugs have been called 'nootropics', 'cognitive enhancers', 'neuroenhancers', or 'smart' drugs. These labels immediately create the belief that the compounds must work, though this is often far from the truth.

There are two main categories of potential cognitive enhancers. The first consists of drugs, often stimulants, that have been prescribed for other medical purposes. In the U.K., buying prescription-only medications without a prescription is illegal, as is supplying them to others for 'off-label' purposes. ('Off-label' means for purposes not prescribed.) The second category of potential cognitive enhancers consists of nutritional supplements and herbal extracts that are legally sold over the counter or on the internet. In the U.K., 'cognitive enhancers' are categorised as foods or nutritional supplements. As such they have to be approved by the Food Standards Agency (FSA). (I will retain the inverted commas around 'cognitive enhancer' as I do not want to imply that they necessarily do what they claim.)

Nutritional supplements are more likely to be approved rather than pharmacological drugs, as they are seen as less risky. A further attraction for herbal products is the unwarranted belief that because they are 'natural' they must be safe. According to the FSA, food supplements are not intended to treat or prevent diseases in humans. Rather, they are intended to correct any nutritional deficiencies. This stipulation affects the claims made by the producers. For example, adverts for supplements often play on our fears that we might be deficient in a particular vitamin or a trace element, such as magnesium. These fears are typically ungrounded. An exception may be vitamin D, as subclinical vitamin D deficiency is widespread, affecting bone health. This deficiency is especially prevalent among the elderly, nursing home residents, hospitalised patients, and those who are obese.

When promoting 'cognitive enhancers', adverts sometimes include anecdotal quotes about their powers. Such personal testimony, even if made by a 'Doctor' (of what?), has no

DOI: 10.4324/9781003537649-10

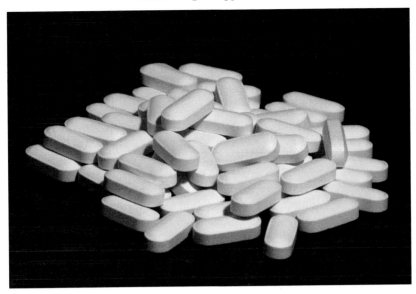

Figure 10.1 The allure of drugs to improve learning and memory.

scientific validity. Quite deliberately, manufacturer's claims are carefully qualified, with terms such as 'may' help. Banner statements such as 'Scientifically Proved' are meaningless without a context – what exactly has been 'proved' and by whom? Was the study rigorous, with proper controls and adequate numbers of participants? There is a lot of hype and self-promotion in this highly lucrative market, so it is all the more important to base any decisions on well-conducted, experimental studies. In a clear message, the U.S. Food and Drug Administration (FDA) warned in 2019 that cognitive enhancement supplements may be ineffective, unsafe, and might prevent a person from seeking an appropriate diagnosis and treatment.

'Smart drugs' – stimulants: There is a boom in the market for 'cognitive enhancers', with the prospect of them becoming common in the workplace. One survey in Germany esti-mated that around 10% of adults had used pharmacological neuroenhancers for non-medical purposes, while an on-line survey across 60 countries put the number at nearer 20%. The numbers among college students are likely to be even higher, given reports that 30% of students at the University of Kentucky have used Attention Deficit Hyperactivity Disorder (ADHD) medicine for cognitive enhancement, in other words, for off-label use.

Some stimulant drugs unquestionably combat fatigue and, can thereby, improve alert-ness. Historically, substances such as ma huang in China (*Ephedra vulgaris*, which contains adrenaline), khat in Northern Africa and Yemen (*Catha edulis*, which contains the stimu-lant alkaloid cathinone), and coca in South America (*Erythroxylon coca*, which contains cocaine) were, and continue, to be used as stimulants. In the more recent past, cocaine was much heralded for its supposed clinical benefits. Sigmund Freud, for example, advocated the drug as a means to boost and maintain physical and mental performance. Sherlock Holmes famously injected himself with a 7% solution of cocaine when in need of mental stimula-tion. Incidentally, the original Coca Cola recipe is thought to have contained extract of coca leaves, although cocaine was completely removed from the drink's recipe in the 1920s.

During World War II, the RAF recommended that exhausted aircrews took ampheta-mine ('Benzedrine') as a stimulant. Likewise, the British Army ordered Benzedrine for the troops fighting in 1942 at El Alamein. However, the clinical promotion of cocaine and amphetamine largely collapsed with the growing realisation that these same addictive drugs can come at a terrible cost. Furthermore, an exhaustive review into the effects of amphetamine in alert individuals found no consistent effects on memory recall, working memory, selective attention, or sustained attention when compared with a placebo control (Roberts et al., 2020). As potential 'smart drugs', cocaine and amphetamine have now been replaced by other stimulants.

One high-profile drug is Modafinil. This stimulant is prescribed for somnolence, the clinical term for excessive drowsiness. There has been a steady increase in Modafinil prescription in the U.K., with growing concerns about off-label use. For instance, the Oxford University newspaper, the Cherwell, reported in 2016 that 16% of students knowingly took Modafinil or a related drug without prescription.

The first task is to determine whether Modafinil can improve memory in healthy adults who are not sleep-deprived. (Arguably more important is whether such stimulants have unwanted side-effects.) An analysis that incorporated multiple studies into the effects of Modafinil on alert participants concluded that there are occasional gains to executive function (Battleday & Brem, 2015). While benefits were sometimes seen for working memory, many studies also failed to see any helpful effects on memory. In general, it was felt that as tests became longer and more complex, Modafinil more consistently conferred a slight cognitive advantage.

A subsequent analysis that amalgamated the findings from a wide array of cognitive tasks still concluded that Modafinil conferred a small positive effect, but this was only seen when the data from many different aspects of cognition were combined (Roberts et al., 2020). While there was some evidence for improved memory updating, there were no apparent advantages for memory recall, sustained attention, or selective attention when compared with placebo. (The lack of effect on attention might at first sight seem surprising, but in these studies the participants were not drowsy.) The conclusion is that Modafinil has marginal effects that can sometimes help narrow aspects of memory in healthy adults who are not sleep-deprived. The fact that these conclusions only emerge after combining multiple studies highlights the inconsistency of many of its effects, in other words, Modafinil is not a reliable nootropic.

The status of Modafinal changes for sleep-deprived individuals. Here, there is clear evidence that Modafinil can combat tiredness, with signs that it can help restore cognitive functioning back towards previous levels. There are, however, concerns that these same effects might create overconfidence. Individuals may believe that their cognitive performance is better than it is in reality. This faulty self-monitoring might, in turn, encourage unrealistic risk-taking. In addition, Modafinil is associated with complaints of restlessness and sleep disturbances, leading to insomnia.

Methylphenidate (MPH – better known as Ritalin) is another supposed neuroenhancer. This drug has long been prescribed for ADHD, but its stimulant properties suggested that it might also boost cognition. Reflecting this belief, the drug has been extensively misused as a cognitive aid by college students. However, when the results of 24 studies into the cognitive effects of MPH in healthy non-sleep-deprived individuals were combined, any benefits of the drug were modest at best (Roberts et al., 2020). Overall, MPH appeared to have small beneficial effects on memory recall and sustained attention but did not aid working memory. It was also apparent that individual responses varied considerably, with any positive actions restricted to a narrow dose range. As a result, it is not clear how individual users might best identify any optimal dose levels.

A general criticism of 'neuroenhancers' when used by healthy individuals is that the brain is already highly effective, so pushing it further with drugs might, at best, have an extremely small effect or might even push it over the top and tip it into a suboptimal state. Indeed, animal studies show that low doses of MPH may occasionally help memory, but higher doses become counter-productive. Also, what might work for one person may not work for another. One reason for this is thought to be individual differences in baseline levels of cognitive performance. Put simply, those individuals with the most to make up, may be those who most consistently show any benefit. One study found, for example, that Modafinil helped those with lower I.Q. scores on a vigilance task, but it had no apparent effect on those with higher I.Q. scores. The same logic applies to levels of arousal. Stimulant drugs, such as Modafinil, have more convincing actions when used to counter negative situations such as a lack of sleep.

Another concern is that 'smart' drugs may have state-dependent effects (see *Context and memory*), so that the subsequent recall of information when not under the influence of the drug may be impaired. Furthermore, because so much of their use is off-label, there are legitimate concerns about dose levels and the appreciation of potential side-effects. The drug Modafinil is, for example, linked to psychiatric symptoms, cardiovascular changes, along with skin and multi-organ sensitivity. It should, therefore, come as no surprise that the British Medical Association (BMA) highlights how improved general lifestyle, such as quality sleep, physical activity, better nutrition, reduced alcohol intake, positive social interaction, and environmental enrichment provides a surer, safer way to reach optimal cognitive performance than so-called 'smart drugs'.

A contentious question is whether the use of such drugs is unethical or cheating ('neurodoping'). In some ways it seems little different from taking a pill to help stay awake to revise the night before an exam. (Not that I would recommend doing that, but if I change the word 'pill' to 'coffee' it becomes more acceptable.) You might also ask what is the difference between taking a cognitive-enhancing drug and receiving personal tutoring, taking additional computer-based training, or the adoption of a healthier lifestyle? Nevertheless, Duke University reportedly took the step of treating the use of 'off-label' drugs as academic dishonesty. Similar anxieties have been raised across U.K. universities, but official policy is currently lacking. These anxieties include potentially rewarding risky behaviour given that the long-term consequences of regularly taking these drugs by healthy adults is largely unknown. Related worries include consuming cocktails of unregulated drugs and their use at unprescribed dosages. These same concerns are further heightened given the potential attraction of these drugs to children and adolescents.

The debate over neurodoping has obvious parallels with the rules concerning sport. Doping has probably been around in sport ever since competitive sport began. One favoured stimulant in more recent times was amphetamine. It is most likely that amphetamine contributed to the death of the British cyclist Tommy Simpson on Mont Ventoux in the 1967 Tour de France. Unsurprisingly, the World Anti-Doping Agency (WADA) currently bans amphetamine and stimulant drugs prescribed for ADHD, including MPH and Modafinil.

The game of chess poses fascinating challenges as its governing body has its own anti-doping rules. There are already intriguing reports that the stimulant drugs MPH (Ritalin), caffeine, and Modafinil affect chess performance. When played under time limits, all three stimulants increased the number of games lost on time rules. Only when considering those games completed was there a modest benefit for Modafinil and MPH (Franke et al., 2017). Seemingly, both Modafinil and MPH increased the thinking time for moves, sometimes causing a player to time out and lose, but on other occasions benefiting them with greater planning time.

Piracetam and related compounds: There is a group of potential cognitive enhancers of which piracetam has been the most studied. These synthetic compounds include oxiracetam, pramiracetam, etiracetam, nefiracetam, aniracetam, and rolziracetam, as well as piracetam. Much of the evidence on the nootropic effects of piracetam comes from animal studies, where there are many reports of improved learning. These animal studies point to piracetam having both neuroprotective and neuroplastic actions. The question is whether these benefits translate to human performance.

Much of that focus has involved looking at the effects of piracetam on existing clinical conditions that impair cognition, especially in the elderly. Some individual studies point to how piracetam might help to combat age-related cognitive decline and dementia, including aiding memory, but others find no such evidence. This inconsistency has led some reviewers to conclude that the published findings do not support the use of clinical use of piracetam for those with dementia or other cognitive impairments. Others hold open the possibility that piracetam might have modest beneficial effects for those with early signs of dementia or cognitive impairment.

There is less published evidence for piracetam's potential cognitive enhancing effects in younger, healthy humans. Nevertheless, piracetam is sometimes used by optimistic students, though this is probably uncommon. One reason may be its low availability. For example, the U.S. FDA has decided that piracetam may not be sold as a dietary supplement, although tests show that it is often added to commercial supplements. While piracetam is barred from prescription in the U.K., it is possible to freely purchase chemical variants such as aniracetam and oxiracetam.

Nicotine: The addictive intake of nicotine is experienced worldwide by an estimated 1.3 billion tobacco smokers. In addition, there is the growing use of E-cigarettes (Vapes). One self-justification for smoking is that it gives a cognitive boost (Figure 10.2). More specifically, one of the commonest reasons smokers give for continued smoking is that it helps them stay focussed. This subjective justification most probably reflects the decline in concentration, attention, and working memory that follows smoking abstinence.

This pattern means that in any experimental study it is necessary to separate any benefits that reflect the relief from nicotine craving from any true positive properties of the drug. This distinction is critical as smoking abstinence, even just overnight, causes anxiety, mood shifts, loss of concentration, depressed working memory, and disturbed sleep. By partially reversing these effects, regular nicotine usage or tobacco smoking becomes reinforcing and gives the illusion of improving memory.

What happens when nicotine is given to a naïve brain? One approach is to test animals that have never experienced the drug. Many rodent studies report that a single dose of nicotine can improve working memory and recognition memory, as well as aid memory consolidation. These outcomes seem plausible as the drug acts directly on the neurotransmitter acetylcholine, which has a multitude of actions, of which one is on hippocampal function.

Once we turn to humans, the story becomes more complicated. As indicated, we need to distinguish those who never smoke from those who regularly smoke. A meta-analysis involving both non-smokers and smokers found that nicotine had positive effects on aspects of attention in the non-smokers, while aspects of working memory were improved in both groups, with nicotine also lifting episodic memory (Heishman et al., 2010). This pattern fits with later studies pointing to how nicotine can enhance some aspects of attention and working memory. While this might sound encouraging for tobacco users, chronic smokers

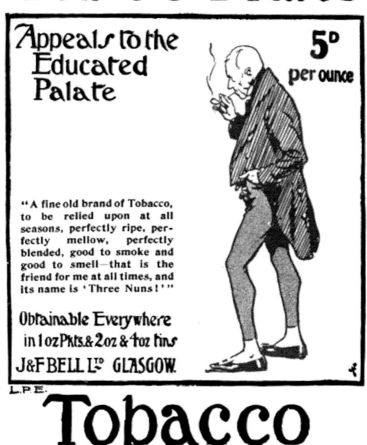

Figure 10.2 An old advert with the implication that tobacco helps you concentrate.

show a loss of short-term memory and long-term memory, as well as difficulties with sustained attention (Conti et al., 2019), along with the need to combat any abstinence.

It has to be remembered that nicotine is highly addictive. Furthermore, the smoke from cigarettes contains a toxic mixture of over 5000 chemicals, of which at least 70 can cause cancer. Unsurprisingly, smoking increases the likelihood of a plethora of life-threatening illnesses, not just numerous types of cancer. There is no safe level of smoking for your health. In reality, regular tobacco smoking is associated with a destructive pattern of cognitive loss that includes memory, as well as an increased risk of Alzheimer's disease.

Vaping (E-cigarettes) is increasingly popular, mainly because it is presumed to provide a purer hit of nicotine. But E-cigarettes still come with over 100 different chemicals, creating a complex cocktail that includes toxic aerosols and potential carcinogens. Animal studies reveal that daily vaping can cause neuroinflammatory responses that reduce memory function. Nicotine can also be toxic to the developing brain. In summary, any positive effects of vaping on cognition are short-lived and are probably far outweighed by the long-term negative effects.

It is both concerning are ironic that a national survey of U.S. youth found that vaping, smoking, and their dual use were associated with self-reported serious difficulties in concentrating and remembering. The earlier the age that people report first vaping, the greater the difficulties. Clearly, nicotine in any form should never be recommended as a memory aid, yet the myth persists.

Caffeine, glucose, and energy drinks: Next, comes one of the best known and widely consumed chemical stimulants, caffeine. The scientific name for caffeine is 1, 3, 7-trimethylxanthine (Figure 10.3). Caffeine intake, from one source or another, has been around for many centuries. One claim is that coffee drinking can be traced back to Ethiopia around 850 ACE. There is a popular legend that a farmer noticed how jumpy and agitated his goats became after eating the berries of the arabica plant. He gave some of the berries to a local monk, who used them to concoct the world's first cup of coffee. After its adoption in the Arab world, coffee was introduced to Europe by Venetian merchants in 1615. The taste spread rapidly, with the first coffee house in London opening in 1652. Going against the tide, the Swedish king Gustaf III (1746–1792) believed that coffee was an evil. To demonstrate its dangers, he is said to have offered two condemned twins an alternative to death. One twin was to drink coffee for life, the other to drink tea. Apparently, the experiment ended when the tea-drinking twin died at the age of 83.

Compared with other stimulants, caffeine is a relatively benign way to increase arousal and reduce fatigue. (As I write this, I have a cup of coffee to hand.) Numerous studies have shown improved performance after caffeine intake on tests of vigilance and sustained response, especially when fatigued. Caffeine can also reduce reaction times and sometimes aid working memory. Other good news is that caffeine intake is associated with a reduction in workplace accidents. Thankfully, we are normally good at self-regulating our caffeine intake to optimise any effects. There is, however, far less certainty over whether caffeine benefits more complex cognitive tasks when we are already alert. It does not, for example, appear to benefit long-term memory, with some studies finding no effect on wider aspects of cognition.

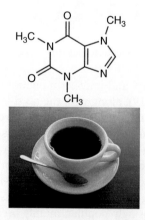

Figure 10.3 Chemical structure of caffeine above cup of coffee.

One concern is that studies of caffeine typically compare the performance of people either with or without the drug. Some researchers argue that any observed differences might stem from the negative consequence of caffeine withdrawal in the drug-free participants rather than any benefits from consuming caffeine. This concern stems from the realisation that caffeine-withdrawal syndrome is a reality, with the potential to cause headaches, fatigue, irritability, depressed mood, difficulty in concentrating, and clouded thinking. The potential confound of withdrawal is particularly relevant to caffeine as the drug is so ubiquitous, being present not only in coffee, tea, and soda drinks, but also in chocolate and a range of other foods. Nevertheless, comparisons between regular caffeine users and non-consumers of caffeinated drinks can still reveal benefits of caffeine on cognitive performance. In other words, the lift sometimes caused by caffeine cannot solely be explained by the reversal of withdrawal effects.

Current evidence shows that caffeine can act as a cognitive stimulant, but its effects are most apparent on reaction time tasks, vigilance, and information processing, along with more inconsistent effects on working memory. It is often more helpful to see caffeine as a cognitive normaliser rather than a cognitive enhancer in those who are already alert. There are also some added concerns that caffeine may have state-dependent effects (see *Context and memory*), potentially making it more difficult to recall information when you switch between a caffeine and a non-caffeine state. As a footnote, because of its stimulant effects, there was a ban on caffeine for athletes between 1984 and 2004. In 2004, the World Anti-Doping Agency (WADA) decided that caffeine did not reach the criteria for exclusion even though it can improve physical performance. Currently, WADA monitors caffeine levels, but they are not acted on, unless the levels are exceptionally high.

Another readily available substance is glucose. This sugar is the energy source for the brain. Studies in both humans and animals repeatedly show that glucose can transiently enhance memory, including episodic memory in humans. This boost has been called the 'glucose memory facilitation effect'. Interestingly, emotionally arousing pictures both increase brain glucose levels and enhance recall, helping to explain the frequent lift in memory for emotional stimuli. (This same lift involves an array of other neural actions, most notably the release of noradrenaline in the amygdala.) While the effects of glucose on memory can sometimes be seen in the young, they are often most evident in the elderly. Despite providing a brief cognitive lift, glucose is not a sensible long-term strategy. Excessive sugar is bad for a great many health reasons.

So-called 'energy drinks' often combine high levels of caffeine with high levels of sugar, along with other additives. In the U.K. they are marketed as either dietary supplements or beverages. These drinks are now very big business. The annual 'energy drink' consumption in the U.S. was recently estimated at 28 litres per person, while in the U.K. it was 12 litres per person. A number of studies have shown that energy drinks can increase subjective alertness, reduce reaction times, and benefit performance on focussed and sustained attention tasks. These drinks can also sometimes improve performance on tests of memory. Much of the arousal effect is thought to reflect their high caffeine levels, although for memory tests both caffeine and glucose probably interact to lift performance. That said, a comparison between Red Bull and Red Bull Sugarfree in young volunteers concluded that the sugar, rather than the caffeine, played a major role in the improved scores for working memory and episodic recognition memory (Wesnes et al., 2017).

Energy drinks have no therapeutic benefit. Neither can they combat the detrimental effects of alcohol on memory. Alarmingly, the popular habit of combining the two is associated with an increased desired to drink and a misperception of levels of intoxication. As a footnote, stated plans by the U.K. government in 2019 to ban the sale of energy drinks to those under 16 years have been repeatedly delayed, despite obvious concerns over the health consequences of consuming excessive amounts of sugar and caffeine.

Nutrition and nutritional supplements: At this point we enter the wild west of nutritional supplements. This is a multi-billion-dollar industry that remains poorly regulated globally and is very adept at marketing. You will, for example, come across terms like 'brain supplements' and 'brain vitamins'. For instance, you might read that magnesium is needed by the brain for normal development (correct). Therefore, a supplement containing magnesium will improve brain health, including your memory. In fact, magnesium deficiency is rare, typically only occurring in those with other illnesses such as diabetes or with some gastro-intestinal conditions. But the adverts play on our fears that we might all be deficient (and we have no direct way of measuring whether this is or is not the case).

Let's begin with one of the few dietary interventions that is of real practical benefit. There is considerable evidence that breakfast is important for children's cognitive performance, helping them to maintain memory and attention across the morning. This beneficial effect is due to micronutrients (minerals and vitamins) as well as macronutrients (such as carbohydrates).

To give one example, a recent British study found that adolescents who always had breakfast attained higher Maths GCSE results than those who skipped breakfast, even after allowing for socio-economic factors (Adolphus et al., 2019). This same association between breakfast and intellectual attainment is seen in countries all around the world. For example, a longitudinal study of Chinese children aged six to 12 found that regular breakfasts were associated with higher I.Q. (Liu et al., 2021). Clearly a proper breakfast is an important start to the day. (By proper I do not mean a sugary cereal, instead I mean items such as eggs, fruit, porridge, nuts, or beans.) The problem is that I write this from the perspective of someone living in an affluent society. This highlights just one of the many inequalities both within a country and between countries, which unwittingly drive differences in I.Q. and academic attainment.

Flavonoids are a group of metabolites produced by a number of plants, some of which provide key constituents to traditional medicines. These compounds have anti-oxidant properties and can reduce neuroinflammation. Studies with animals also suggest that flavonoids can stimulate hippocampal neurogenesis. Whether any of these properties translate into real-life differences is far more contentious.

Flavonoids are present in grape skins, which helps to explain newspaper claims that red, but not white, wine might have beneficial effects on aging. (Red wine is fermented with grape skins, white wine is not.) The bad news is that alcohol, probably at any level, is injurious, so this is not a good strategy.

Perhaps chocolate, which also contains flavonoids, can stake a stronger claim? The good news is that cocoa flavonoids can, in the short term, improve memory. Dark chocolate contains higher levels of cocoa flavonoids than other chocolates (white chocolate has no flavonoids), enabling comparison studies that help to separate out any contributions from glucose. For example, eating a 35 g dark chocolate bar (70% cocoa) improved memory recall two hours later when compared with consuming a 35 g white chocolate bar (Lamport et al., 2020). Likewise dark chocolate can aid visual working memory. Indeed, a range of studies support the view that cocoa flavonoids can aid cognition in young adults, possibly through increasing brain blood flow. It is also worth remembering that chocolate also contains small amounts of caffeine, along with generous amounts of sugar.

In addition to dark chocolate and red wine, a range of other foodstuffs contain flavonoids. Examples include blueberries, green tea, and soy as well as with extracts from the ginkgo tree (*Ginkgo biloba*). Coloured beans such as speckled beans and black beans contain particularly high levels of flavonoids, while white beans have only low levels. One detailed analysis combined the findings from multiple studies that employed different flavonoids supplements, most often from soy, but also from ginkgo, pine bark extracts, and cocoa. Many of the volunteers in these studies were elderly subjects who had taken the supplements for many weeks and months. The researchers could only cautiously conclude that there may be a weak, positive link between flavonoid consumption and cognitive function (Macready et al., 2009). They found evidence that flavonoid compounds could sometimes aid executive function and explicit memory, including working memory and episodic memory, but did not assist semantic memory. Other, later analyses emphasise how the habitual intake of dietary anti-oxidants is only inconsistently associated with improved cognitive performance. There seem to be marginal positive effects, but they may be restricted to certain types of memory and only appear under narrow, as yet unspecified, conditions. These results are a far cry from the advertiser's push that more anti-oxidants must equate to enhanced brain function.

Ginkgo extract has long been promoted for its supposed health-giving properties, creating inevitable interest in its long-term impact on cognition (Figure 10.4). Perhaps surprisingly, chronic consumption of ginkgo typically fails to produce memory enhancing effects in healthy adults. This may come as even more of a surprise if you read the manufacturers' claims. An unusually thorough double-blind study followed over 3000 older adults who took a 120-mg dose of *ginkgo* twice a day for six years (Snitz et al., 2009). There was no evidence that ginkgo delayed the rate of memory decline in these elderly participants. Likewise, there was no evidence that taking ginkgo twice a day prevented the onset of Alzheimer's disease. Ginkgo is not the 'brain herb' it is often marketed as.

Another popular compound, already mentioned, is ginseng. This is usually given as a powder or tea, both derived from the roots of *Panax ginseng* (Figure 10.4). The Ministry of Food and Drug Safety of Korea officially recognises that ginseng might have memory

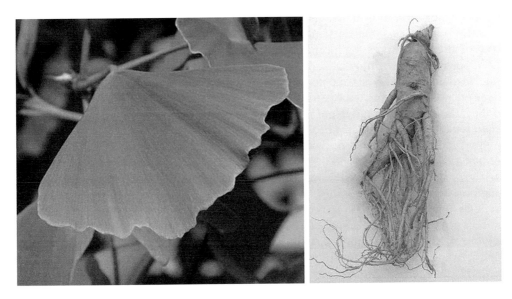

Figure 10.4 Highly distinctive (and unique) leaf of Ginkgo biloba alongside Panax ginseng root.

improving effects. Nevertheless, an initial review of chronic ingestion by healthy subjects could only conclude that the effects on cognition were 'suggestive'. A later analysis also concluded that when ginseng is taken over multiple days the pattern of effects on cognition remains mixed, with selected benefits to working memory but negative effects on reaction time. While there is evidence that a single dose of ginseng could improve performance on tests of long-term memory, these effects were only found within a narrow dose range. Echoing this finding, a later review concluded that single doses of ginseng in healthy volunteers can have both positive and negative effects on cognition. Consequently, within the narrow, optimal dose range, improvements in working memory and long-term recall might sometimes occur, but at the risk of poorer performance at other doses. It is very unclear how an individual might determine their correct dose level.

There has been much interest in whether ginseng can somehow protect against neurodegenerative conditions such as dementia. While there have been a series of such studies, mainly from Korea, that report positive findings, an authoritative Cochrane review (2010) concluded that there was no high-quality evidence about the cognitive benefits of giving ginseng to patients with dementia, but neither did ginseng cause adverse effects. While a later study found some evidence that 24 weeks of ginseng might improve aspects of visual memory in those with Mild Cognitive Impairment (Park et al., 2019), the effects were borderline and there was no impact on the Mini-Mental Status Examination (MMSE), a standard tool used to assess this disorder. Taken together, we currently lack quality evidence that ginseng combats memory loss.

Fish oils, and in particular omega-3 fats, have been a source of interest for decades. They are known to be required for normal brain and eye development. Furthermore, omega-3 fats are classified as 'essential'. This means that the body cannot make them from scratch. For these reasons, pregnant mothers may be prescribed supplementary omega-3 fats. While these fatty acids can be helpful in a number of clinical conditions, the question here is whether they can improve memory in healthy individuals.

Meta-analyses from 2012 and from 2015 combined multiple studies into the cognitive effects of omega-3 fats. Both analyses both found no overall evidence that omega-3 fats benefit memory in healthy individuals. There was, however, some evidence that those with cognitive impairments, but not diagnosed with dementia, might show some benefits on levels of attention, processing speed, and immediate recall. There were, however, no apparent beneficial effects for those already with dementia. The most recent meta-analysis again concluded that omega-3 fats had no benefits for overall cognition but did find modest positive evidence when memory measures were pooled (Alex et al., 2020). Even so, the majority of the individual studies still found no effects of omega-3 fats on memory, highlighting the tenuous nature of any potential benefits.

A search on the internet quickly reveals an almost endless list of foods and herbal supplements claimed to aid cognition, including memory. The ancient Greeks noticed the uncanny resemblance between walnuts and a miniature brain. This similarity gave rise to long held beliefs that walnuts must be good for the brain. Like several other nuts, walnuts are high in levels of omega-3 fatty acids. Encouraging evidence comes from reports that walnuts can improve the memory of rodents, but when carefully put to the test in healthy volunteers, no reliable memory enhancing effects of a walnut-supplemented diet have been found. Another supplement is from the herb bacopa. (Bacopa is the name for a genus of water plants, with *Bacopa monnieri* being the most popular supplement.) Single doses of bacopa appear to have little benefit, though there is tentative evidence that more chronic bacopa consumption might aid memory retention and working memory (Neale et al., 2013).

To this ever-growing list are a variety of mushrooms heralded for their memory enhancing powers. A prominent example is lion's mane (*Hericium erinaceus*), which contains bioactive ingredients that can affect the brain (Figure 10.5). (This mushroom is not to be confused with the lion's mane jellyfish, *Cyanea capillata*, made famous by the Sherlock Holmes story.) Studies with animals do reveal that extracts from *Hericium erinaceus* can promote nerve growth in culture. But this is a far cry from aiding human memory in any useful way. You may also see claims that lion's mane extract can benefit people with Dementia or Mild Cognitive Impairment, but these claims are from studies that lack statistical power. There is a need for much better, larger studies. Just because many mushrooms contain anti-oxidants it is not safe to say that these equate to meaningful brain benefits. Finally, a very different product, chewing gum, has also attracted claims that it might improve cognitive performance. A review of relevant studies only highlighted the mixed outcomes, so the jury is still out.

Repeated words of warning: I have to add a final note of caution before you rush out to eat dark chocolate, take a couple of pills, consume mushrooms, or buy a supplement. Because these products are sold as nutritional supplements, there are legal limits in the U.K. concerning what the sellers can claim. One way round this is to promote customer reviews as positive evidence for the product. These anecdotal accounts can sound very persuasive. But the only way to determine whether a particular supplement or pill benefits cognition is through carefully controlled experiments. Because of so many inconsistent experiments, the most meaningful conclusions come from meta-analyses that combine multiple studies. This large-data approach is needed as any positive effects are almost always small and inconsistent. To summarise, drugs or food supplements offer little, if any,

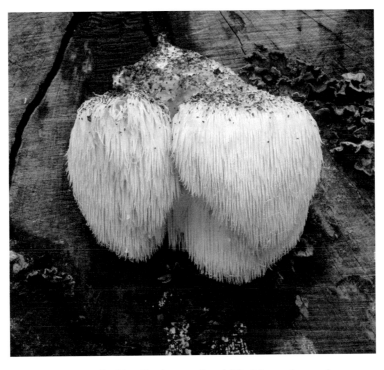

Figure 10.5 The extraordinary looking lion's mane fungi (Hericium erinaceus).

meaningful benefit to a healthy individual. On top of this, some drugs have the potential to cause negative 'side-effects'.

It is safe to conclude that the cognitive benefits of purported 'neuroenhancers' are, at best, modest and very often seem remarkably well-hidden. As caustically noted when reviewing Methylphenidate and Modafinil, *"expectations regarding the effectiveness of these drugs exceed their actual effects"* (Repantis et al., 2010). Likewise, in 2015, the British Medical Association concluded when reviewing stimulant drugs, that *"The benefit for real people, performing everyday work tasks in the real world is dubious"* (Nicholson et al., 2015). The situation has not changed since then.

Electrical brain stimulation: It sounds like the stuff of science fiction – a device that you can hold close to your head to stimulate parts of the brain to improve memory. In fact, there is a very long history of applying electrical currents to the head. Almost 2000 years ago, Scribonius Largus advocated applying a live electric ray fish to the head as a cure for headaches. This remedy was later extended to haemorrhoids, gout, depression, and epilepsy. By the 19th century, the peripheral application of electrical currents had been introduced for anaesthesia. Often forgotten was the fad for 'Medical Batteries', which were sold in their thousands during the latter part of the 19th century and early part of the 20th century. These devices provided electrical stimulation for the head region. While Medical Batteries were claimed to combat a wide range of medical disorders, they do not seem to have been promoted as cognitive enhancers.

One current method (my apologies) of external brain stimulation is called Transcranial Magnetic Stimulation (TMS). During TMS a focal, transient magnetic pulse is applied with a coil in order to stimulate neurons in the targeted brain area (Figure 10.6). Repetitive TMS has been used experimentally to try and help those with impaired memory, including those with Mild Cognitive Impairment and Alzheimer's disease. It has also been used to see if it is possible to enhance memory in healthy people. To do this, you need to decide which part of the brain to stimulate, including which hemisphere, as well as the optimum stimulation intensity.

In healthy adults, the effects of TMS stimulation of the prefrontal cortex are very mixed, but some studies claim improvements in the learning of face/word combinations and other paired-associates (Phipps et al., 2021). It is possible that prefrontal cortex TMS stimulation may also help to restore appropriate memory representations in other brain regions, such as in the hippocampus. Meanwhile parietal cortex stimulation may improve word recognition, aspects of long-term recollection, paired-associate learning, and learning face/word pairings. However, just as many TMS studies have found no beneficial effects, while in a few other studies there was a deterioration in cognition. These different outcomes highlight the need to identify the ideal combination of stimulation parameter, brain location, and memory task.

More promising are the effects of TMS in people with Mild Cognitive Impairment or Alzheimer's disease. Following ten or more sessions of repetitive prefrontal TMS in people with mild Alzheimer's disease, improvements have sometimes been reported for a variety of specific memory tasks, as well as for more global assessments of cognition such as the Mini-Mental Status Examination (MMSE) (Phipps et al., 2021). Related analyses focussing on Mild Cognitive Impairment have concluded that repetitive TMS over multiple sessions could improve overall global cognition as well as aspects of memory. As with nootropics, there appears to be a 'baseline effect', so that it is easier to boost a system that is functioning poorly. What is not clear, is whether any such gains may improve quality of life and whether they might be long-lasting.

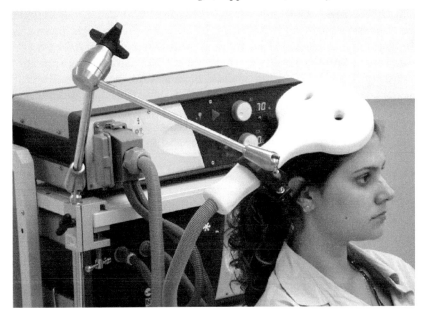

Figure 10.6 Transcranial magnetic stimulation (TMS) applied by the coil held outside the skull.

Another methodology is direct transcranial current stimulation (tDCS). In tDCS a weak, direct electrical current is passed into the brain from an external device. Given its ease of administration, versatility, and minimal side-effects, there has been much interest in its potential. The occasional side effects include sensations such as tingling or burning but they are rarely severe and seem to carry no serious health risks.

Like TMS, some tDCS studies report improvements in working memory in healthy participants following prefrontal cortex stimulation, while others see no effects. Perhaps unsurprisingly, meta-analyses have concluded that the evidence is mixed, and that any benefits to working memory are capricious. Meanwhile, recent reviews covering episodic memory have found no overall effects of tDCS stimulation in healthy volunteers.

These inconsistent results have not deterred home brain stimulation. Starting from around 2010, a do-it-yourself brain stimulation community (DIYers) emerged, using tDCS devices. DIYers fall into two camps: those who wish to enhance cognition and learning, and those trying to combat psychiatric disorders, such as depression. This movement has been encouraged by the availability of tDCS devices on the internet, including self-assembly kits. A feature of this DIY community is how they often share their tDCS experiences in the hope of refining their protocols.

There are inevitable concerns about DIY tDCS. These include how users may want to push the boundaries, leading to lengthy sessions of repetitive stimulation. Other concerns are that our brains might operate as 'a net-zero' system, boosting one facility may come at the cost of diminishing another. When measuring any tDCS effects, individual DIY users rely heavily on subjective feelings of improvement and fail to include proper control conditions. For this reason, their methods would never stand up to scientific scrutiny. Despite justified concerns, there is general consensus that tDCS poses no major health risks when used in ways that match published experiments. The expectation is that we will see a rise and refinement of such devices over the near future.

Just as with 'cognitive enhancing' drugs, there are ethical issues over electrical brain stimulation. One potential area of concerns is its use competitive sports. Brain stimulation devices are currently not included in WADA's Anti-Doping Code 2021 (WADA is the World Anti-Doping Agency), yet studies suggest that tDCS can improve accuracy in pistol shooting, basketball, and golf putting, while also combatting the adverse effects of mental fatigue in professional swimmers (Au, 2022). Perhaps unsurprisingly, there is evidence of tDCS use by Olympic athletes and professional sports teams. One of WADA's criteria for banning is that it violates 'the spirit of sport', a rather fuzzy concept. While tDCS may arguably fall foul of this criterion, to be banned, a substance needs to fail at least one other criterion.

Not wishing to step into the realms of science fiction, but human brain/computer interfaces have already been developed to assist vision for the blind, as well as the motor movements of those who are paralysed. The concept of 'brain chips' has already arrived. Entrepreneurs like Elon Musk see a future in which implanted brain/computer interfaces can assist or boost cognition, including providing memory. The ethical ramifications are endless.

11 The value of sleep

There is only one thing people like that is good for them; a good night's sleep.

Edgar Watson Howe

Why sleep?

Sleep is vital for the well-being of all vertebrates, as well as many invertebrates, but how much sleep an animal takes varies hugely. This fact is well worth remembering when considering the complex topic of sleep and learning. Sleep serves many functions. Reasons to increase sleep include saving energy, the removal of unwanted metabolites, and having a secure hiding place from predators. These reasons are further increased in those animals that rely on foods that are only available for short time periods within each day, such as at dawn and dusk.

In contrast there are many reasons to increase wakefulness and decrease sleep. Reasons include making time to forage for food, avoiding predators, heating up the body, and finding a mate. You will not, therefore, be surprised to discover that different mammals take very different amounts of sleep. A lion, which is a top predator, may sleep and rest for 20 hours a day, while a wildebeest, a favourite prey of the lion, sleeps for just four or five hours a day.

These comparisons tell us that the sleep patterns of different species are set by opposing pressures, with contributions to learning and memory being just one of many demands. As a child we are told that elephants never forget. (Some aspects of their memory, such as their large-scale mapping of the environment, is highly impressive.) You might, therefore, be surprised to discover that elephants take only four hours of sleep a day, while armadillos and koalas will sleep for 20 hours a day. I personally doubt that armadillos and koalas have unusual amounts of data to process every night. I might also add that sloths have had a bad press. Many internet sites state that they sleep for around 16 hours each day, but studies of wild sloths show that it is more like nine or ten hours.

The message from this brief introduction is that sleep has multiple functions, and while supporting learning and memory may be one of them, it does not determine how long an individual species normally sleeps. Nevertheless, sleep restriction is bad for cognition, with effects that include losses of short-term memory and attention. Sleep also affects long-term memory, impacting on both explicit and implicit memory.

You may find mention of the term 'sleep quality'. Good sleep quality occurs when you fall asleep within 30 minutes of getting into bed. During 'good sleep' you are also expected to sleep through the night, waking up no more than once. Adults should take seven or more hours of sleep each night. In contrast, newborn babies require around double that amount.

DOI: 10.4324/9781003537649-11

Over the following 20 years or so we gradually require less sleep until we reach adult durations (Figure 11.1). But just as you can have too little sleep, you can take too much sleep, so that both shorter and longer sleep patterns are associated with poorer cognition.

Sleep and memory: There are many potential reasons why sleep might be good for learning and memory. Probably the most obvious is that the tiredness caused by sleep loss impairs *subsequent learning* and retention. There is, however, the additional possibility, that sleep *after learning* helps memory consolidation and subsequent retention. Both reasons turn out to be correct. Sleep helps to prepare the brain for upcoming learning, while also strengthening recently acquired new memories.

Sleep is standardly divided between rapid eye movement sleep (REM sleep) and non-REM (NREM) sleep. These two components have different patterns of brain activity. During REM sleep there is desynchronised cortical activity that has some similarities to what happens during wakefulness. Vivid dreams are most closely associated with REM sleep, and we normally have several bouts of REM sleep every night. By waking people during bouts of REM sleep it is possible to confirm that we all have multiple dreams every night. These bouts of REM sleep are concentrated in the second half of the night.

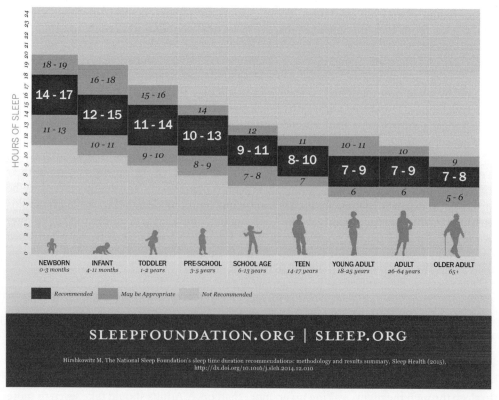

Figure 11.1 Recommended durations of nightly sleep for different age groups from the National Sleep Foundation.

Sleep, and in particular REM sleep, has long been associated with the acquisition of visuomotor skills and their consolidation. These tasks make demands on a form of implicit learning called procedural memory (Figure 1.3). Procedural memory tasks used in sleep studies include learning key press-tone combinations, mirror tracing, novel motor sequences, pursuit rotor tasks, adapting to lenses that distort the visual field, Morse code training, and learning to trampoline. REM sleep is thought to have a leading role in supporting the progressive acquisition of such skills, which may take days or even weeks to master. One of the contributing factors is the upregulation of myelin-related genes during sleep, which then enhance appropriate brain pathways (see *W for White matter learning*).

Immature mammals, including human babies, experience considerably more REM sleep than their adult counterparts. This REM dominance points to an important role in brain maturation, including white matter wiring and tuning. This contribution makes it all the more incredible that some mammals almost completely dispense with REM sleep. Whales and dolphins experience slow-wave sleep in one hemisphere at a time, with little or no REM sleep. The principal reason for this highly unusual sleeping pattern is that these marine mammals are 'conscious breathers', they decide when to breathe. Unlike us they do not have a continual breathing reflex. So, they sleep with one hemisphere awake in order to breathe at the right time, while also scanning for predators and obstacles. As far as we know, birds that sleep on the wing adopt a similar sleep strategy.

The other division of sleep is non-REM (NREM). During NREM sleep the brain's electrophysiological profile changes so that the EEG signal is more synchronised. One result is the appearance of slow waves, leading to the term 'slow-wave sleep'. These slow waves dominate much of NREM sleep. Dreams can also occur during NREM sleep, but these often lack the narrative, movie-like feel of REM dreams, being more thought-like, less emotional, and less bizarre.

Of the two divisions of sleep, NREM has been more closely associated with supporting explicit memory, including the consolidation of episodic information. At the neuronal level, it is thought that during slow-wave sleep the hippocampus is able to replay waking events. That same 'replay' helps the consolidation of hippocampal-neocortical information transfer and strengthens the relevant cortico-cortical connections.

To understand these consolidation processes, attention has focussed on what are called 'sharp waves' and 'ripples'. These terms refer to the synchronised activity of hippocampal neurons that occurs during NREM. These activity patterns are thought to stimulate the transfer of explicit memory-related information from the hippocampus to the neocortex. One possibility is that NREM contributions to memory may be especially significant during the initial stages of learning. In contrast, REM sleep may have a later role, helping to stabilise the changes acquired during NREM sleep. This is, however, just one of many models of how REM and NREM sleep can separately and jointly influence explicit memory, and we are a long way from reaching a consensus. For example, it has also been suggested that the gradual, progressive learning of schemas, which contribute to explicit memory, may rely heavily on REM sleep. (A schema is formed by grouping together related facts or experiences.)

Sleep is famously related to creativity and problem solving. Well-known anecdotes include how the structure of the benzene ring was solved by August Kekule following a dream of a snake eating its own tail. It is also said that the chemical elements in the periodic table were correctly classified by Dmitri Mendeleyev in a dream. Studies show that sleeping on a problem can help to find the solution. This effect could be because the period of sleep reduces interference from erroneous solutions or that sleep encourages the replay of potential solutions. Comparing easy with difficult word problems showed that sleep was especially helpful when solving the difficult problems. This pattern suggests that sleep allows the brain to replay information to test for weak, less obvious solutions, as well as replaying those with strong associations. While some studies find that REM sleep might be especially helpful for flexible cognitive processes such as solving anagrams, others find that increasing levels of slow-wave sleep (NREM) are associated with innovative problem solving. These seemingly different findings may highlight differences in the type of problem and the types of cognitive processes needed to reach a solution. These are fascinating issues awaiting more definitive answers.

Poor quality sleep: It is clear that having sufficient, good quality sleep is desirable for many reasons. Insomnia is a global problem. It is estimated that around one third of the population suffers from insomnia, with around 10% having a specific insomnia-related disorder. Factors associated with an increased risk of insomnia include being female, advancing age, smoking, and depression. Perhaps unsurprisingly, insomnia is associated with a variety of psychiatric and other medical conditions.

We should also spare a thought for new parents and those who work night shifts. They suffer a loss of total sleep and a decrease in sleep quality. Also, the majority of students experience chronic sleep disturbances. There are many causes, but one of them is how changes to circadian rhythms in adolescence push back in time the onset of sleeping. This shift leads to difficulties with getting up in the morning and a resulting loss of overall sleep. This chronic loss of sleep matters as it is associated with a wide range of negative consequences, including lower academic success. Poor sleep quality in adolescence is also associated with a loss of cognitive control and greater risk taking. These are some of the reasons why schools have occasionally experimented with later start times.

There are various steps you can take to improve your sleep quality. These steps include having a regular routine of when and how you go to bed, taking exercise during the day, and learning to clear your thoughts when trying to sleep. Your bedroom should be quiet, dark, and cool. You also want to avoid large meals close to bedtime.

Having good sleep quality is sometimes more about avoiding the many things that disrupt sleep. An obvious candidate is the stimulant caffeine. The problem is that caffeine has a 'half-life' of four to six hours, meaning that its levels only reduce by a half across this time. This means that you may still have half of the caffeine you initially consumed as long as six hours after a coffee or an 'energy drink'. Alcohol is also bad news as it disturbs REM sleep, especially in the second half of the night. It also causes people to wake up after a few hours of sleep, leaving them in a restless, wakeful state. To clear the alcohol from your body before sleeping you many need to stop drinking for some hours. (On average you remove alcohol at the rate of one unit per hour – a 330 mL bottle of beer and a small glass of wine are both about 1.5 units, the equivalent of 90 minutes.)

Watching TV is a very common bedtime ritual. The problem is that TVs emit additional blue light, as do computer screens and smart phones. At school we learnt that the eye contains two, and only two, types of photosensitive cells, namely rods and cones. Remarkably, in 2002, another class of retinal cells (sometimes called 'photosensitive retinal ganglion cells') were found to respond to light. These ganglion cells contain melanopsin, a chemical that is particularly sensitive to blue light. Although few in number, these cells have some profound effects, including synchronising our 24-hour biological clocks (our circadian rhythm).

One action of these ganglion cells, when stimulated, is to suppress the release of the hormone, melatonin. This chemical helps to regulate our sleep-wake cycle, so its unnatural suppression by blue light adds to wakefulness. This action takes us back to the perils of late-night TV, smart phone, or computer usage. This is also one of the reasons why those on shift-work, who try to sleep during the daytime, find good sleep quality so elusive. Given the nature of their work, which can include time zone shifts, it is also unsurprising that aircrew can suffer chronic fatigue, as well as sleep problems.

Traditionally, many people in hot Mediterranean countries, the Middle East, China, and India would take a break in the afternoon, a break that often included a nap. There is renewed interest in the value of a daytime nap. Studies show that such naps are especially beneficial for procedural learning. In one example, participants learnt a motor task in the morning with their left hand. Those taking a nap of 60–90 minutes that same day demonstrated enhanced performance of that motor skill in the evening. But the benefits of napping for a variety of explicit memory tasks are also now being increasingly reported. An interesting comparison between cramming factual knowledge and taking a 60-minute nap in the middle of learning found equivalent initial gains in learning but that napping resulted in better retention a week later (Cousins et al., 2019). Other studies have examined how long a nap needs to be for it to benefit memory consolidation. Current evidence suggests that a nap as short as six minutes can help.

The content of dreams and their forgetting: By matching life diaries with dream diaries, it is possible to show that elements of recent life events are sometimes re-experienced in dreams. More unexpectedly, there is often a 'dream-lag'. When aspects of recent experiences are found in REM-associated dreams, this typically does not happen immediately. Instead, there is a lag of a day or more, up to around seven days. This delayed re-exposure of events seems to be more common for especially salient occurrences.

One major obstacle when trying to make sense of dreams is that we are so bad at remembering their content. The memory expert Allan Hobson estimated that he recalled less than 1% of his dreams. Furthermore, what we do remember are often tantalising fragments. Rather than recalling a series of dreams every morning, we may sometimes remember just the last dream. Even then, its contents are usually fleeting, quickly becoming increasingly hard to describe.

People do vary in the ability to remember their dreams. With motivation and practice it may be possible to improve dream recall, but this normally means remembering more fragments of just the last dream. Even with training, multiple dreams are still lost every night. This transience is all the more surprising given that dreams are often full of vivid imagery. Although bizarreness and emotionality are associated with a greater likelihood of dream recall, we still fail over and over again to remember the content of our dreams.

An added challenge is that it is next to impossible to confirm if we can accurately recall the content of our dreams. We are almost certainly prone to confabulation (making up missing bits) as we struggle with images and narratives that do not fit our waking lives. Consequently, when we reconstruct our dreams it is likely that we straighten out many of the details that do not fit our expectations. This means that the accuracy of our dream reports remains highly questionable. Although there can be links between the pattern of our eye-movements and the content of our dreams, it is not possible to reconstruct the details of a dream from eye-movements alone. In other words, we cannot verify a dream report. That said, there have been attempts to reconstruct dream content from fMRI signals. Although there is a long way to go, it may eventually prove possible.

To investigate dream content, researchers have tried to deliberately reactivate past events within a dream. One method is to play cues during REM sleep that are associated with a previous learning experience. The hope is that the current dream will incorporate elements of the past experience that has been cued. In one example, people learnt a flying task using Virtual Reality (Picard-Deland & Nielsen, 2022). Sound cues associated with the flying task were then played to those same people during REM sleep. This cueing was sometimes effective in evoking aspects of the Virtual Reality experience within REM dreams when it was given a few days after training. This delay was consistent with the 'dream-lag' seen in other studies.

These aspects of dreaming bring us back to the curious issue of why dreams are so poorly remembered. One possible explanation begins by considering the state of dreaming. Dreams are akin to mind-wandering as both are internal states. We employ a process called 'reality-monitoring' to help us locate the source of a memory. In this case, to distinguish internal thoughts from external events.

Dreaming, however, occupies a unique status as we can see and feel things that are not being experiencing externally. Furthermore, dreams may contain autobiographical elements and are often set in a complex context, features consistent with external events, despite being internal. When recalling a memory, we may rely on reality-monitoring to exclude possible competitors. This normally helpful process may create obstacles as our dreams share features with external episodic events yet are stored in very different ways, as they are internal.

Another class of explanation again starts from the assumption that our neurocognitive state is dramatically different when dreaming and when awake. While undoubtedly correct, this assertion is really just a re-description of the problem and not an explanation. We do, however, know that an intact hippocampus is needed for typical dreaming. Studies of amnesics with bilateral hippocampal tissue loss found that they dream less frequently, and their dream content was less episodic-like in nature, lacking rich imagery (Spanò et al., 2020). It appears that the hippocampus normally contributes to dreams by enhancing episodic-like content yet, paradoxically, its actions do not ensure the recall of dream content. Similarly, we know that during REM sleep the cortex is active. Regions including the medial prefrontal cortex, anterior cingulate cortex, and amygdala all show increased regional cerebral blood flow during REM sleep. Clearly, the failure to subsequently recall our dreams is not due to the brain shutting down when asleep. At present, we have a fascinating mystery with lots of potential clues that needs solving.

One of these clues comes from the in-between world of 'lucid' dreaming. About half of us have dreams in which we are aware that we are dreaming. During a lucid dream, people can sometimes intentionally perform certain actions and even be aware of their waking lives. Lucid dreams, which occur during REM sleep may, for example, permit more controlled eye-movements. Remarkably, a pre-arranged sequence of eye-movements has been used by sleepers to signal the onset of a lucid dream. The limited fMRI data indicates that during a lucid dream more cortex is activated than in usual (non-lucid) dreams, including parts of the anterior prefrontal, parietal, and temporal cortical regions. The hope is that lucid dreams offer another route to understanding what is happening during a dream and uncovering some of its mysteries.

Can we learn while asleep? Many of us secretly hope that we might learn a foreign language while sleeping. The desirable ability to learn while asleep has been given a scientific name – 'hypnopaedia'. In 1927, Alois Saliger invented the 'Psycho-Phone' to help sleep learning. He claimed that during sleep we are highly receptive to suggestions and so might better ourselves during this otherwise blank period. It might be added that Alois Saliger had a chequered past, so a bit of cynicism about his claims might be in order. Sleep learning also features in the famous book 'Brave New World' (1932), where it is used to impart moral and ethical lessons.

To test any claims of sleep learning it is vital to confirm that someone is indeed asleep when learning. Electroencephalography (EEG) is standardly used to make this judgment. An EEG records aspects of brain activity, making it possible to distinguish states of arousal and sleep. An encouraging start to the possibility of sleep learning is the discovery from EEG records that our sleeping brain reacts differently to the sound of our own name, when compared with other names. This difference reveals that our sleeping brain can process and categorise words. Furthermore, our face muscles can respond to words when sleeping, suggesting brief periods akin to consciousness.

Two questions now need to be answered. The first is whether we can explicitly recall something that we heard when asleep. The answer to this first question is no. We are unable to remember verbal information heard while asleep when subsequently given an explicit memory test. It is important to add that this failure to learn is found when being asleep is confirmed by EEG. Consequently, learning a foreign language while sleeping remains the stuff of dreams.

The second question is whether any new learning can occur when asleep. The answer is yes, implicit learning is possible. Many of the experimental tests of implicit learning during sleep involve priming. One example is semantic priming. Repeatedly hearing a word when asleep facilitated the ability of some individuals to later distinguish words with similar meanings. While explicit recall of the test word was not possible, semantic priming demonstrated that its meaning had been processed and retained. Not all studies have, however, found evidence of sleep learning in the form of priming. One explanation for these differences might reflect the need to present the information at the optimum sleep stage, such as during slow-wave peaks.

In an ambitious priming task, pairs of words and non-words were repeatedly played to people during slow-wave sleep (Züst et al., 2019). Using a test of implicit memory, participants were later asked to guess whether the non-word, e.g., 'tofer', would fit into a shoe-box. People's guesses were found to be biased by the real word pair. For instance, if the word paired with tofer was 'house', participants were more likely to guess that a 'tofer' would not fit in a shoe-box. While the authors generously described this as 'vocabulary learning', this implicit learning remains far distant from learning a new language.

Other examples of implicit memory learning acquired during sleep include classical conditioning. Pleasant and unpleasant odours have been paired with different tones when participants were asleep. Later, when sniffing to the sound of the training tone, participants' pleasant/unpleasant reactions reflected their sleep conditioning. As might be expected, the subjects had no conscious awareness of the learning experience.

So, hypnopaedia is possible, but very restricted in its nature. There are no convincing demonstrations of new explicit memories for events taking place during confirmed sleep, though implicit memory learning is possible. Although, as described, both priming and classical conditioning can take place during sleep, many studies have failed to demonstrate implicit learning. The reasons remain uncertain, but one factor is likely to be the stage of sleep at the time of the implicit memory learning.

12 Imagination, future memory, and prospective memory

It's a poor sort of memory that only works backwards.

Through the Looking Glass, Lewis Carroll (1871)

Future memory

Remembering the future: One of the most remarkable revolutions in how we think about memory has been the change from looking back to looking forward. It might seem to make no sense to talk about our memory for things that have not yet happened, but Psychologists now readily refer to 'future episodic memory', as unlikely as that initially sounds. Just as we can time-travel back in our minds, so we can envisage future events. This switch in perspective was perfectly captured by the author Terry Pratchett of Discworld fame who wrote *"People think they live life as a moving dot from the past to the future, with memory streaming out behind them like some kind of mental cometary tail. But memory spreads out in front as well as behind"* (Lords & Ladies, 1992).

At the heart of this revolution is the idea that past episodic memories and simulated future events share core attributes. Both seem to contain similar sensory and contextual attributes, and both appear to revolve around oneself. Try to remember this morning's breakfast and then imagine tomorrow's breakfast. There will be many shared attributes. A parallel approach is to compare brain activation patterns for past and future 'memories'. Such experiments reveal a common network of brain areas for both recalling past episodes and imagining the future.

The brain regions activated by both past episodic memories and future simulations include the hippocampus and the adjacent parahippocampal cortex. Other areas jointly activated include lateral parts of both the temporal lobe and the parietal lobe, as well the dorsolateral prefrontal cortex. Simulating the future can also bring about additional activity in some prefrontal and parietal brain areas. This extra activity probably reflects how simulations require additional cognitive effort to direct and explore possible alternative futures.

The assembly of areas activated by episodic simulation overlaps with much of the brain's 'default mode network'. This network received the title 'default' because it becomes engaged when people are *not* performing cognitive tasks, e.g., between trials in a brain scanner. Consequently, the default mode network is activated when we are mind-wandering, such as between test trials in a brain scanner. The fact that the default mode network and the episodic simulation network show considerable overlap should not be so surprising as during mind-wandering we move around both real and imagined scenarios.

DOI: 10.4324/9781003537649-12

Can amnesics remember the future? Like so many things, the idea that past and future episodic memories rely on shared mechanisms can be traced back to Endel Tulving. Partly from his observations of amnesic patients, he concluded that a key property of episodic memory is mental time travel, which logically must be able to take you to the future as well as to the past. One of those amnesics was K.C., who suffered catastrophic memory problems due to the brain injuries he incurred in a motorcycle accident (Rosenbaum et al., 2005). As a result, K.C. could neither access his episodic memory for past events nor imagine future events. These problems meant that K.C. lacked an awareness of both past and future time. When he was asked to think back to what happened yesterday, or to think forward to what he may do tomorrow, he said that his mind goes blank, making it difficult to separate the past from the future.

"Imagine you are lying on a white sandy beach in a beautiful tropical bay"
"Imagine you are standing in the main hall of a museum containing many exhibits"

These are two of the fictitious scenarios given to a group of five amnesics with hippocampal pathology. Although the amnesics patients understood the task and appreciated aspects of the scenarios, such as hearing seagulls by the imagined beach, their stories were superficial (Hassabis et al., 2007). The amnesics struggled to create a coherent spatial context and their descriptions lacked personal feelings and experiences. The challenge of imagining future events has since been reported in other amnesics. As a result, there is agreement that many amnesics have difficulties with both past and future memories.

From such observations, the 'constructive episodic simulation' hypothesis emerged (Schacter & Addis, 2007). Rather than just serving past events, episodic memory also supports the creation of simulated future events, using past experiences to create possible future scenarios (Figure 12.1). This hypothesis also highlights how semantic knowledge must contribute to the process. For example, if you are asked to imagine camping on an island, you will access learnt schemas concerning camping and islands to create a plausible future. The flexibility of episodic memory then helps you to create a unique, fictitious experience.

Episodic foresight or What will I do this morning now I see that it is raining? The re-orientation of memory, from the past to the future, has led to much speculation about the properties and significance of episodic foresight. Descriptions of the 'remembering–imagining system' emphasise how this system ensures that we are prepared for future eventualities. While other species have mechanisms for general preparedness, our more flexible cognitive abilities make it possible to anticipate multiple possibilities, as well as eliminate unlikely scenarios. The link between the 'remembering–imagining system' and current memory is thought to create a peak of effective activity at the present moment ('now'), with a decreasing awareness of the recent past and the near future that affects memory accessibility. An intriguing thought is that the 'remembering–imagining system' may supply our dreams with not just past, but also future, events.

The ability to construct possible futures is highly adaptive. Foresight is integral for appraising potential risks and contingencies. Such appraisals integrate current schemas with episodic simulations, helping us anticipate and cope with the complex world around us in order to plan the next hour, day, or weeks. This re-alignment of cognition from the past to the future is paralleled by the growing appreciation that sensory processing is not passive. Rather, our sensory experiences are actively modified by future predictions based on past experience. Likewise, much of our decision-making assumes that we live in a largely

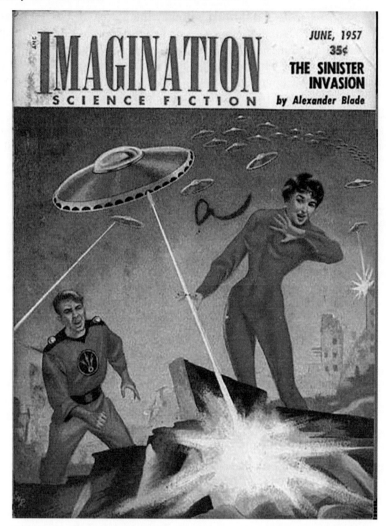

Figure 12.1 Future thought can come in all forms.

predictive world. By taking elements from past experience and running future simulations, this same cognitive machinery can promote creativity and reach novel solutions. Indeed, we might start to wonder if the primary adaptive function of explicit memory is to guide future actions rather than recollect the past.

This re-formulation raises the question of how we distinguish real from imagined memories to avoid believing our fantasies. This distinction is important, as becomes clear when this ability goes awry. For example, key symptoms of schizophrenia, such as delusions, seem to reflect just such a failure. Consequently, it is useful to consider how we might separate real from imagined 'memories'. Our ability to distinguish external from internal memories is called source monitoring.

In most instances, real memories have added sensory detail, greater contextual precision, and are more plausible, often creating a sense of familiarity. Meanwhile, imagined scenarios may contain memories of the internal cognitive operations that helped us to create and refine that same imagined situation. That said, the differences between real and imagined memories will often remain subtle because when recalling a past episodic memory we retain both true elements of the original experience and create imagined elements driven by our expectations and schema relevant for the situation. For this reason, both episodic memory and future thinking will often reflect much of the same underlying process, constructive episodic simulation.

Do other animals possess mental time travel? These same considerations raise fascinating questions about whether mental time travel is unique to humans. Endel Tulving believed that mental time travel and, hence, episodic memory is only present in humans. This belief has not stopped the many ingenious attempts to demonstrate episodic memory in other animals. Given their lack of language, these attempts are typically based around determining whether an animal can simultaneously acquire the what? where? and when? of a unique event. These three attributes are integral to episodic memory, along with mental time travel.

Behavioural tests show that a range of species including scrub jays, ravens, great apes, and some rodents can all pass the three-attribute test. But, because it is not possible to interrogate animals verbally to confirm mental time travel, the more cautious term 'episodic-like memory' is often used to describe these learning abilities.

Given how challenging it has been to test episodic memory in animals, determining whether any animals possess future time travel may be almost impossible. Testing for what looks like future planning is not sufficient. Numerous bird species migrate, but we would not explain this genetically-determined behaviour by an ability to anticipate the outcome of the long-distance journey. Instead, we need to consider examples of flexible behaviour that reflect an anticipated what-where-when triplet of information.

Food storage ('caching'), a behaviour shown by some bird species, offers unique insights into their memory capabilities. The Olympic champion of food caching is probably the pinyon jay, an American member of the crow family. An individual bird may cache 20,000 pinyon pine (*Pinus edulis*) seeds during a single autumn and then use these caches to feed itself through the following six-month period, displaying remarkable spatial memory. Some European birds, such as the coal tit and willow tit, also cache food, while other related species, such as the great tit, do not. Those tit species that cache have a relatively larger hippocampus, a brain structure critically involved in spatial memory. Remarkably, in species such as the willow tit, the action of seasonal hoarding may promote enlargement of the hippocampus, with the production of new neurons.

In a series of ingenious studies, Nicky Clayton showed how some crow species, such as scrub jays (Figure 12.2), are not only adept at storing and relocating food items (where), but also display knowledge of the nature of the food (what) and how long ago (when) it was cached. Furthermore, their ability to decide whether to cache perishable or non-perishable food can seem to resemble foresight. Remarkably, experienced scrub jays will move cached food to new site if observed by another scrub jay when first hiding the food (to stop that other bird from stealing their horde). This behaviour is learnt by experience as it is flexible and not innate. Other studies add to the impression that scrub jays can spontaneously plan for tomorrow when deciding what to cache and where.

A very different source of evidence for future thinking comes from recording neuronal activity in the rodent hippocampus. Many hippocampal neurons fire when the animal is in a specific location. Such neurons are called 'place cells'. Furthermore, some hippocampal neurons show 'prospective coding' as they seem to anticipate where the animal is going to go, reflecting current and future memory demands. Examples include neurons that predict whether the animal will subsequently turn left or right in a maze.

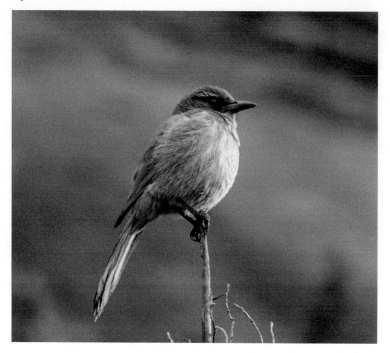

Figure 12.2 The scrub jay possesses episodic-like memory, but can it plan?

Just as remarkable, place cells sometimes fire in sequence, seemingly replaying a route previously traversed by the animal. This neuronal replay can happen even after the animal has been removed from the location of that route. Consequently, this same memory replay provides evidence of 'displacement', the ability to describe something not currently present. In this way, hippocampal replay may contribute to navigational planning and decision making, in addition to memory consolidation, reflecting its potential to support mental time travel.

Non-human primates and future intelligence: If we believe that there is no seismic leap in the evolution of *Homo sapiens* it is reasonable to assume that some form of imaginative time travel exists in other, related animals. By this argument we should first focus on the great apes, given our shared ancestry. Anecdotal evidence of foresight is provided by the sad story of the chimpanzee Santino who resided at the Furuvik Zoo in Sweden (Figure 12.3). Santino appeared to horde hundreds of rocks in his enclosure so that he could later throw them at visitors. He even broke up chunks of concrete to create better missiles. For his impudence Santino was castrated. In 2022 he escaped from his enclosure but was then shot and killed. *Homo sapiens* does not come out of this story very well.

In the natural world, chimpanzees will carry hammer stones to break open nuts in trees several hundred yards distant. They appear to deliberately select appropriate stones for the particular task and then select the most direct route to the source of nuts. While this behaviour might seem to fit the criteria for foresight, if it is driven by current hunger, it is not in anticipation of a future need, rather it is a consequence of present drives and needs. For similar reasons, the interpretation of other ape behaviour that seems to anticipate future need has often been disputed.

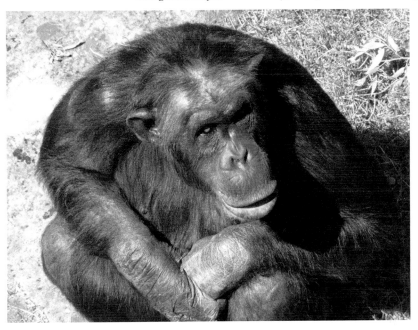

Figure 12.3 Santino the rock-throwing chimpanzee.

A different approach is based on Endel Tulving's 'spoon test'. He recounted the following Estonian children's story.

> … a young girl dreams about going to a friend's birthday party where the guests are served delicious chocolate pudding, her favourite. Alas, all she can do is to watch other children eat it, because everybody has to have her own spoon, and she did not bring one. So the next evening, determined not to have the same disappointing experience again, she goes to bed clutching a spoon in her hand.
>
> (Tulving, 2005)

The point of the story is that the girl both reflects on her disappointing experience (episodic memory) and make provision for the future possibility of being re-invited (episodic foresight). Behavioural tests based on the logic of the 'spoon test' have been given to both children and great apes. Four-year-old children can solve these problems, but three-year-olds often struggle (Scarf et al., 2014). While monkeys also fail, great apes sometimes succeed. Although solving this test may indicate foresight, their lack of language means that the apes require extended training before tackling the final, critical problem. The lengthy training may encourage less imagination-based solutions.

There remains intriguing descriptions of what has been called animal Machiavellian intelligence. For example, monkeys appear to sometimes employ deception to circumvent problems posed by their social hierarchies. Take the case of a young monkey unable to reach a good food source because it is being monopolised by adults. The youngster lets out a scream, causing his high-ranking mother to come to his aid, thereby, displacing the other monkeys and providing access for the youngster. If this behaviour represents true deception then it indicates foresight.

Romantics and killjoys: The descriptions of possible Machiavellian intelligence by monkeys serves as a prompt to what is called Lloyd Morgan's canon (1903), which describes the need to avoid anthropomorphic explanations when simpler accounts exist. *"In no case is an animal activity to be interpreted in terms of higher psychological processes if it can be fairly interpreted in terms of processes which stand lower in the scale of psychological evolution and development."*

As Conwy Lloyd Morgan observed, the fact that his terrier Tony could open the garden gate does not mean that Tony understands latches or levers and how they work. Rather, Tony learnt by a series of actions that occasionally achieved the desired goal, opening the gate. The successful actions were rewarded and so became more frequent. No moment of insight was required. With this description, Lloyd Morgan had metaphorically poured cold water on George Romanes.

On 17th October 1878, the journal Nature published a letter by George Romanes with the request for *'any well-marked instances of the display of animal intelligence which may have fallen within their own notice or that of their friends'*. Anecdotes poured in. His 1884 book 'Animal Intelligence' showed how Romanes came to believe that birds could show sympathy and even pride. His countless second-hand anecdotes included pigs shaking apple trees to bring down fruit, horses deciding that they need shoeing and spontaneously heading off to the blacksmiths, and monkeys that had learnt the mechanical principles of the screw. While these stories are beguiling, they provide no details of how the animal arrived at that behaviour. A pig that bumps into an apple tree, bringing down ripe fruit, finds that behaviour being rewarded, so increasing the likelihood that tree-bumping will be repeated. No higher intelligence is required.

Likewise with monkey Machiavellian intelligence. We cannot infer that the outcome was planned without understanding previous occasions when the young monkey screamed or its consequences. To help resolve the problem, we can consider more formal experiments that try to test whether monkeys possess a 'theory-of-mind'.

Theory-of-mind describes the ability to behave as though you can understand and take into the account the mental state of others, sometimes called 'mind-reading'. It seems likely that some great ape species can solve some tests for a theory-of-mind. For example, by tracking eye movements, apes appear to anticipate that a person will go to a food cache located where that person last saw it, even though the ape knows that the food is no longer there. There are also claims that some crows and parrots display what is likened to a theory-of-mind. As already mentioned, scrub jays will adjust their food caching when other birds are watching, by removing the food to another location. They are more likely to do this when in the presence of a bird they regard as dominant. Despite this remarkable behaviour, the researchers acknowledge that this need not reflect a humanlike theory-of-mind.

Not wishing to be a spoilsport, the diversity of species claimed to have a theory-of-mind does raise alarm bells. Instead, animals with excellent manipulative skills, a propensity to imitate, allied to an ability to break down actions into components substages, may well pass nonverbal theory-of-mind tasks, even though they lack the propositional representations that underpin human theory of mind. Consequently, there remains an unresolved dispute between the 'romantics' and the 'killjoys', the former willing to ascribe some animals with complex cognitive abilities including episodic memory, a theory-of-mind, and spontaneous tool production. The reality is likely to lie somewhere in between the two views, but according to Lloyd Morgan's canon, the burden of proof should remain with those claiming advanced cognitive abilities for animals.

To test spontaneous foresight, it may well be necessary to look for examples of problem-solving that are quite different to anything previously encountered by the animal. One intriguing suggestion is the forked-tube test (Redshaw & Suddendorf, 2020). The challenge is to catch a food item dropped into the top of an inverted Y-shaped tube (one top entrance, two bottom exits) (Figure 12.4). If you put your hand under one of the two exit tubes you will only catch the food on half of the trials. It is thought that spontaneously solving this task by simultaneously using both hands, putting one under each exit spout, involves imagining future timelines. When this task is given to monkeys or chimpanzees they typically only cover one exit, failing to anticipate the best solution, covering both exits.

In contrast, most four-year-old children, and some three-year-olds, spontaneously cover both exits of the forked-tube test (Redshaw & Suddendorf, 2020). Meanwhile, two-year-olds typically cover just one exit. Comparisons between different cultures suggest that humans universally begin to acquire the ability to prepare for alternative futures around the age of three, consistent with when children start to solve Tulving's 'spoon test'.

What can be agreed is that human powers of imagination far exceed those of any other animal, assuming that it exists in other animals. One obvious explanation is that language provides that greater power and flexibility. Indeed, if language is essential for mental time travel then it implies that episodic future thinking is unique to humans. This same argument can, however, be reversed, so that mental time travel becomes a prerequisite for language development. This same reversal then opens up the potential for imagination in other species.

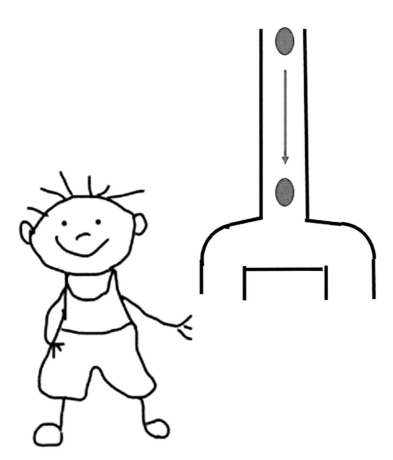

Figure 12.4 Forked-tube test. What is the best strategy to catch the falling sweet?

Prospective memory

I am particularly poor at remembering the upcoming birthdays of my brothers and sisters. I even manage to forget to send a card to my sister with whom I share a birthday. The previous section considered episodic foresight, which involves imagining the future. The ability to remember when to carry out future actions has a different name, it is called 'prospective memory' (Figure 12.5). When someone says 'I have a bad memory' they are often referring not to their memory for past events but to their failure to carry out planned, future actions. (Just today, I bought eye drops that I have to take every two hours for the first two days, then every four hours for the next three days – a daunting test for my prospective memory.)

Future tasks might include joining a work meeting or class, taking medication, attending a dentist's appointment, posting a letter, or remembering to 'save' material that we are writing on a computer. Prospective memory 'crimes' include forgetting to switch your phone off when in class, at the theatre, or in church. Other prospective memory crimes include forgetting Valentine's Day or your wedding anniversary.

Prospective memory is important. We need it to deliver our future actions, even when juggling multiple goals. It allows us to structure our time economically. Our prospective memory can also affect how others see us. There is a big difference between being seen as conscientious and well-organised, rather than being unreliable and unstructured. An extreme example of failed prospective memory is that of the Liverpool man who, in 2013, realised at the last moment that he had forgotten to book his wedding venue. In his panic,

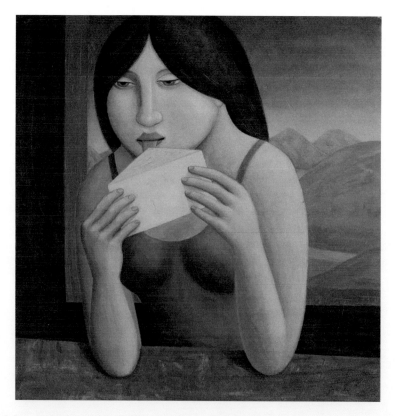

Figure 12.5 Remembering to post a letter. A classic challenge for prospective memory.

he made a hoax bomb call to stop the wedding from going ahead. His plan was uncovered, and he was sentenced to 12 months' imprisonment.

The challenge of prospective memory: Despite its importance in everyday life, prospective memory remains poorly understood. Early studies tried to model naturalistic problems, such as asking people to return postcards they had received or to phone the experimenter on specified days. A serious limitation is that it is hard to determine what strategies individuals used to complete their tasks. For example, did people use a diary and, if so, how often did they consult it. Laboratory tests can be designed to control reminder cues, but they are often artificial in nature, e.g., asking people to carry out a series of future actions during or at the end of the test session. This challenge feels very different to the many real-world demands on prospective memory.

Prospective memory is complex as you need to remember to carry out the delayed intention, recognise the appropriate context in which to act, and then remember to make the correct action. Prospective memory is also unusual as a time estimation is often part of the memory for the task to be executed ('time-based' prospective memory). This timing signal can be self-generated, for example, remember to do something in five minutes or it can be more reliant on external cues, for example, remember to do something at 9.30 pm. But in the second case you still need to remember to check the time, preferably close to the desired moment. However, some prospective memory tasks are not time dependent. An example would be remembering that the next time I go to work, I must take in some coffee. This variant has been called 'event-based' prospective memory, as it is the event of preparing to go to work that provides the reminder cue.

Solving prospective memory problems: There is much interest in how we solve prospective memory tasks. For some tasks, when memorising the goal, we also set up an on-line monitoring process to enable retrieval. The drawback is that the monitoring process remains switched on, making it cognitively demanding, especially if there is a long interval before the action has to be initiated. More often it feels as though the need to perform the desired task just 'popped' into our mind. One explanation is that we form a link between the action and a potential, future reminder cue, so that when that cue appears you retrieve the prospective task. An example would be planning that after lunch I will go to the library. This class of solution involves event-based prospective memory.

As you might expect, we tend to be better at prospective tasks in the near rather than the far future. Another aspect is the importance of the task to be performed. The failure to renew your passport could prove catastrophic, while forgetting to buy pepper when passing the shop is not a calamity. Experiments have tried to manipulate task importance by attaching monetary rewards, emphasising the significance of the task, or providing social motives. Perhaps not surprisingly, if you are told that your name will go into a lottery you are more likely to remember to send back a postcard. Other studies using food or money reward have often, but not always, found better prospective memory when the task is deemed important. But, increasing the significance of a future action brings the risk that you will devote excessive cognitive resources to the prospective task, leading to the disruption of other, current cognitive tasks.

The reverse problem is seen when you have to perform a demanding cognitive task. Consider driving in rush-hour traffic. The high mental load leaves you less able to monitor prospective memory, causing you to forget to stop to buy some milk. Put simply, if you are cognitively overloaded, you will struggle to remember your mental list of future actions. This is because prospective memory makes its own cognitive demands, on top of current demands. Consequently, having constant mental to-do lists soon becomes detrimental.

An obvious area of high 'mental load' is childcare, where there are endless tasks to be overseen and anticipated. (In concentrating on writing this paragraph, I find that I just forgot to attend a planned Zoom meeting – there is a certain irony.)

With increasing age, people tend to perform worse on both time-based and event-based prospective tasks set in the laboratory. This increased difficulty for older people seems most frequent for time-based tasks, which rely on internal monitoring. The situation for prospective memory outside the laboratory, where it really matters, may, however, be somewhat different. Here, important factors include the ability to use external aids, such as a diary or calendar, as well as one's motivation. Because older people tend to believe that they make more memory mistakes, they are more likely to supplement their prospective memory with external cues. As a result, naturalistic studies of prospective memory sometimes show better performance with increasing age.

Failing prospective memory: It has long been known that damage to prefrontal cortex can leave people unable to plan and organise future tasks. Examples include cooking a meal, where different components have to be incorporated at different times. Consequently, it is thought that our prefrontal cortex plays a critical role in prospective memory. Careful comparisons between the effects of different frontal brain lesions have highlighted the especial importance of the most anterior part of the prefrontal cortex (known as area 10) for prospective memory. Complementary research using fMRI points to a complex array of frontal-parietal cortex networks that are thought to support the various components of prospective memory.

Because prospective memory makes multiple cognitive demands it should be no surprise that it is severely affected in many illnesses, including various dementias and Parkinson's disease. This same vulnerability means that is often affected in the early stages of a neurological disease, an important reason for including tests of prospective memory when screening for cognitive loss. Indeed, prospective memory may sometimes be more sensitive than tests of past memory for detecting the initial stages of dementia. (Clinical measures for prospective memory include the Royal Prince Alfred Prospective Memory Test, the Cambridge Prospective Memory Test, and Memory for Intentions Screening Test.) A further reason to assess prospective memory is that its loss severely affects quality of life, including the ability to live independently.

As mentioned, there is a long list of neurological and psychiatric disorders that impair prospective memory. Indeed, it is almost more difficult to find a disorder that does not affect prospective memory. Because of the importance of prospective memory for daily life, a number of compensatory mechanisms are recommended. These include the use of memory notebooks, electronic prompts from your smartphone, the placement of written reminders on surfaces, creating a more fixed, daily routine, and having a stable environment. Other guidance is to focus on how you process and memorise any initial task instructions. This advice includes the use of greater elaborative encoding, often in conjunction with visualisation. Such guidance rather presupposes that the person has insight into their loss of prospective memory, something that may, alas, be lost.

13 Recognition memory and illusions of familiarity

Recognition memory

Who is he? ....(Do I know him from work; is he a movie star, a TV commentator, the milkman?).
Eventually the search may end with the insight, That's the butcher from the supermarket!

George Mandler (1980)

In a hypothetical encounter on a bus, George Mandler described a familiar challenge that taxes recognition memory. Throughout our lives, we automatically judge whether the people we meet or the events we encounter are novel or familiar. This ability is of enormous survival value. Detecting something novel in your surroundings might signal a new opportunity, such as a potential food source, or it might signal the presence of a fearsome predator. Meanwhile, detecting what is familiar may lead to past information about how best to react. Clearly, novel/familiar decisions need to be solved accurately and rapidly.

It is helpful to first clarify the term 'recognition'. In everyday language 'recognition' often refers to the identification of something. (For instance, I recognise that a particular tree is an oak rather than a sycamore.) In contrast, the term 'recognition memory' is used to describe those processes that make it possible to determine whether a stimulus is the same (familiar) or different (novel) to one previously experienced. (I recognise that oak tree as the one we saw earlier today.)

Recognition memory is often spectacularly effective. I previously mentioned how people could correctly recognise as familiar over 90% of 2500 pictures of objects shown earlier that day. In a separate study involving 10,000 pictures it was concluded that our capacity for picture recognition memory is almost limitless. Given these achievements, it is perhaps not surprising that recognition memory consistently outperforms recall. We are, for example, far better at distinguishing familiar faces from our school days than recalling their names.

Occasionally our recognition memory can be fooled. We struggle to distinguish a mirror-imaged picture from the original orientation. This Achilles heel even applies to famous masterpieces (Figure 13.1). When students were asked to determine the correct orientation of a famous painting they had presumably seen before, they performed at chance. In other words, they found the task almost impossible. Another way to generate recognition memory errors is to first ask people to imagine seeing specific objects. Participants then start to believe that they have seen those same objects when they occur in a recognition memory test.

When I walk into a familiar room I might notice that all of the furniture is present, but it has been re-arranged. This scenario creates a slightly different challenge for recognition memory as all of the elements are familiar, but their composition is novel. This class of

DOI: 10.4324/9781003537649-13

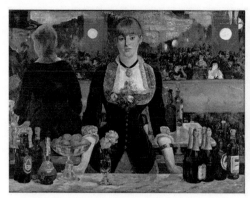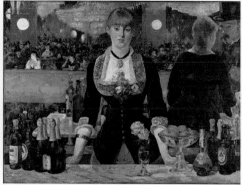

Figure 13.1 The bar at the Folies Bergère. Edouard Manet. Which is the original?

problem has been called 'associative recognition'. To solve these more complex problems, our brain needs to recruit additional areas.

Models of recognition memory: Alas, my ability to recognise other people is not perfect. Years ago, at a wine reception in the Villa Borghese in Rome, I noticed a striking-looking woman walking towards me who seemed familiar. We met, hugged, and kissed each other on the cheek. I knew we had met before (I don't hug everyone), but I had absolutely no idea who she was. I am embarrassed to say I spent the rest of the reception avoiding her. Only years later did I find out who she was and how we had previously met.

I am sure that I am not the only person who has experienced recognition memory without any accompanying knowledge, leaving just a feeling of familiarity. This was the situation described by George Mandler on initially seeing the local butcher in an unfamiliar place (on a bus). At first, he realised the person was familiar but could not understand why. Only subsequently did he realise why he knew him, confirming his recognition judgement. These two different elements (recognition with or without accompanying knowledge) turn out to be pivotal in understanding how we solve the problem of novelty/familiarity detection. (The painting on the right is the original image of the Bar at the Folies Bergère.)

Experiences similar to mine at the Villa Borghese led Mandler to the belief that recognition memory consists of two independent components. Such explanations are referred to as 'dual-process' models of recognition memory (Figure 13.2). One process can be called 'familiarity' or familiarity-based recognition. This process is rapid and seemingly effortless, but the familiarity signal is the only conscious information you have. Consequently, the signal lacks associated information, such as who is this person or what is their name – just as I had experienced in the Villa Borghese or Mandler initially described for the butcher on the bus.

The second component of dual-process models can be called 'recollection' or recollective-based recognition (Figure 13.2). This process involves the active retrieval of episodic-like information about the target, such as their name, their profession, or where you last met. This remembered information helps us to verify our recognition judgement. When the villain Auric Goldfinger supposedly says, "*So we meet again, Mr Bond*", Goldfinger's recognition of 007 is confirmed by by the recollection that his adversary's name was Bond. Similarly, George Mandler eventually recalled that the man's profession was a butcher, confirming his recognition. The assumption is that familiarity-based and recollective-based information provide separate, additive evidence that we use when making recognition decisions and

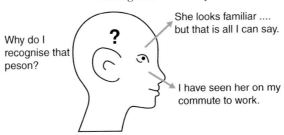

Figure 13.2 Dual-process models of recognition assume that two independent processes help to solve the question of whether something is novel or familiar. One process conveys a feeling of familiarity (or not). The second process involves associated information about the object or person.

determining our confidence in those decisions. We are more confident when using recollective-based information as we have access to allied data that strengthens our decision.

There are, however, simpler explanations of recognition memory, namely 'single-process' models. These models see familiarity and recollection as two sides of the same memory coin. As this explanation requires fewer components, just a single-memory store, it is more economical. In this alternative account, weaker memory traces are perceived as familiar, giving a sense of 'knowing' the target but little else. Meanwhile, stronger memory traces are perceived as though they are 'remembered' as they provide better links to other information. These stronger traces are accompanied by greater confidence.

Testing between single-process and dual-process models: There has been much debate over which is the better explanation for recognition memory. To resolve this controversy, two key questions need to be answered. The first is whether recognition and recall can be separated (dissociated) from each other. Single-process models assume that recall and recognition draw on the same memory store. Consequently, it should not be possible to dissociate recall from recognition.

Question one: Can recall and recognition be separated?

Much of the relevant evidence comes from studying people with amnesia. Following brain injury, people with anterograde amnesia struggle to learn and remember new episodic information (see Chapter 17). As a consequence, they cannot recall what they did this morning or what they said a few minutes ago. Nevertheless, a subset of amnesics seem to show a consistent sparing of recognition memory (Brown et al., 2010).

One such group are those with damage to a brain tract called the fornix. The fornix is a major brain pathway that carries information to and from the hippocampus, which is vital for memory. While amnesics with fornix damage struggle to recall new episodic information they often show relatively preserved recognition memory. Likewise, memory loss associated with damage to a related brain structure, called the mammillary bodies, disrupts the recall of episodic memory but spares recognition memory (Tsivilis et al., 2008).

Proponents of single-process models argue that this apparent dissociation of recall from recognition merely reflects how tests of recognition memory are usually easier than tests of recall. (I began this section pointing out how recognition memory typically outperforms recall.) Consequently, any memory sparing in these amnesics will disproportionately benefit tests of recognition memory as they are easier to solve, requiring less information. To address this problem, it is necessary to give tests of recall memory and recognition memory that are equally difficult. When this is done, patients with fornix damage or mammillary body damage still show a sparing of recognition memory (Tsivilis et al., 2008), as predicted by dual-process models.

Other relevant evidence arose from the discovery that neurons outside the hippocampus can signal the familiarity of stimuli , i.e., from brain sites not thought to be central for episodic memory. These recognition neurons, which are especially numerous in the parahippocampal region, decrease their activity when a stimulus is repeated, so signalling familiarity. When the parahippocampal area is removed in animals, recognition memory is severely impaired. This result is consistent with the idea that this region supplies us with information about novelty/familiarity while the brain apparatus for recollection is largely preserved.

Question two: Can familiarity-based recognition and recollective-based recognition be separated?

Dual-process models assume that the two routes to recognition are independent of each other, creating parallel processes. It is, for example, argued that those amnesics with spared recognition memory retain access to familiarity-based signals. This is theoretically possible because, as explained above, sites outside the hippocampus provide novelty/familiarity signals. Meanwhile, single-process models assume that no such separation between familiarity-based recognition and recollective-based recognition is possible.

Various cognitive tests have been designed to try and separate the two recognition processes. The simplest method is to ask subjects whether they feel that a recognition judgement is solely based on a sense of familiarity ('know') or whether it involves recollected information associated with the target ('remember'). Another approach assumes that recollective-based recognition judgements are associated with greater confidence than familiarity-based judgements.

Based on these tests, it is found that recollective-based recognition is the more disrupted when forced to make fast decisions, when attention is divided, and when semantic encoding is varied. Recollective-based and familiarity-based recognition are also differently affected by aging, as the elderly become more reliant on feelings of familiarity. In contrast, familiarity is more sensitive to changes in response criterion and forgetting over short retention intervals (Yonelinas, 2002). As different factors can affect these two processes in opposing ways, the implication is that familiarity and recollection are independent. While this distinction sounds persuasive, without independent measures of familiarity and recollection there remains a risk of circularity, such that you define familiarity and recollection differences by the task outcomes, not by an independent standard.

A more compelling solution would be to find out if some patients exist with impaired recollective-based recognition but spared familiarity, while other patients show the opposite pattern, impaired familiarity but intact recollective-recognition. It is almost impossible to see how these opposing profiles, called a double-dissociation, could be predicted by a single-process model. I have already described how patients with fornix and mammillary body pathology can show near-normal recognition but poor recall. Subsequent analyses showed that these same patients have preserved familiarity-based recognition but deficient recollective-based recognition (Vann et al., 2009).

Although very rare, patients do exist with the opposite profile, impaired familiarity but intact recollective-recognition (Bowles et al., 2010). The patient N.B. consistently performed at high or normal levels of recollection but repeatedly showed diminished familiarity. The patient's pathology is notable as it was centred in the parahippocampal region – the same area in which animal studies first uncovered neurons that distinguish novel from familiar stimuli. Furthermore, N.B. shows sparing of the hippocampus, a site needed for recollective-based recognition.

Another source of evidence comes from looking at EEG and fMRI brain activity patterns associated with familiarity-based and recollective-based recognition in normal volunteers. Put simply, do these two processes have different brain activity fingerprints? The answer is yes. Many studies now show how certain brain areas are differentially activated by familiarity-based and recollective-based recognition, creating double-dissociations best explained by dual-process models.

Other signals for familiarity: When we see the face of a friend, our sense of familiarity is boosted by our accompanying emotions. Emotion can interact with recognition memory in other ways. Faces that elicit arousal are better recognised months later. Also, words that have a positive or a negative emotional valence are better recognised than neutral words.

In addition to emotions, priming can sometimes contribute to feelings of familiarity. Prior exposure to a stimulus affects the fluency with which that same signal is later accessed – an example of priming. While it seems intuitive that increased fluency should contribute to recognition memory, the evidence is not straightforward. For instance, some dense amnesics show intact perceptual priming yet remain at chance when given recognition memory tests. This finding reveals a failure of perceptual priming to support recognition memory.

Counter-evidence comes from how normal participants can perform above chance when given very difficult recognition memory problems involving kaleidoscopic patterns. Critically, the participants may report no subjective awareness of a recognition signal, yet still do better than chance. The implication is that their guesses were aided by priming. Furthermore, brain imaging studies of conceptual priming show that fluency can interact with cortical signals for familiarity, thereby influencing recognition. From such evidence it now appears that priming can sometimes aid recognition, but when it does and when it does not remains poorly understood.

Finally, it is worth returning to *why* we have mechanisms for distinguishing novelty. When interacting with the environment we need to detect whether something is new, so that we can attend to it and learn about its significance as rapidly as possible. Delay could prove fatal. For these reasons, having rapid novelty/familiarity signals in the brain would make very good sense as speed matters when reacting to something that might prove to be life-threatening. Consistent with this demand for speed, brain areas capable of distinguishing novel from familiar, such as the parahippocampal region, are among those that provide the first full identification of incoming stimuli. By processing information before the hippocampus, familiarity can precede recollective data. We also now know that our cognitive systems are attuned to novelty, typically increasing attention, and prioritising learning resources to such stimuli. For this reason, rates of learning are often steepest for novel stimuli.

It's like déjà vu all over again: This line, attributed to the baseball coach Yogi Berra, brings us to the issue of false feelings of familiarity. The most frequently experienced is *déjà vu* ('already seen'). *Déjà vu* refers to the overwhelming sense of having previously experienced an event, even though this feeling is somehow wrong. Surveys show that the large majority of the population experience *déjà vu*, though its frequency decreases with age. The likelihood of *déjà vu* appears to be raised by stress and fatigue. Related phenomena include *déjà vécu*, which describes the sense of repeating a sequence of events. Consequently, *déjà vécu* is a protracted *déjà vu*, more akin to Groundhog Day. There is also the phenomenon of *jamais vu* ('never seen'), the experience of feeling unfamiliar with a person or situation even though they are very familiar.

When Penfield directly stimulated the brains of people with epilepsy (see *The case for permanent episodic memories, Chapter 4*), he sometimes reported dreamy states that included *déjà vu* and *déjà vécu*. Since then, other neurosurgeons have described similar experiences caused by direct brain stimulation. These experiential states are most associated with activation of medial temporal lobe structures, including the hippocampus and adjacent parahippocampal region.

Déjà vu appears to be especially associated with stimulation of the parahippocampal region. Feelings of *déjà vu* can also form part of the aura that precedes seizures for sufferers of temporal lobe epilepsy. These epileptic *déjà vu* experiences are often similar to those experienced by the normal population. From such observations it has been suggested that *déjà vu* arises from a feeling of familiarity due to erroneous parahippocampal signals. This interpretation builds on the finding from animals that neurons in this same brain area change their firing rate for familiar stimuli. Meanwhile, *déjà vécu* may prove to be associated with abnormal hippocampal activity, giving the sense of a real recollective narrative. A related possibility is that faulty parahippocampal activity not only evokes *déjà vu* but can sometimes recruit event memory via the hippocampus.

A more cognitive explanation is that *déjà vu* occurs when we have an unrecalled memory of a past experience that relates to the current situation. A potential element of the unrecalled memory is the sense of what will happen next. This feeling of premonition has been recreated using virtual reality, the results pointing to a link between the sense of knowing what will happen next and feelings of *déjà vu*.

That leaves *jamais vu* (never seen), which is less common than *déjà vu*. I have to confess that I often feel that my students suffer collectively from *jamais vu*. They frequently deny covering a topic even though they sat through the relevant lectures. Like *déjà vu*, *jamais vu* can occur in normal people but it is also associated with temporal lobe epilepsy. One speculation is that faulty signals from deep in the brain help switch novelty detection, leading to the erroneous perception that people and events are novel, when in reality they are familiar. (For other disorders of familiarity see *D) Duplicates, delusions, and familiarity disorders.*)

14 Brief memory stores

Sensory memory

The more brilliant the lightning, the quicker it disappears.

Avicenna (980–1037)

Sensory memory

Glance around. How do you absorb and remember all that sensory information? The truth is that you do not. Instead, we possess brief sensory memory stores that operate automatically. There are separate stores for vision, sound, and touch that each hold sufficient information just long enough to help us interrogate aspects of the world around us.

Vision – Iconic Memory: Give a child a lit sparkler on Guy Fawkes night, and he or she will wave it in the air, fascinated by its glowing trace (Figure 14.1). Why does it even have glowing trace? That same visual persistence fascinated the Hungarian mathematician, Jan Segner. In 1740 he attached a glowing ember to a rotating wheel and asked the simple question, how fast must the wheel rotate for the trail of light that follows the ember to become a full circle? From this experiment, Segner estimated that there must be a brief visual store lasting around one-tenth of a second.

That brief sensory store is called iconic memory. The name comes from the Greek word for image (icon), which accurately captures the nature of this visual store. The beauty of iconic memory is that it contains a visual representation that lingers just long enough for us to extract more detail, should we need to do so. But, we had to wait over 200 years after Segner for a psychologist to find a way to study the nature of this visual store.

Imagine I ask you to very briefly look at the nine letters (below) then look away. Your glance should be so brief that you cannot rehearse the information. Now report back as many of the letters as possible.

```
H    P    W
Y    J    C
T    L    B
```

In 1960 George Sperling realised that because the iconic store is so brief, its contents might disappear during the time taken to verbally describe those same contents. Consequently, it would be impossible to measure the capacity of iconic memory. His solution was the 'partial report' procedure. (I confess, that as a student I struggled to follow this procedure and understand how it solved a tricky problem – I will try to do better now.)

DOI: 10.4324/9781003537649-14

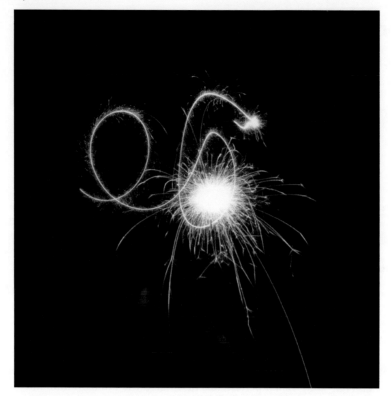

Figure 14.1 A moving lit sparkler leaves a brief visual trace.

Let us say you remember four of the nine letters displayed above (44%). Is this your real capacity? In fact, it would be an underestimate if the time taken to report those four letters reaches the time limit of this brief store. In other words, any remaining letters you initially stored would now be erased from memory by the additional time taken to report those extra letters. Sperling solved this problem by asking subjects to report only the letters from either the top, middle, or bottom row – hence, 'partial report'. By having to report fewer letters the erasure problem caused by the time to say the words is much reduced. The trick was to signal from which row to retrieve the letters *just after* they were removed from sight.

Imagine that you report two out of the three letters in the signalled row. Because you did not know in advance on which row to focus, your score of two reveals that you retained six out of the nine letters (67%). (Six because it is two from each of the three rows). The partial report benefit (67% versus 44%) exists because you had sufficient time to report the letters before they vanished.

As this is a temporary visual store, the partial report benefit will disappear if the row signal is delayed too long after the display is removed – for by then, the letters will have disappeared from memory. In practice, Sperling found this critical time limit to be about one second. Less than that, there was a partial report advantage. Longer than that, the advantage disappeared. In other words, he found clear evidence of a brief visual store that lasts for around one second.

Iconic memory is thought to combine two different aspects of visual persistence. The first, 'sensory persistence', reflects properties inherent in the early stages of visual processing, such as tested by Segner and the rotating ember. This component is regarded as 'pre-categorical', consisting of raw visual data available for up to around 200 msec. The terms pre- and post-categorical are used to separate brain activity that occurs before and after a visual stimulus is identified for what it is. One element of this pre-categorical sensory persistence is neuronal activity in the primary visual cortex (V1) where transient information may be extended by attention. (It is called primary visual cortex as it is the first part of the cerebral cortex to receive incoming visual stimuli.) Two surprising properties of this visual persistence are that the longer the stimulus lasts, the shorter its persistence (inverse duration effect), and the more intense the stimulus, the briefer its persistence (inverse intensity effect).

The second component of iconic memory is 'informational persistence'. This component is presumed to reflect later stages of visual processing. Sperling's partial report method principally tested this later, post-categorical component which, in turn, provides information for short-term memory.

The brevity of iconic memory helps us to detect visual change in the world and assists in motion detection. At the same time, sensory persistence ensures a continuous stream of visual moments as we explore the world. Quite naturally, the maintenance of information in iconic memory was thought to explain why the world looks stable when we blink – nothing happens and so the visual information persists over the brief period. Surprisingly, this explanation now looks wrong. Instead, blinking during the partial report procedure does interfere with iconic memory, probably by altering processing in the visual system. The effect even has been given the glorious name 'cognitive blink suppression'.

The terms 'flicker fusion frequency' or 'flicker fusion threshold' both refer to how rapidly a light has to go on and off to appear continuous. It is set by the part of the visual system that is the slowest to refresh after being activated. Many factors affect flicker fusion frequency, but for black /white contrasting images it can be around 50-60 flashes per second. The refresh time for colour images is, however, longer. Because of the brief sensory persistence in our visual system, modern films appear continuous despite consisting of separate frames. In contrast, old silent movies feel staccato because they were shot with hand-cranked projectors that only took around 16–18 frames per second. To make them appear more continuous they were often sped up, explaining why the actions of Charlie Chaplin and Buster Keaton look so hurried.

Nowadays, films have 48 or 72 frames per second, so that the time gaps become invisible to our visual system and motion appears continuous. To reach this higher rate, each frame from a series of 24 per second is repeated twice (giving 48 frames per second) or even three times (giving 72 frames per second). Each frame is so brief that we do not spot the repeat, nor do we spot any gap between images. Repeating consecutive frames is also favoured in cartoons, as creating each frame is very laborious. Here, 12 drawings might be shown in consecutive, duplicate pairs, giving 24 frames per second, creating illusions of near-continuous movement. The same trick of duplicating frames is used in stop-animation, as seen in the films starring Wallace and Gromit (Figure 14.2).

Audition – Echoic memory: The corresponding, brief sensory store for audition is called echoic memory. Like the poor Greek nymph Echo, who was forced to always repeat the last few words she heard, echoic memory retains the traces of the last things you hear. Like iconic memory, echoic memory consists of more than one process. It differs, however, from iconic memory in being longer lasting. This difference can be seen if you compare the ability to recall spoken numbers or recall numbers presented visually. When spoken, the final item to be heard is very often recalled. When seen, the last item is often forgotten.

This difference reflects how echoic memory outlasts iconic memory, leaving the last spoken item still available. The longer duration of echoic memory may help to counteract a key

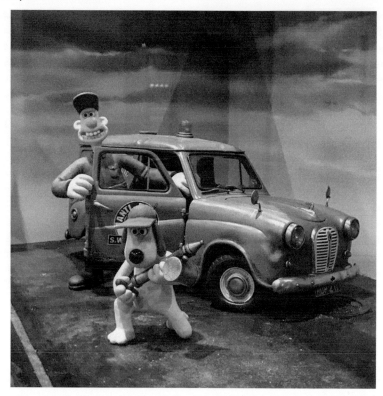

Figure 14.2 Multiple still shots of Wallace and Gromit, who are made from Plasticine clay, are sequenced to create the illusion of movement ('stop-animation').

difference in the properties of sound and vision. A visual stimulus can often be re-inspected, in other words, looked at again. In contrast, auditory information is typically received just the once. This property increases the value of having longer, temporary storage for sounds.

To make sense of the auditory world we often need to distinguish between a crowd of different sounds. Just think of the challenges posed by a noisy environment such as a pub, restaurant, or open-plan office. To help separate different sounds we try to distinguish their various sources. Prior to echoic memory, there is a tiny signal persistence in the auditory system. We use the very small differences in the arrival times of the same sound reaching our left and right ears, along with their differences in intensity, to locate the source of that sound. A sound to the side will have the largest arrival time difference.

To use this sound difference information, we must have an extremely brief store to help hold and then match sounds. By then identifying the locations of different sound sources, we can begin to separate the cacophony around us. This vital ability allows us to form and segregate what are sometimes called 'auditory objects', allowing us to separate and discern multiple sound items in our environment.

This initial form of sound localisation depends on comparing the arrival times of the same noise in the left and right ears. Consequently, animals with larger head sizes are, on average, better sound-locators, although other factors such as ear shape and moveable ears come into play. As a bird-watcher, the ability to locate where a bird is calling from is invaluable, not that I have moveable ears. Meanwhile, animals with small heads and, hence, ears close together cannot use this time difference information for sound localisation.

For example, birds' heads are typically too small to use this method, so instead they monitor pressure differences on their ear drums, sometimes combined with rotating their heads.

As an aside, there is a fascinating interplay between when a bird wants its call to be located and wants it to remain hidden. A bird making sounds that are difficult to locate by a predator, such as a sparrowhawk, will gain an advantage. But sometimes, the tables are turned. A potential prey may signal to the sparrowhawk that it has been detected and so an attack will be unsuccessful, resulting in a waste of energy. This is just what happens when small birds 'mob' a predator, such as an owl or a hawk (Figure 14.3). What is so fascinating is that the small birds make loud calls that are acoustically structured to make them easy for other birds to locate and join in with mobbing the predator.

It is now time to return to echoic memory. To appreciate echoic memory, consider how we sometimes find ourselves asking a friend to repeat what they just said, while simultaneously realising that you can still 'hear' their last words. When bird-watching I am only too familiar with someone else rapidly identifying a bird call that I had 'missed', only to realise that I can still catch an echo of the call. When listening to music, we enjoy chains of notes, relying on echoic memory to appreciate their combined appeal. But, when individual notes are spaced out beyond the duration of echoic memory, even the most famous of tunes can become unrecognisable. Astonishingly, most people do not recognise the first four notes of Beethoven's Fifth Symphony when each note is separated by three to five seconds.

Partial report methods have been used to estimate the duration of echoic memory. For this, numbers or letters are simultaneously heard from different locations. Their offset is rapidly followed by a signal giving the location of just those auditory stimuli to be recalled.

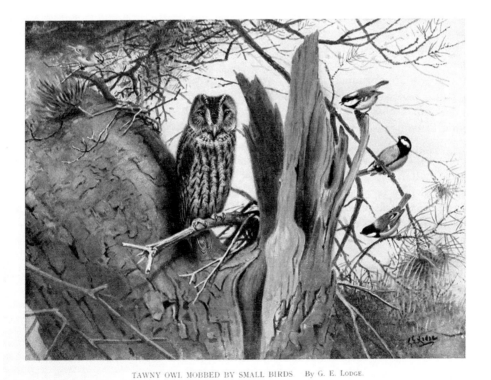

TAWNY OWL MOBBED BY SMALL BIRDS   By G. E. Lodge.

Figure 14.3 Painting of tawny owl being mobbed by small birds (G. E. Lodge, 1922).

The partial report benefit lasts for signals up to a few seconds after termination of the heard numbers or letters but is often lost by around the fourth second. In other words, by this measure, echoic memory lasts up to four seconds.

In practice, other methods can give longer duration estimates for echoic memory. An example is when participants are asked to read a book and, at unexpected intervals, see a light signal telling them to report whether they have or have not heard a low tone produced at variable intervals prior to the light signal. The problem is that methods to measure the duration of echoic memory often mix together a very short (largely perceptual) and a longer (largely mnemonic) component. Those methods that give the longest estimates probably reflect additional spillover into working memory.

The very short perceptual component of echoic memory lasts for about 200–350 msec and is thought to be pre-categorical as it reflects a low level of initial analysis prior to complete identification. Evidence for this brief sensory component comes from phenomena like 'backward masking'. Imaging hearing two consecutive tones. The ability to remember the first tone is reduced if it is closely followed by a second tone, which backwardly erases (masks) the first tone. If the interval between the tone and the following 'mask' is too long, this masking effect is lost as the first tone is established in the other, longer component of echoic memory. Other investigations of this very brief store have looked at the auditory equivalent of following a lit sparkler. A number of such methods give a range of duration estimates that, together, reveal a brief auditory store lasting up to 350 msec that is essentially sensory in nature.

There is also a more durable component of echoic memory. For example, our ability to retain and then comprehend ambiguous speech points to an auditory store that is much longer than 350 msec. Likewise, the modality effect described above shows how echoic memory outlasts iconic memory, which can itself persist up to a second. (If you remember, in a spoken list the final item to be heard is very often recalled as it still persists. For a visual list the last item is often forgotten.) Other duration estimates come from playing repeating sequences of scrambled notes. If the sequence is less than three seconds we can detect that it is a repeat loop, presumably because we can hold it long enough in echoic memory to compare the past with the present sounds.

A different way of studying this longer component of echoic memory comes from 'dichotic' listening tasks. Imagine hearing two different passages of speech, one in your left ear, the other in your right ear. (This is called dichotic listening.) You are told to attend to (shadow) just one ear. What happens when unexpectedly you are asked to identify details from the unattended ear? People can tell if the words are the same in both ears, but only if the unattended ear is less than a few seconds in advance of the attended ear. Any longer, and the words in the unattended ear are lost. The various types of shadowing task again point to an auditory store lasting up to four seconds.

Touch – Haptic memory: As the poet John Keats wrote *"Touch has a memory"*. He was, of course, correct as we possess a brief store for feelings of touch, called haptic memory. This form of memory involves both touch and joint information, the latter arrives when we manipulate an object.

Like iconic and echoic memory, haptic information is prone to rapid decay. Partial report procedures adapted from those used to measure iconic memory have been adopted. Typically, different numbers of skin sites are stimulated simultaneously, and the task is to say how many places were touched. The results suggest a sensory duration of only a second. Comparisons of how we adjust to picking up the same or different object give slightly longer duration estimates of haptic memory, reaching up to two seconds.

15 Brief memory stores

Short-term memory

All things are transient.

Buddhist teaching

What is and isn't short-term memory?

In the film '50 First Dates' (2004) the lead character, played by Drew Barrymore, suffers from Goldfield's syndrome, which means that because of her short-term memory loss she can never remember the events of the previous day. In 'Memento' (2000), a much darker film, Guy Pearce's character is also described as suffering from short-term memory loss. Yet, no cognitive psychologist would ever consider that either character lacked short-term memory. (Neither, for that matter, does Goldfield's syndrome exist.) Indeed, for the purpose of the film's dialogue it would rapidly become impossible if the lead character suffered a loss of short-term memory. Amongst other things, we depend on short-term memory to follow a conversation.

But it is not just films that get it so wrong. When I searched the internet for examples of short-term memory the following immediately popped up 'Examples of short-term memory include where you parked your car this morning, what you had for lunch yesterday, and remembering details from a book that you read a few days ago'. Not one of these examples remotely corresponds to short-term memory.

Put simply, short-term memory holds a changing store of information for a brief period of time. This information, drawn from our sensory memory stores, is 'on-line', meaning it is consciously available. This same information has the potential to enter long-term memory. However, the contents of short-term memory are typically lost in seconds, not minutes, hours, or days. Without refreshing or deliberate overwriting, that upper duration of short-term memory is often only around 15–30 seconds.

A familiar example of a short-term memory task is digit span. For this task, you remember a list of numbers in the correct order. Most people have a digit span of around six to nine numbers. Digit span is invariably illustrated by referring to the problem of remembering a telephone number. Rather surprisingly, this challenge can be traced back to a measles epidemic in 1879.

One of the world's first telephone exchanges was installed in 1878 in Lowell, Massachusetts. Subscribers were initially identified by their names, but a measles epidemic hastened the switch to number codes, so that new operators could be trained more quickly. Ever since, we have had to remember chains of numbers. During that time, telephone numbers have grown. Currently, the maximum telephone number is 15 characters, well beyond normal digit span.

DOI: 10.4324/9781003537649-15

In addition to words and numbers, there is a short-term memory span for spatial locations. In the Corsi block-tapping task you see an array of nine blocks located on a test board. The tester taps a sequence of different blocks, which you then repeat. For many people, the longest sequence they can reliably replicate is around five. The electronic game 'Simon' is also designed to challenge your short-term memory. The toy emits a sequence of tones and lights, and the player then repeats the sequence on the device (Figure 15.1). If you succeed, the sequence becomes increasingly long and complex. (Apparently there is a Swedish game with the name 'Follow John', a name I particularly like. It is a 'follow my leader' type game in which the players remember and mimic the physical actions of their leader, John.)

Some of the initial evidence for the existence of short-term memory came from studies of anterograde amnesia. In this condition, the person cannot, after a short while, retain new information (see Chapter 17). Nevertheless, the same amnesics often displayed an intact digit span and Corsi block span, as well as being able to follow complex conversations. In other words, they retained a brief memory store well beyond sensory memory. It is for this reason, there is typically no apparent loss of I.Q. in amnesia, even though I.Q. tests make substantial demands on immediate memory. This spared ability only becomes possible if we assume that a temporary memory store remains intact in these amnesic patients, namely, short-term memory, even though long-term memory is devastated.

At this point, it is almost obligatory to mention the famous amnesic patient H.M., surely the most studied single case in all of psychology. More will be said about H.M. in the section on amnesia. For now, all that matters is that, following brain tissue removal, which included the hippocampus, H.M. showed a profound, permanent inability to acquire new long-term memories. Nevertheless, his I.Q. did not decline while his digit span remained a respectable six digits. His intact short-term memory is highlighted by what Brenda Milner

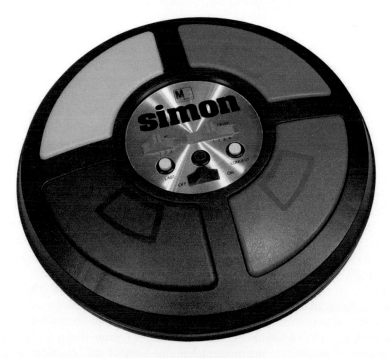

Figure 15.1 The game 'Simon', which taxes short-term memory.

said about H.M. "*His comprehension of language is undisturbed: he can repeat and transform sentences with complex syntax, and he gets the point of jokes, including those turning on semantic ambiguity*" (Milner et al., 1968).

A question that arises is what causes forgetting from short-term memory. A popular explanation is that time is the critical agent, causing trace decay and leaving any content less temporally distinct and, hence, harder to retrieve. It has also been argued that temporal decay as a cause of forgetting distinguishes short-term from long-term memory. There are, however, other explanations for forgetting within short-term memory. One candidate is 'interference'. Interference occurs when similar competing items exist, with the potential to disrupt or displace those in short-term memory. This competition can come in many forms including overwriting by earlier or later items, confusion at retrieval, and interference when refreshing an item. As interference is a cause of forgetting from long-term memory this property would not help to distinguish the two memory stores.

Short-term memory and the concept of working memory: Let me give you a simple problem: Hold the letters **E N Y** in your head, then, starting at the beginning of the alphabet, find the common four-letter word ending in those three letters. Please give it a go. You immediately see how this problem engages far more than just maintaining the phonological representation of the three letters. You need to retain E N Y while you try the letter A, then B, then C, and so on, all the time drawing on prior knowledge from long-term memory to decide whether you have found the solution. Consequently, you have to hold and execute a number of task rules while also maintaining the relevant information. (By the way, you may find the solution to the problem harder than you might initially think.)

This same problem highlights how we can actively engage with the contents of short-term memory, in order to compute sums, weigh up decisions, test ideas, or shuffle our thoughts around. These control functions (often called 'executive' functions) relate to how information is sorted and controlled by reference to task goals, i.e., the bigger picture. To incorporate these control functions into short-term memory, the concept of 'working memory' emerged. While both terms, short-term memory and working memory, co-exist, there is growing preference for working memory. One reason is that this conceptualisation helps to capture the complexity of our cognitive interface with the world.

Here, I will follow the guide of Alan Baddeley (2012) who, along with Graham Hitch, introduced the original concept of working memory in 1974. Baddeley regards short-term memory as a simple temporary store of information, while working memory implies both the storage and manipulation of that information. In this way, working memory subsumes short-term memory but adds features to create a more active system. A simple span task, such as repeating back a list of numbers, is seen as just requiring short-term memory as the information is merely held and repeated. In a complex span task, such as digit span backwards, the order of the numbers is reversed in your head before repeating. Complex span tasks require working memory as they involve both the storage and the control of information. (Just in case you didn't find the solution to the **E N Y** problem, the answer is deny.)

The capacity of short-term memory: In a landmark paper from 1956, George Miller proposed that the capacity of short-term memory is 7±2 items, though as we will see, that estimate has since been reduced. The opening lines of George Miller's paper are as arresting as any introduction to a scientific paper. He wrote

My problem is that I have been persecuted by an integer. For seven years this number has followed me around, has intruded in my most private data, and has assaulted me from the pages of our most public journals. This number assumes a variety of disguises, being sometimes a little larger and sometimes a little smaller than usual, but never changing so much as to be unrecognizable. The persistence with which this number plagues me is far more than a random accident. There is, to quote a famous senator, a design behind it, some pattern governing its appearances. Either there really is something unusual about the number or else I am suffering from delusions of persecution'.

That number was, of course, seven.

That opening paragraph has stuck with me for decades because of its sheer brilliance. Incidentally, seven decades before Miller's famous paper, Hermann Ebbinghaus (1885) highlighted the magic number seven for serial learning, stating *"What number of syllables can be correctly recited after only one reading? For me the number is usually seven"*.

There has been endless debate over the capacity of auditory short-term memory. Based on digit span it should be around 7±2 items. However, word-span is consistently smaller. Part of the problem is that an 'item' is not a fixed thing. Take the two words 'water' and 'rail'. To most people they represent two distinct items, but to a bird-watcher they join to give a species of bird, a water rail, making a single item. This example highlights how prior, individual knowledge affects short-term memory capacity.

Read out the following sequence of letters and then try to recall them in the correct order: BTORSPBNNR. If you try to do this letter by letter it is almost impossible. But the task becomes much easier if you can group the letters. I would immediately group them as BTO (British Trust for Ornithology), then RSPB (Royal Society for the Protection of Birds), and then NNR (National Nature Reserve). This gives me three 'items' and not ten. The ability to group items together is called 'chunking', and so it might be better to think of the capacity of short-term memory in 'chunks'. But as we have just seen, chunking depends on past learning and is, therefore, individual. Even so, current best estimates place the capacity of auditory short-term memory at around 4±1 chunks.

To see why short-term memory capacity is not seven but closer to four items, we can return to that problem originating from 1879, remembering a telephone number. Real telephone numbers invariably exceed our digit span of 7±2. For this reason, we often group digits in twos and threes. To help, we introduce pauses to separate the groups and retain their order. Furthermore, the numbers within a group may be compressed to form a chunk. Take the numbers six and four. They could be regarded as two distinct digits, but they could also become '64', combined because 64 is eight squared or it is the age (according to the Beatles) when you become truly old. This is why our digit span appears longer than the short-term memory capacity of 4±1 chunks. For the same reasons, frequent digit sequences lead to better immediate serial recall than less frequent ones. Likewise, our word-span is greater for words than non-words, and also for words in our own language rather than in a foreign language. The explanation is that it is much harder to group non-words or foreign words.

Postcodes (or zip codes) pose interesting challenges for our short-term memory. The good news is that U.K. postcodes retain the potential to be chunked because the pairs of letters and pairs/triplets of numbers often combine, aiding memory. Canadian zip codes are, alas, the stuff of nightmares. These codes alternate between single letters and single numbers, e.g., T6E 5J8. This arrangement makes grouping almost impossible, leaving them incredibly hard to remember. The task is made all the more challenging as we find it especially difficult to remember random sequences of letters. This difficulty reflects our unfamiliarity with random sequences given that letter order is normally constrained by spelling rules.

While we spontaneously chunk suitable information to increase our memory span, with training chunking can produce remarkable results. As already described, expert chess players group pieces in perceptual chunks, so aiding their memory of board positions. Similarly, car experts have a more extensive short-term memory for car images, reflecting more effective processing. You might recall the college student who, with considerable practice, raised his digit span from a typical seven to an incredible 79. He achieved this feat by grouping the digits as times (minutes, seconds, milliseconds) and relating those to the times for athletic achievements, with which he was already fascinated. This process, which also invokes long-term memory, allowed him to repeat lists of up to around 20 digits. He then mastered a method of grouping these chunks to create higher-order super groups. His achievements highlight the close interactions between long-term memory and short-term memory, a process that has been formally incorporated into models of working memory.

Up to now, the focus has been on auditory short-term memory, but we also have visual short-term memory. Its duration outlives iconic memory, but its capacity is limited. Importantly, we can interact and interrogate the contents of visual short-term memory in ways not possible for iconic memory. The capacity of visual short-term memory is usually estimated at around three or four objects, though that capacity depends on the complexity of the objects. As the complexity increases, capacity decreases. Conversely, that capacity can be increased if visual features are simplified.

It is natural to think of short-term memory for auditory or visual information, but we should also consider other modalities. One example is tactile (haptic) information. Touch sequences on different fingers can be recalled using finger movements, giving a serial span of 5±1, with memory properties similar to those in auditory and visual short-term memory. Other attempts to measure the properties of haptic short-term memory include testing the ability to discriminate novel from familiar geometric objects by touch alone or retaining non-verbally where you have been touched on the arm. In addition, we have a separate olfactory short-term memory that may have a capacity of up to six smells.

16 Brief memory stores

Working memory

The true art of memory is the art of attention.

Samuel Johnson (1759)

Working memory – the mental blackboard

We need working memory to think. Working memory is often likened to a mental blackboard, providing a temporary workspace for planning, reasoning, and problem-solving. The blackboard is then erased to help tackle new problems. Because we use working memory to hold and juggle information in our head, problems can arise when additional, competing information also gains access to working memory. (I am sure I am not the only person who switches off the car radio when confronted by challenging driving conditions; in this way, I can devote my working memory to the principal task and not share it with sounds from the radio.) Unsurprisingly, working memory and attention are intimately linked.

Working memory is effortful as it involves consciously holding and manipulating information. If I ask you to multiply three by our in your head you will rapidly, and without effort, respond 12. If I ask you to multiply 13 by 14 in your head you will probably adopt a much slower, effortful process that involves temporarily holding numbers and then returning to them. (You might, for example, multiply 13 by 10, hold the answer 130, then multiply 13 by four to give 52, and then add the two answers to give 182.) Solving this harder task requires working memory.

Problem solving also requires working memory. One classic example is the 'river crossing' challenge. This ancient problem, dating back at least to the ninth century, can involve a farmer, a fox, a goose, and a bag of beans. All parties must cross the river in a boat that only holds two, but the pairs on the bank must be compatible, in other words, not eat each other. This means that the fox cannot be left with the goose, or the goose with the beans. Other variants include 'the three jealous husbands', who must never be left with the wrong partner! (Figure 16.1). For these problems, working memory makes possible both the temporary maintenance and manipulation of the relevant information.

Working memory is not only critical for problem solving, but also for the switching and scheduling of job priorities when multi-tasking. This broad conception of working memory reflected the desire to move away from single-storage models of visual and verbal short-term memory. One consequence is that the properties of working memory take it far closer to what is called 'fluid intelligence'. This likeness helps to explain the power of working memory to predict future academic performance in children (see *Infant and children's*

DOI: 10.4324/9781003537649-16

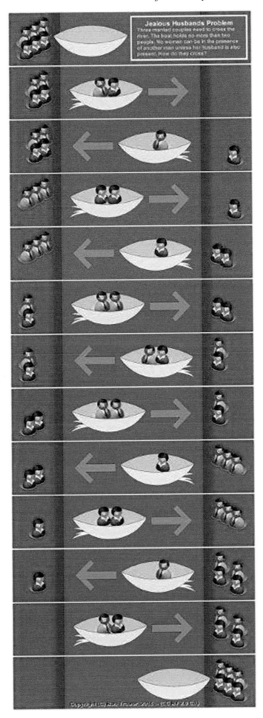

Figure 16.1 First six of 11 river crossings to solve the jealous husband's problem. Three married couples have to cross the river. The boat holds no more than two. No woman can be in the company of another man unless her husband is present.

memories; *four and beyond, Chapter 2*). As already noted, some of the elements of working memory rely on the prefrontal cortex, which matures slowly, so that this type of memory does not reach full capacity until adolescence and beyond.

Demonstrating working memory: One of the reasons why working memory was first introduced is our ability to perform simultaneous reasoning and memory tasks. Imagine you are asked to solve a series of logic problems. You are told that 'A is not preceded by B'. Is the example 'BA' true or false? You need to pause and think (it's false). The extraordinary thing is that people can still solve this reasoning task while simultaneously having to retain and repeat a six-digit number, e.g., 739142. Not surprisingly, the reasoning task now takes longer, but it is still possible (Baddeley, 2012). Traditional views of auditory short-term memory assume that the two problems must compete for the same space, so that solving both tasks becomes impossible as the system is overloaded. To explain this ability, parallel storage components were incorporated.

The simultaneous reasoning/memorising problem described above is an example of a 'complex span' task. These tasks add a demanding, secondary cognitive element to the basic memory span problem. In this way, complex span tasks require people to engage in some processing unrelated to the memory task, yet still maintain the memory. For this reason, they have also been called 'storage plus processing' tasks. Such tasks embody key aspects of working memory.

A previously described complex span task is 'digit span backwards' (Figure 2.3). For this task, you repeat back a string of numbers, but in reverse order (you may hear 39518 but repeat back 81593). Another complex span task involves mentally holding a sequence of letters, e.g., R, S, L, Q, T, then solving a simple mathematical problem $(8/2) -1 = 1$? before repeating back the string of letters. This 'storage plus processing' design is again seen when people are first given a string of letters to hold in mind while at the same time reading a sentence that may or may not contain an obvious error. All of these complex span tasks highlight the step-up in cognitive demand from short-term memory to working memory.

Another family of working memory problems are called '*n*-back' tasks, where *n* is a variable number (Figure 16.2). Imagine you hear a list of random letters. The first challenge is to hold in mind the constantly changing letters in their correct order. The second challenge is to say whether the item currently presented is the same as the item presented a specific number (*n*) of items back in the list. For a three-back task you would indicate a match when hearing GBUG but then no match for the following letter P, as you now have BUGP, and P did not appear three items back (Figure 16.2). The items used in this type of task can be letters, words, digits, symbols, or locations. The relatively modest correlations between performing

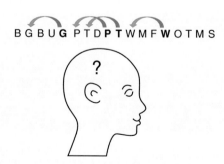

Figure 16.2 For an auditory n-back task of three, the person indicates those letters repeated (bold) from three back in the list.

n-back tasks and other working memory tasks reflect how there are multiple process within working memory, which contribute in different ways, creating different bottlenecks.

These descriptions of complex span tasks sound very artificial, with little real-word applicability. In fact, similar cognitive demands happen all the time. We are constantly multi-tasking, juggling different types of information. The many children who tackle their homework while watching television are unwittingly creating complex tasks in which two sets of serial information are being monitored and processed. (The internet informs me that half of all teenagers admit to watching television while doing homework.) As soon as the homework becomes a little more complex, that assignment becomes harder and takes longer to complete. Again, around three-quarters of teenagers apparently do homework while listening to music. To appreciate why this matters, we first need to understand the 'phonological loop'.

The structure of working memory: In its original conception, working memory contained three distinct components, each with different functions. These components were the phonological loop, the visuospatial sketchpad, and the central executive (Figure 16.3). A fourth component, the 'episodic buffer', was added by Alan Baddeley decades later. These are 'fluid' systems, so that the contents of each store are subject to continual change. A key feature is that these various components are not held in isolation, they work together in an integrated manner. Later refinements emphasised the many effects of long-term memory on working memory. For this, three key influencers, episodic memory, language, and visual semantics were identified (Baddeley, 2012). These three long-term memory influencers all rely on 'crystalised', stable information, contrasting with the fluid contents of working memory.

The phonological loop: The first of the three original components is the phonological loop. This brief memory subsystem specialises in holding speech-based sounds, though the same system can assist lip-reading and signing. Reflecting these properties, the phonological loop may have evolved in order to support language processing. Despite its modest storage capacity, the phonological loop holds information in the correct temporal order. This property is vital for processing language. Information within the phonological loop is rapidly lost by trace decay and is either rapidly overwritten and replaced, or refreshed by subvocal rehearsal, in other words, by speaking inside your head. This refreshment process helps to set the capacity of the phonological loop as it approximates to the number of words you can say subvocally in around two seconds.

The phonological loop is not, however, the sole retainer of verbal information. If you tie up the phonological loop by repeating words out loud, digit span only falls by about two

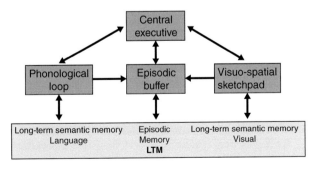

Figure 16.3 The relationships between the various stores that comprise the Working Memory Model (based on Baddeley, 2012).

items, as other components help to share the load. Nevertheless, the properties of the phonological loop help to provide a coherent account of a number of short-term verbal memory effects. These memory effects include the impact of word length (short words give longer memory spans), phonemic similarity (which causes confusion and interference when words sound similar), the irrelevant speech effect (see below), and articulatory suppression (what happens if you tie-up subvocal rehearsal, e.g., by saying 'the, the, the' repeatedly).

Background sound effects: Words or word-like sounds can directly enter the phonological loop. This means that background conversations can occupy working memory whether you like it or not. This intrusion is called the irrelevant speech effect. This same effect helps to explain some of the drawbacks of working with background chatter or music, such as in an open-plan office. Background speech consistently reduces memory span, irrespective of whether the speech is in your own or a foreign language, or even if it consists of nonsense words. This disruptive effect on working memory can, however, be greater when hearing familiar, rather than unfamiliar, background speakers (Kreitewolf et al., 2019). A disruptive effect is also found for background vocal music but is much diminished for instrumental sounds, i.e., for sounds lacking words.

This intrusive effect is not, however, confined to words. Background tones that are modulated in ways that resembles speech are also disruptive. In fact, speech and non-speech sounds can have equivalent disruptive effects on verbal memory when they make similar changes between successive sounds. For this reason, the disruption has been described by Dylan Jones as the 'irrelevant sound' effect or the 'changing state' effect, rather than the irrelevant speech effect.

Although the effects of irrelevant speech appear greatest when the task involves remembering the serial order of items, other tasks can be affected. One example is proofreading for errors in text. While the degree of disruption does depend on whether the background speech is meaningful, it is not dependent on its volume. However, the impact of background speech is reduced if the perceptual demands of proofreading are increased, forcing the reader to make closer inspection of the text. Examples included changing from this font (Times New Roman) **to this font** (Haettenschweiler), or visually masking the text. By increasing task engagement, the reader is shielded from irrelevant speech effects.

As you might expect, the impact of background conversation increases with the number of speakers, but it soon reaches a maximum disruptive effect with about five unattended speakers. What you might not expect is that any disruptive effect begins to decrease with additional background speakers. This means that with a crowd of background conversations, as in an open-plan office, the irrelevant speech effect starts to diminish. This has been called the babble effect, and it occurs when individual background words lose their salience in the mass of chatter. That said, background chatter still disrupts serial working memory tasks, and attempts to counteract its effects with masking sounds, such as waterfalls, have not yet been successful.

Before shielding ourselves from any background noise pollution, we should remember that the greatest impact of irrelevant speech is on the retention of serial stimuli. When hearing a list of words to remember by free recall, a background foreign language had no apparent impact as word order does not matter. Clearly, there are disruptive effects of unwanted background speech, but they are moderated by the type of cognitive challenge and its complexity. As a practical guide, it is best to avoid background speech or vocal music when problem solving, doing homework, or writing a book.

There are understandable concerns about the potential impact of background noise on the classroom. For instance, multi-talker background babble has been shown to disrupt a range of working memory tasks in young children. In addition, a number of studies have confirmed that noise pollution, such as that from background trains, traffic, and aeroplanes, has detrimental effects on children's cognition (Thompson et al., 2022). Reading and language skills, along with attention, are affected. While a host of factors could contribute to this relationship, the impact on working memory is one contender. A clear lesson is the need for good sound insulation.

The visuospatial sketchpad: The next component of working memory is the visuospatial sketchpad. (The same store is often called the visuospatial 'scratchpad', a term derived from computer memory storage.) The term sketchpad refers to a set of temporary notes or sketches. Consequently, this store briefly retains the spatial representation of incoming information. That information is typically visual. One of its functions is to handle and manipulate visual imagery. Solving the river crossing problem, with its farmer, fox, goose, and beans, is a task that heavily taxes the visuospatial sketchpad.

Another example is when mentally rotating the spatial features on a map. If you are travelling South and the map is held the right way up (North at the top), the journey is planned and tracked using reverse turnings, so that left becomes right and *vice versa*. This particular ability shows alarming individual variability, helping to explain many past navigational disputes, now often solved by satellite navigation (Sat Navs). Somewhat predictably, orienteers, but also gymnasts, have superior mental rotation skills to non-athletes. Finally, tactile (haptic) information may also access the visuospatial scratchpad. At first this may seem surprising, but blind readers using Braille seem to translate the touch information into a spatial format.

The central executive: The central executive helps to regulate attention, make decisions, guide the storage of information, and interface with long-term memory. It is thought to rely heavily on the actions of the frontal lobes of the brain. This broad functionality allows the central executive to support the other working memory components. Given these top-down actions it is no surprise that the central executive can start to resemble a 'homunculus' – a clever little person in the head that does all our thinking. This is a lazy way of explaining memory and needs to be fought. So, to gain a more systematic view of what the central executive provides, subjects are often given concurrent cognitive tasks to see how one task impacts on the other. Spared abilities can reflect the contributions of the central executive. It is this approach that has helped to reveal central executive roles in attention, decision-making, and task-switching, functions appropriately given the generic term 'executive'.

The episodic buffer: This was the last store to be incorporated within working memory, being added years after the original formulation. This buffer is another store with limited capacity that interacts with the rest of working memory. However, in addition, the buffer links working memory to perception and long-term memory (Baddeley, 2012). One of its presumed functions is to allow features from different sources to be bound into chunks or episodes. As we have repeatedly seen, brief memory stores do not operate in isolation, they have two-way interactions with long-term memory. It was partly in recognition of this reciprocity that the episodic buffer was added to the array of components, which together comprise working memory. Like the central executive, the episodic buffer is presumed to have limited capacity and be attention demanding.

The capacity of working memory: There are two main models to account for the capacity of working memory. The 'slot model' assumes that the maximum number of objects that can be held in working memory is set by a finite limit. This means that there is a maximum number of independent object slots. Consequently, working memory is all-or-none: an object either gets into a memory slot and is remembered or it does not, and fails to be remembered.

In contrast, the 'resource model' presumes a fixed amount of common resource that can be flexibly distributed across working memory, according to demand. This means that defining capacity by numbers of objects will not generalise across different tasks. The resource model argues that, in theory, there is no upper ceiling to the number of items that can be stored, but if you increase the numbers you have to decrease the precision of their representation. Consequently, there is a trade-off between the quality and quantity of working memory representations. A further, related idea is that working memory capacity is not simply about how many items can be stored in each component but, just as critically, reflects individual differences in the ability to control attention and maintain information in an active, accessible state.

The word length effect and its curious implications in Wales: We can now return to some of the memory phenomena that arise from the working memory model. As you will recall, the phonological loop is specialised for verbal information. Its contents decay but can be refreshed by subvocal articulation, in other words, saying things to yourself. Evidence for articulatory coding includes the 'word length effect'. This effect describes how words that take longer to say have a smaller word span than words that can be said more quickly.

To take an extreme example, a list of words such as catapult, anteater, cellulose, tapioca, bungalow, spinnaker, and tornado, will result in a shorter word span than one composed of single syllable words such as cat, ant, cell, tap, bun, spin, and tor. This is, of course, not a fair comparison as the longer words contain more syllables and, hence, potentially more information (and are less frequent). The critical test is what happens when the number of syllables and phonemes are matched, but one set of words (e.g., harpoon, coerce) takes longer to articulate than a comparison set of words (e.g., bishop, phallic). Memory span is superior for those words that are quicker to say. From such studies it was concluded that a subject's span approximates to the number of words that can be read in about two seconds. This is one of the reasons why young children have a smaller working memory capacity, their subvocalisation speed is slower.

The word length effect has some surprising implications. One of these is that different languages will produce different digit spans, reflecting the times taken to articulate those numbers. In Chinese, the digits 0-9 are naturally said more rapidly than in many other languages. As might be anticipated, Chinese speakers have a longer digit span than the speakers of various European languages (English, Finnish, Greek, Spanish, and Swedish), which themselves do not differ in their digit spans. China also tops the Gold Medal table of the International Mathematical Olympiad, which has been held since 1959. Clearly, there are many reasons for this, but having a larger digit span is not a bad start.

Word length effects on mathematics may happen much closer to home. Nick Ellis observed that the average digit span for Welsh-speaking children appeared lower than the test norms, which were based on English speaking children (Figure 16.4). At first sight this difference seemed to make no sense. He then decided to find out whether it takes longer to articulate the digits 0-10 in Welsh (dim, un, dau, tri, pedwar, pump, chwech, saith, wyth, naw, deg) than in English (nought, one, two, three, four, five, six, seven, eight, nine, ten). For the same length of time, he found that bilingual speakers could say six digits in English but only five when using Welsh (Ellis & Hennelly, 1980). In other words, the same list of numbers took longer to speak in Welsh. Reflecting this difference, the average digit span for these same bilingual speakers was 5.8 in Welsh, but 6.6 when using English.

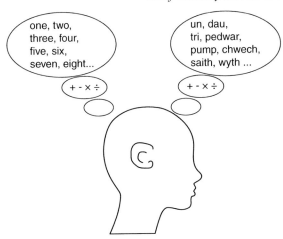

Figure 16.4 Digit span can vary across languages, reflecting the time it takes to say the various digits.

One reason why understanding these reading time differences might matter is that digit span contributes to some intelligence tests, creating disadvantages where none should exist. Furthermore, these reading time differences might affect mental calculations. For simple calculations (e.g., two × 14) we immediately reach the answer but for others (e.g., eight × 142) we have to hold and manipulate the digits in our head, drawing on working memory. For this, we typically use internal speech to help reach the solution. (You can test this by trying to multiply 8 × 142 while simultaneously saying 'the, the, the, the' repeatedly). Consistent with the digit span difference for Welsh numbers, Nick Ellis found evidence that Welsh speaking children were slower and made more errors on those sums that made considerable demands on working memory.

The Welsh psychologist Dylan Jones has since refined our understanding of these language effects. In particular, he found that the times taken to pronounce individual numbers did not differ between the two languages. Instead, it was the lengthier pauses between individual Welsh numbers that led to longer reading times. It is this co-articulation difference that may principally impact on digit span. This finding helps to explain some of the initial results of Nick Ellis, as he asked subjects to read lists of numbers, so the longer times in Welsh may have principally come from the gaps placed between digits.

Challenges to the working memory model: It should come as no surprise that the working memory model has been criticised. An early suggestion was that the 'levels of processing' account removed the need for distinct short-term and long-term memory processes, creating a unified picture. In fact, this was not the belief of the originators of 'levels of processing'. They maintained the idea of both long-term and short-term memory systems, but also emphasised the engagement of long-term memory on short-term memory (Craik, 2002). Within the working memory model, this important role is largely taken on by the central executive and the episodic buffer. There remains, however, the concern that the working memory model has become overcomplex and contains elements such as the central executive and the episodic buffer that are increasingly difficult to define and isolate.

Another challenge is that rather than consisting of multiple stores, working memory might be thought of as the focus of attention across a wide domain of information types. A related view is that working memory is the label we give to long-term memory that is activated by attention. These attention-based views can, however, still be assimilated within the multi-component working memory model as they reflect attributes of the central executive and episodic buffer.

While these criticisms each have their proponents, the concept of working memory remains centre stage. One reason is that it creates a framework to explore real-world situations involving complex decisions. A related reason is that measures of working memory correlate with other intellectual abilities, surpassing other measures, including short-term memory. This reason has, for example, galvanised research into working memory and education (see *Infant and Childhood Memory, Chapter 2*).

Working memory and the brain: Neuroscientists have long assumed that temporary changes in neuronal transmission enable short-term memory, but for some information these changes become structural and more permanent, forming long-term memories. To study memory mechanisms at this level, we are often reliant on animal research. But there is a big problem. How do we independently know that a phase of animal learning corresponds to short-term memory without employing a circular argument – it is short-term because we cannot find stable structural changes.

Working memory became the preferred term as it could be defined using the analogy of a mental blackboard that can be erased and then re-used. Consequently, the term working memory is used to describe animal memory tasks in which a piece of information is briefly required but then discarded before using a new piece of information on the next trial to solve the same category of problem.

I vividly remember as a child how the bus conductors would wind out each ticket from a machine strapped to their body. Their challenge was to remember, for the rest of the journey, who had tickets, but then discard all of that information when beginning the next journey. Exactly the same logic is used when testing animal working memory. One example of this logic is the radial-arm maze devised by David Olton.

Imagine a maze with eight arms radiating out from a circular centre. A sweet is then placed at the end of each arm. Next, a rat is placed in the centre, from which it can run down every arm to reach the reward. The most effective foraging strategy is for the rat to run down each arm to collect the sweets but not to visit an arm more than once as there will be no reward on the second visit. Consequently, the rat should maintain an updated list of arms already visited and those yet to visit. But, after being removed from the maze that information needs to be rubbed off the animal's mental blackboard, just like the bus conductor. The next time the rat is returned to the re-baited radial maze it can start with a clean slate when trying to subsequently remember those arms to visit and then avoid. Exactly the same type of radial-maze task has been used to test spatial working memory in children showing, for example, that young girls are often better than boys and that this spatial memory skill is not fully proficient until around seven years of age.

This conception of animal working memory galvanised studies on the prefrontal cortex. Again, using the mental blackboard analogy, imagine seeing a signal that briefly comes on and then off. Your task is to turn and face that signal, but you cannot turn towards the signal until after it has been switched off. Maintaining the information during this holding delay creates the working memory component. The spatial location of that signal moves from trial to trial, so that information from the previous trial is of no current benefit and needs to be wiped off the mental blackboard. Neurons within the prefrontal cortex were discovered that seem to hold information during the critical delay periods in ways that correspond to working memory demands. Furthermore, removing those same prefrontal brain areas impaired performance on working memory tasks. The initial interpretation was that the prefrontal cortex holds the working memory store.

That initial view has since been much modified. Instead, the prefrontal cortex is now seen as akin to the central executive, having both memory capabilities and top-down control processes that operate both in the short and the long term. Different types of mental control may involve different parts of the prefrontal cortex. These same executive processes then operate across much of the rest of the brain, so that the substrates for working memory can appear widely distributed across the neocortex. This means that the attributes of working memory are not clustered in one brain site, rather they are distributed across multiple brain areas, yet differ subtly for different task demands. For example, spatial tasks activate more dorsal parts of the posterior cortex while non-spatial tasks activate the ventral posterior cortex.

17 Losing memory

Real amnesias and simulated amnesias

I've a grand memory for forgetting!

Kidnapped, Robert Louis Stevenson (1886)

A sudden loss of memory

Amnesia holds an undeniable fascination. It is easy to see why. For fiction writers the condition creates instant tension and mystery. The loss of one's memory seems like one of the cruellest twists of fate. For psychologists, amnesia provides some of the strongest evidence that we possess fundamentally different forms of memory. For neuroscientists, the sudden loss of memory provides unique insights into how the brain encodes, stores, and retrieves information. This understanding depended on identifying those brain sites responsible for different kinds of memory loss. On top of this, we need to appreciate that there are many different types of amnesia, including some that don't even exist.

Amnesia in fiction: The dramatic device of having a lead character with amnesia has a long history. At least ten silent movies before 1926 involved characters with memory loss. Wikipedia lists well over 200 films that feature amnesia, including 'The Muppets Take Manhattan', 'Desperately Seeking Susan', and 'Finding Dory'. Sadly, these depictions remain far removed from most amnesic conditions. In a U.S. survey, 83% of respondents mistakenly thought that 'People suffering from amnesia typically cannot recall their own name or identity' (Simons & Chabris, 2011). It is tempting to blame films such as 'The Bourne Identity' for the misplaced associated between amnesia and the loss of identity. In reality, a loss of identity, often associated with a period of wandering, may be seen in a 'fugue state' – but this is a very rare type of psychogenic amnesia.

Already highlighted for its misuse of the term short-term memory, the lead character Lucy in the 2004 film '50 First Dates' has recurrent amnesia so that within each day she has no recollection of the previous day. This fictional contrivance (Goldfield's syndrome) bore no resemblance to any known amnesic condition. But there was a remarkable twist. In 2010, patient F.L. suffered a car accident. Afterwards she seemed to demonstrate a similar pattern of retaining memory within a day but losing it by the following day (Smith et al., 2010). After careful examination it was felt that F.L. exhibited a unique form of functional amnesia. The nature of F.L.'s memory loss was thought to have been influenced by her knowledge of how amnesia was depicted in '50 First Dates', although it was not believed that she deliberately fabricated her apparent amnesia.

Organic amnesia: The term organic amnesia refers to the loss of memory following an insult to the brain. In other words, the amnesia has a physical cause. The many potential

DOI: 10.4324/9781003537649-17

causes of organic amnesia include strokes, tumours, brain trauma, a lack of oxygen to the brain, viral encephalitis, and vitamin B1 deficiency. By contrast, in 'psychogenic' amnesia the severity of the memory loss far exceeds any apparent brain disruption.

Organic amnesias are divided into two, often overlapping, categories (Figure 17.1). Anterograde amnesia is the failure to learn or recall personal events that occurred *after* the brain trauma. Consequently, the core deficit is a failure to acquire and maintain new memories. Sadly, this form of organic amnesia is often permanent. Meanwhile, in retrograde amnesia there is a loss of autobiographical memories from *before* the onset of the amnesia. This loss can involve both episodic memory and aspects of semantic memory. In many cases of retrograde amnesia there is a partial return of seemingly lost memories. Varying levels of both anterograde and retrograde amnesia often co-occur in the same person, but occasionally someone only suffers from anterograde or retrograde amnesia.

Despite their various causes, different organic amnesias share important features. One diagnostic feature is the preservation of I.Q. To meaningfully measure I.Q., it is necessary to have an effective short-term memory, which is also typically spared. To complete the various challenges in an I.Q. test it is also necessary to comprehend the instructions and interact with the testers. The sparing of these cognitive abilities sets amnesia apart from dementia.

How bad can it get? Though not representative, I shall begin with the tragic case of Clive Wearing. He unwittingly provides disturbing insights into what follows after an almost complete loss of past, present, and future memories. Yet, in spite of his profound memory loss, he shows those aspects of cognitive sparing that help to define amnesia. Thankfully, the completeness of his combined anterograde and retrograde amnesias is not typical of organic amnesia.

Clive Wearing was an eminent musician (he coordinated much of the music on BBC Radio 3 for the day of Charles' and Diana's wedding in 1981). At the age of 46, he suffered extensive brain damage caused by herpes simplex encephalitis. This illness occurs when the cold sore virus enters the brain, something that thankfully rarely occurs. Clive suffered a catastrophic loss of his past memories, along with an inability to learn and remember any new events. He retained a few prominent facts such as who he was, where he went to school, and where he studied music, but most of his life history was erased. Consequently, he lost almost all of his autobiographical memories for the 45 years prior to his illness. Despite everything, his I.Q. remained in the normal range (though undoubtedly less than before his illness), and his short-term memory was spared.

As he had no apparent past, Clive believed that he had just become conscious for the first time. It was the only logical explanation for his predicament. He would repeatedly write this deduction in his diary, only to later strike it out, as by then he could not recall making the earlier diary entry. He was able to recognise and remember his wife Deborah,

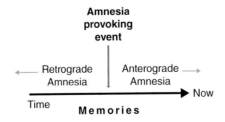

Figure 17.1 Amnesias are distinguished by being anterograde (new memories not formed or lost) or retrograde (past memories are lost).

but he always greeted her as if they were being re-united for the first time in years, even if she had only briefly stepped out of the room. Despite his devastating loss of memory, he retained implicit memory skills, such as playing the keyboard and being able to conduct a choir from sheet music. But he could not remember performing these skills. In doing so, Clive highlights the loss of explicit memory that contrasts with the sparing of implicit memory, a feature of amnesia. My few words cannot begin to do justice to the tragedy of Clive Wearing, which is poignantly detailed in 'Forever Today' by Deborah Wearing (2005).

Anterograde amnesia

The core deficit in anterograde amnesia is a failure to acquire and recall new episodic memories (Figure 17.2). Consequently, conversations and day-to-day experiences are rapidly forgotten. The amnesic will fail to recall what they have just done and where they have just been. Most, but not all, amnesics will also have difficulties with recognition memory. In contrast, factual (semantic) knowledge, including vocabulary, is retained, along with short-term memory. Consequently, on first meeting it can be surprisingly difficult to realise that you are chatting with an amnesic. This is especially true if the person is prone to 'confabulation'. Confabulation is the filling in of missing holes in one's memory, which some amnesics will do almost effortlessly. This habit is most common when the brain pathology includes the prefrontal cortex.

Many people with anterograde amnesia are painfully aware of their memory problems, but some lack this insight. The latter condition may be a mixed blessing. Being unaware of your amnesia makes it far harder to take practical steps to cope with the many day-to-day challenges, but a lack of insight is also likely to be less distressing. I used to visit two amnesics in the same Northumberland hospital. Neither had any insight into their condition and both displayed confabulation. The two amnesics were friends and would sit together on the same bench endlessly talking to each other. Neither could remember past the last sentence, and both freely confabulated. They seemed surprisingly content in their unreal world.

The failure of amnesics to remember recent events can even include eating meals. The famous amnesic H.M. apparently ate a second meal within a minute of finishing the first. This happened not because he was still hungry, but because he had forgotten the first meal. A more controlled study of this behaviour confirmed that anterograde amnesics would indulge in multiple meals, 15 minutes apart (Higgs et al., 2008). Again, this behaviour stemmed from a failure to remember the previous meal. At the same time, the amnesics did

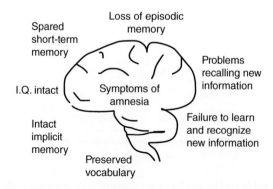

Figure 17.2 Core symptoms of anterograde amnesia.

show a form of learning called sensory-specific satiety. They reported a normal decline in the subjective pleasantness of the food as they reached the end of each meal.

Another consequence of anterograde amnesia is a failure to appreciate the passage of time. The amnesic H.M. could reproduce time intervals up to 20 seconds but, thereafter, he consistently underestimated longer intervals. By extrapolation, it was estimated that H.M.'s equivalence for one hour was three minutes, one day was 15 minutes, and a year was three hours.

This time-monitoring problem is not unique to H.M. as other amnesic struggle at estimating durations beyond 20–30 seconds. Temporal monitoring seems to be especially problematic in cases of the amnesic Korsakoff's disease. A particularly poignant example was described by Oliver Sacks in 'The Man Who Mistook his Wife for a Hat' (1985). His 'Lost Mariner' was capable of little or no new explicit learning and could not recall past decades of his life. When Oliver Sacks unwisely gave him a mirror he was bewildered and distressed. The mariner believed he was still 19 years old yet saw an aged person looking back at him in the mirror.

While people with anterograde amnesia struggle to acquire new facts (semantic knowledge), this ability is rarely completely lost. The amnesic H.M. demonstrated limited factual learning, such as the names of a few people who became famous after the onset of his amnesia. Examples included Billie Jean King and Woody Allen. He also knew that John Glenn was an astronaut who went to the moon. It appears that with sufficient repetition, anterograde amnesics can acquire some new facts. One helpful technique, 'errorless learning', is designed to stop errors during initial learning.

Amnesia is not global: When I was a student, anterograde amnesia was seen as 'global'. That is, all aspects of long-term memory were affected. We now know this is wrong. Over and over again it has been shown that amnesics can acquire and retain new implicit memories. One example is the reading of mirror-imaged words, a perceptual skill that gets quicker and quicker with practice (Figure 17.3).

Other visuomotor skills, such as learning to draw when looking in the mirror and 'rotary pursuit', a motor task that involves keeping a marker above a moving target, can also be acquired, and retained, at seemingly normal rates in people with anterograde amnesia.

Further examples of spared implicit memory in anterograde amnesia include priming, along with classical conditioning (Figure 17.4). Priming occurs when re-exposure to an

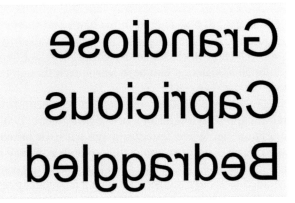

Figure 17.3 The ability to improve at reading mirror-imaged words remains intact in those with amnesia.

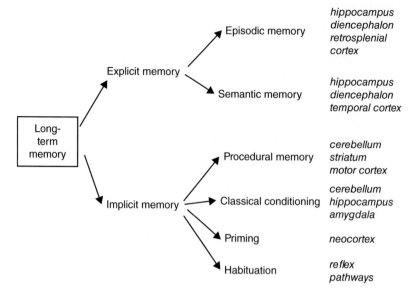

Figure 17.4 Memory systems in the brain and the various critical structures for each memory type.

item results in its faster or more effective processing, along with the greater likelihood that the item will spontaneously come to mind following a cue. Tests using degraded images of previously seen words or the starting letters of previously seen words both show that amnesics are able to provide the appropriate answer when asked to guess, even though they cannot recall the earlier image or word in a formal, explicit memory test.

To examine classical conditioning, two amnesics first heard a signal, immediately followed by an unexpected puff of air into the eye (Weiskrantz & Warrington, 1979). Both amnesics successfully acquired the conditioned response, blinking to the auditory signal alone, i.e., in the absence of the air puff. In stark contrast to their successful classical conditioning (implicit memory), neither amnesic could remember participating in the experiment and could not describe what had happened (explicit memory). That study was inspired by the curious observation of Édouard Claparède, a Swiss neurologist. Claparède regularly met an amnesic woman, who repeatedly failed to remember him. On one occasion in 1911, the neurologist hid a sharp pin in his hand and then vigorously shook the woman's hand, pricking her. The following day the woman failed to remember meeting Claparède, but she was reluctant to shake hands, withdrawing her hand without knowing why. A fearful conditioned association had been learnt even though the actual experience could not be recalled.

Despite the sparing of old implicit skills and the ability to acquire new skills, problems can arise when amnesics apply such skills in a new environment. Two experienced drivers acquired anterograde amnesia. When tested in a simulator or tested on the road, their driving skills appeared normal and they could still remember driving rules and the meanings of road signs (Anderson et al., 2007). But both had difficulties when being given route directions, and they failed to avoid a collision following a sudden, unexpected situation in the simulator. The heightened risk of an accident may result from a poorer ability to anticipate future scenarios while driving (see Chapter 12, *Imagination, future memory, and prospective memory*).

The sparing of all types of implicit learning in anterograde amnesia reveals how this division of memory is reliant on a different set of brain structures from those required for explicit memory (Figure 17.4). This division helps to explain why other properties of implicit and explicit memories often appear so different, including their respective vulnerability to various neurological conditions, including dementia, as well as their different sensitivity to some drugs. At the same time, the driving study described above serves as a reminder that these divisions of memory often work in tandem.

The next challenge is to pinpoint those brain sites responsible for organic amnesia. Identifying the brain sites responsible is not only clinically important but also provides unique insights into how the brain processes and stores episodic memories. Alas, the long search for the neurological origins of anterograde amnesia is littered with misadventure.

The causes of anterograde amnesia – a series of tragic endings: To begin, I need to introduce a modest cast of brain sites (Figure 17.5). To help, Chapter 20 explains the nature of some of the brain names that will occur.

Anterograde amnesias can arise from damage in more than one brain region. The two brain regions most closely associated with anterograde amnesia are the temporal lobe ('temporal lobe amnesia') and the diencephalon ('diencephalic amnesia'). The medial part of the temporal lobe includes the hippocampus and parahippocampal region. The second area, the diencephalon, is a subcortical brain region. Within the diencephalon, the two areas that are most relevant to this story are the anterior thalamus and the mammillary bodies (Figure 17.5).

The thalamus can be likened to a midfielder in a football team – a player who does an enormous amount of work in distributing the ball back and forth, but their vital contributions often go largely unnoticed. So it is with the thalamus, which distributes information back and forth to the cortex. In the case of the anterior thalamic nuclei, their work is mainly with the cingulate cortex (Figure 17.5). Meanwhile, the mammillary bodies sit at the base of the brain within the back of the hypothalamus, another major part of the diencephalon. The mammillary bodies, which form two bumps at the base of the brain, have been the subject of a rather bizarre spelling debate (see *Chapter 20*).

Our tragic journey begins with the French neuroanatomist Felix Vicq d'Azyr who provided some of the most accurate 18th century depictions of the brain. In 1786, Vicq d'Azyr uncovered a brain pathway that would help to unlock diencephalic amnesia. He described the mammillothalamic tract, a pathway that links the mammillary bodies to the anterior thalamic nuclei. In his honour, the mammillothalamic tract is still sometimes called the

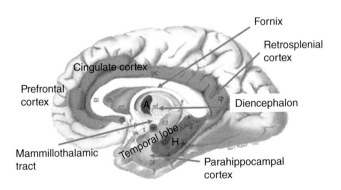

Figure 17.5 Location of some key brain sites implicated in memory and amnesia.

bundle of Vicq d'Azyr. He is, however, probably better remembered for being the last physician to Queen Marie-Antoinette. Vicq d'Azyr lost close friends to the guillotine, including
Antoine Lavoisier, but somehow avoided it himself. He did, however, die during the Terror,
plagued by nightmares and dread.

Exactly 100 years after Vicq d'Azyr published his anatomical descriptions, a German
neuroanatomist died under mysterious circumstances that have since fascinated a nation.
Bernhard von Gudden was an eminent psychiatrist and brilliant neuroanatomist. He also
did much to improve the condition of patients held in institutions. However, he is best
remembered for an entirely different reason. He was appointed to a team tasked with determining the mental state of Ludwig II, King of Bavaria, also now known as 'the Dream
King'. On the 13th June 1886, Bernhard von Gudden took a walk with Ludwig by the side
of Lake Starnberg near Munich. Neither returned. Both Bernhard von Gudden and Ludwig
II drowned (Figure 17.6). It remains a mystery as to whether it was murder, an accident, or
suicide.

Before his untimely death, Gudden described in new levels of detail the pathway that
links the hippocampus to the mammillary bodies. This pathway is called the fornix. Only
much later was it discovered that the fornix directly links those temporal lobe and diencephalic sites responsible for amnesia. Meanwhile, Gudden's name will always be remembered by neuroanatomists as he has that most precious of accolades, a part of the brain
named after him (Gudden's tegmental nuclei).

The next major advance came with the first formal description of an amnesic syndrome.
Credit is normally given to the Russian neurologist Sergei Korsakoff (Korsakov) who, in

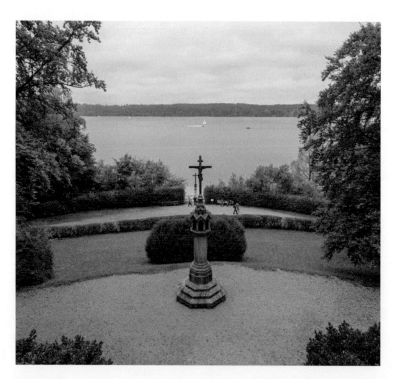

Figure 17.6 Memorials to Ludwig II in front of Lake Starnberg (where Bernhard von Gudden also
    drowned).

1889, described how some alcoholics suffer a permanent memory loss. Several years later (1897) at a conference in Moscow the name 'Korsakoff's disease' was adopted for this amnesic condition, a name that remains to this day (sometimes also called Korsakoff's syndrome or Korsakoff's amnesia).

Given this accolade, it may be surprising to discover that Korsakoff was not the first to describe this amnesic condition. Almost a decade earlier, in 1878, the physician Robert Lawson, who was the Medical Superintendent at a hospital in Exeter, described the same alcoholic amnesic syndrome. The condition is, however, never called Lawson's syndrome and his earlier observations are largely forgotten.

The naming story is further complicated as six years before Korsakoff, in 1881, Carl Wernicke described a condition in alcoholics characterised by mental confusion, aberrant eye movements, and motor difficulties. These transient Wernicke symptoms were often a prelude to the more chronic, Korsakoff 's amnesia. For this reason, some amnesic patients are still described as suffering from the Wernicke-Korsakoff syndrome. Sadly, Carl Wernicke was to die in a bicycling accident in 1905.

Korsakoff's disease provided the first opportunity to directly link memory loss with brain pathology. The breakthrough was made in 1896 by Hans Gudden, the son of the drowned Bernhard von Gudden. Post-mortem analyses of Korsakoff cases revealed consistent neuronal loss in the mammillary bodies, brain structures that sit at the base of the diencephalon. This link between mammillary body pathology and Korsakoff's disease has since been confirmed but, as subsequent cases were to show, mammillary body damage is only part of the explanation for diencephalic amnesia.

Temporal lobe amnesia: The sequence of tragedies now shifts to the study of temporal lobe amnesia. The Russian neurologist Vladimir Bekhterev is credited as the first person (in 1900) to suspect that hippocampal pathology causes memory loss. Bekhterev is the forgotten rival to Ivan Pavlov as both developed theories of conditioned reflexes. Some of Bekhterev's other work remains enormously influential. For example, he identified Ankylosing Spondylitis, sometimes known as Bekhterev's disease. His many achievements were, however, ruthlessly suppressed after his sudden death on the 24th December 1927. Many believe that Stalin personally ordered Bekhterev's death following unguarded remarks concerning the dictator's mental health. It is thought that Bekhterev unwisely described Stalin as paranoid. Within two days he was dead, possibly poisoned. The tragedy does not end there as during the 1930s his children were arrested and sent to a concentration camp in Siberia, where they died.

Bekhterev's suspicions about the hippocampus were proved correct, though it took almost another century to show that hippocampal damage is sufficient to cause anterograde amnesia. At this point in the story, we should describe the tragic case of H.M. (or Henry Mollaison as we discovered after his death in 2008). H.M. is often seen as the archetypal amnesic, and it would be remiss to ignore his many important contributions. However, as so much has already been written about H.M., including several books, I will only highlight the most relevant facts.

In 1953, William Scoville surgically removed tissue from parts of the right and left temporal lobe of H.M. in an attempt to treat his epilepsy. At the time, H.M. was 27 years old. While the surgery reduced his seizures, it had permanent, unwanted consequences. In 1955, Scoville invited Brenda Milner to Hartford, Connecticut to study H.M. in more detail. The rest, as they say, is history. The most striking change in H.M. was his profound, permanent anterograde amnesia. After a brief interval he consistently failed to remember whom he had just met, what was just said, and where he had been. This amnesia contrasted with his preserved short-term memory, skill learning, and I.Q., along with his semantic knowledge from before the surgery. These contrasting effects proved immensely important in establishing divisions across memory, including short-term memory versus long-term memory, and explicit memory versus implicit memory.

The causes of temporal lobe amnesia: H.M. is often credited with providing the first convincing evidence that the hippocampus is vital for forming new episodic memories (though Scoville and Milner sensibly avoided making this claim). In reality, H.M. was one of nine patients who received bilateral removals of medial temporal lobe tissue thanks to William Scoville. Almost all of the other patients suffered from schizophrenia. Tragically, the experimental psychosurgery did not lessen their psychosis. But, like H.M., some of these psychotic patients were left with severe memory problems. Importantly, it was not H.M.'s surgery that highlighted the potential significance of the hippocampus, rather it was the comparison made across all nine patients. The severity of their individual memory problems seemed to match the amount of hippocampal tissue Scoville thought he had removed. What made H.M. unique was the fact that he was epileptic and not psychotic. Unlike the other eight patients it was possible to explore his cognitive abilities over the following decades. Furthermore, after Brenda Milner's findings on H.M. were publicised, it became evident that similar surgeries should never be repeated. This ensured H.M.'s unique status.

It is important to appreciate that Scoville removed far more than just the hippocampus from H.M. Consequently, the search was on for amnesic patients with more selective temporal lobe pathology. Hypoxia, the shortage of oxygen to the brain, is a frequent consequence of cardiac arrests. It is also the case that hypoxia can lead to brain damage causing long-term memory loss. Because the hippocampus is very sensitive to oxygen loss, pathology in this structure was presumed to be the cause of the amnesia sometimes seen in survivors of cardiac arrests. Individual analyses helped to establish that while the brain pathology caused by hypoxia is often diffuse, in some patients with anterograde amnesia it appears largely restricted to the hippocampus.

Other conditions can give rise to temporal lobe amnesia. Examples include diseases such as herpes encephalitis, autoimmune limbic encephalitis, and meningitis. In all of these conditions, when anterograde amnesia is present the hippocampus appears to be involved. In addition, the more extensive the temporal lobe damage, the denser the amnesia. At one extreme, sufferers of autoimmune limbic encephalitis can develop an unusually discrete hippocampal pathology, resulting in a relatively mild anterograde amnesia. But as hippocampal formation damage increases, so does the severity of the amnesia.

It is widely agreed that the hippocampus is of especial importance for the initial encoding and consolidation of episodic information, although its contribution to memory retrieval is more controversial (see below, *Retrograde amnesia*). However, additional damage to other temporal lobe sites, such as the cortex in the parahippocampal region, increases the severity of the amnesic syndrome.

Diencephalic amnesia: It is now time to return to diencephalic amnesia. (The diencephalon largely comprises the thalamus and hypothalamus). This amnesic condition can arise after strokes or tumours within the thalamus. However, Korsakoff's disease remains the most studied form of diencephalic amnesia. Although this disease is strongly linked to alcoholism, the brain pathology is largely caused by a deficiency of vitamin B1 (thiamine), reflecting the inadequate diet of many alcoholics. Excessive alcohol makes a bad situation worse as it is both neurotoxic and impedes vitamin (especially thiamine) uptake.

The particular significance of dietary thiamine is highlighted by the deficiency disease, beriberi. This association was sadly seen in allied Japanese prisoners of war, who often suffered from beriberi, provoking Wernicke and Korsakoff symptoms. When given vitamin supplements most people recover from the acute Wernicke stage but, for some, the subsequent amnesic syndrome is permanent. In a successful attempt to reduce the high incidence of alcoholic Korsakoff's disease in Australia, it became mandatory from 1991 to add thiamine to bread flour.

Thiamine deficiency can also happen in childhood, due to repeated vomiting and gastrointestinal disease. Also, around 20% of those diagnosed with Anorexia Nervosa may suffer from severe thiamine deficiency, thereby running the risk of neurological damage and memory loss.

Korsakoff's disease usually involves both anterograde and retrograde memory loss. There may also be a slight reduction of short-term memory, while confabulation and a lack of insight are common. These additional features are thought to reflect the frontal lobe deficits often seen in this condition. For the same reason, the disease can cause difficulties with executive function, difficulties that are greater than those seen in chronic alcoholics who do not have Korsakoff's disease.

A carefully controlled post-mortem study of Korsakoff's disease found that atrophy of the anterior thalamic nuclei, along with the mammillary bodies, was the best predictor of the anterograde amnesia (Harding et al., 2000). These same two structures are joined by the mammillothalamic tract, i.e., the bundle described by Vicq d'Azyr (Figure 17.7). On top of this core pathology, Korsakoff's disease often causes additional damage to other thalamic sites, along with parts of the prefrontal cortex. These additional sites inevitably add to the cognitive deficits seen in this syndrome.

Because Korsakoff's disease can affect a large list of brain sites, attention turned to other causes of diencephalic amnesia to help pinpoint the most critical locations. By comparing amnesic patients with thalamic strokes against patients whose thalamic strokes spared memory, it was possible to isolate the best neurological predictor of amnesia. Repeated studies using this method have concluded that mammillothalamic tract damage

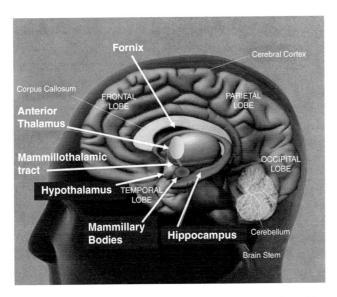

Figure 17.7 Side view of the human brain showing key brain sites implicated in amnesia. The hippocampus and its major tract, the fornix, are in the centre.

is the best predictor of any memory loss. Together with the findings from Korsakoff's disease, it now seems clear that the mammillary bodies, in conjunction with the anterior thalamic nuclei via their interlinking pathway (the mammillothalamic tract), jointly support episodic memory. These findings did, however, leave uncertain whether focal damage confined within these interlinked sites is sufficient to cause anterograde amnesia. Two freak accidents have helped to answer that question.

In 1960, then aged 22, an American airman (N.A.) was stationed in the Azores. During a mock dual, a miniature fencing foil entered his right nostril, crossing to the left nostril, and entering the brain. The foil cut through the left mammillothalamic tract and reached the thalamus, leaving the airman with a loss of new verbal memory of moderate severity (Teuber et al., 1968). Although his memory loss persisted, it was far less severe than that in Korsakoff's disease.

Related evidence comes from the equally unfortunate case of B.J. (Dusoir et al., 1990). During a fight in a bar, B.J.'s assailant picked up the nearest weapon, which was a snooker cue. By accident or design, the assailant thrust the snooker cue up B.J.'s nose so that it rested in the base of his brain. In doing so, both the left and right mammillary bodies were largely destroyed, but little else. Thankfully B.J. recovered but he was left with an anterograde amnesia that affected the recall of new episodic information but largely spared recognition memory. Over time, the severity of his amnesia subsided.

Further evidence comes from patients with tumours that affect the mammillary bodies. Comparisons show that mammillary body volume consistently predicts memory performance, the smaller the mammillary bodies, the greater the difficulty with episodic memory recall (Tsivilis et al., 2008). Both cases N.A. and B.J., along with these tumour patients, help to show that damage to the mammillary bodies and the mammillothalamic tract is sufficient to cause anterograde amnesia but the resulting memory loss may be mild, and it often affects memory recall far more than recognition memory. The mildness of the memory disorders shows that additional thalamic damage is likely to exacerbate the amnesic syndrome. To understand why, it is necessary to consider the relationship between different amnesic syndromes.

Unifying temporal lobe and diencephalic amnesias: An obvious question is whether temporal lobe amnesia and diencephalic amnesia are part of the same, larger syndrome. Reasons to believe so include how the core cognitive deficits in temporal lobe amnesia are strikingly similar to those in diencephalic amnesia. Furthermore, the most critical site for temporal lobe amnesia (the hippocampus) is directly connected to two key sites for diencephalic amnesia (the mammillary bodies and the anterior thalamic nuclei). This connection is via a pathway called the fornix (Figure 17.8). The implication is that the two major anterograde amnesias arise from disrupting the same common system.

The French neurologists Jean Delay and Serge Brion are often credited with first proposing an integrated memory circuit from the hippocampus via the fornix to the mammillary bodies and then onto the anterior thalamus, thereby incorporating the tracts described by Bernhard von Gudden and Vicq d'Azyr (Figure 17.7). (Delay and Brion borrowed this circuit from James Papez, who had previously argued that it was necessary for emotions.) Subsequently, this memory circuit was extended to include the return projections from the anterior thalamus to the hippocampus, some of which relay in an area called the retrosplenial cortex (Figures 17.5 and 17.8). This cortical area is of considerable interest as bilateral retrosplenial damage can also cause anterograde amnesia. Sadly, Jean Delay's career was much affected when, in May 1968, a group of about five hundred students attacked his Paris offices to ultimately force his removal. The rioting students

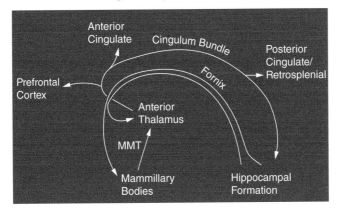

Figure 17.8 Circuitry interlinking brain sites responsible for temporal lobe and diencephalic amnesia. (MMT, mammillothalamic tract).

professed an abhorrence of his use of pharmacological treatments, reflecting their antipsychiatric beliefs.

A critical test of Delay & Brion's 1969 theory, which directly linked temporal lobe amnesia with diencephalic amnesia, is to determine whether fornix damage causes amnesia. The fornix is the pathway that joins the hippocampus to those diencephalic sites that also cause amnesia. Their model predicts that fornix damage would cause amnesia.

From the study of tumours that impinge on the fornix, it became clear that severance of the fornix does indeed cause anterograde amnesia. Further support for a unified memory system came from analysing a large number of amnesic patients with a seemingly diverse array of brain pathologies (Ferguson et al., 2019). It was found that the various sites of amnesia-related pathology were consistently linked anatomically to a common brain area – the area running from the back of the hippocampus to the retrosplenial cortex. Together, these findings signify a core network that interlinks multiple brain sites which support episodic memory. Key elements of this network are the hippocampus, the fornix, the mammillary bodies, the mammillothalamic tract, the anterior thalamic nuclei, and the retrosplenial cortex. Other important contributors include the prefrontal cortex, the parahippocampal region, and parts of the lateral parietal cortex.

Space, episodic memory, and amnesia: Research with rodents has shown that the same core network of brain sites is vital for spatial navigation and spatial learning. In 2014, John O'Keefe received the Nobel Prize for his discovery of nerve cells in the rat hippocampus that signal location, so called 'place cells'. These place cells, along with other spatial signalling cells, have since been found all around the temporal – diencephalic memory network. Linking these rodent spatial signals to human memory became conceptually easier with the discovery that rodents can reactivate sequences of hippocampal place cells that correspond to past routes. This hippocampal 'replay' is thought to help maintain hippocampal memories and aid decision making. The belief is that brain sites for spatial memory and navigation have been appropriated for episodic memory in the human brain.

Building on the brain's spatial systems makes intuitive sense given the importance of context (place and time) within episodic memory. Just try and recall what you had for breakfast. The relevance of identifying the place and time in your mind underlines their significance. It is thought that the hippocampus combines item information with simultaneous context (place and time) information. A close variant on this idea is to swap the term 'place' for 'scene', to help emphasise the importance of the hippocampus and its extended network for the construction of both new memories and the retrieval of past episodic memories, both of which deploy scene-building. If this viewpoint is correct, then pathologies causing anterograde amnesia should often overlap with those causing retrograde amnesia.

Retrograde amnesia

Falling off a horse is never a good thing, I should know. But for a 26-year-old nanny (L.T.) described by Narinder Kapur it proved disastrous. The resulting head injury caused a severe retrograde amnesia. When tested 18 months after the accident, she had no memories of her time together with her fiancé of almost nine years, nor could she recall holidays or funerals attended before the accident. She had only sketchy information about houses lived in and schools attended. Almost all past episodic memory was lost, though some factual autobiographical information remained. She also retained implicit memory skills such as playing the piano and driving a car but could not remember her driving test. Fortunately, her ability to remember new events was good, helping her to rebuild some of her lost life.

The severity and duration of retrograde amnesia varies enormously from case to case. The loss of past memories can extend back for decades, or it may just cover the last few minutes. While past episodic memories are the most vulnerable, there can be an additional loss of personal information. Consequently, autobiographic details are often more affected than shared semantic (factual) memory. Personal identity is not, however, lost.

As seen in the nanny L.T., aspects of memory survive. People with retrograde amnesia do not normally need to re-learn how to speak, walk, write, drive a car, or use a knife and fork. Such sparing is found even in extreme cases such as Clive Wearing. Likewise, short-term memory typically remains intact. The persistence of the amnesia varies enormously from person to person. In some cases, it is permanent, in others it resolves. All of this variability reflects how there are different causes of retrograde amnesia, with different patterns of pathology and varying consequences.

Measuring retrograde amnesia: Why did Eyjafjallajökull became world famous in 2010? Studying retrograde amnesia is not easy. With anterograde amnesia you can administer new learning tasks and measure precisely which new learning abilities are lost and which remain. To appreciate someone's retrograde memory loss you need to test for events that occurred before the onset of the amnesia. This presupposes that the tester knows what the person had or had not previously learnt. If you don't remember Eyjafjallajökull it may mean that you never knew or that you once knew but have subsequently forgotten.

Testing for retrograde amnesia often involves giving structured autobiographical interviews about past significant events such as birthdays, school events, holidays, and weddings. Other approaches include asking about famous public events, recognising past movie titles, or naming photographs of famous people from the past. A macabre method is the Dead or Alive test. Here the subject decides the fate of famous individuals, e.g., is Olivia Newton-John dead or alive; is Barbara Streisland dead or alive? For obvious reasons, the task needs constant updating.

When assessing retrograde amnesia by looking at past news items it is important to avoid using people or events that have remained in the public gaze, as that information could have been re-learnt after the brain insult. One obvious example would be the tragic death of Princess Diana in 1997. A related problem applies when trying to date precisely how far back the retrograde amnesia extends. For this you need date-stamped information that only had a short shelf-life. One ingenious approach was to test people for their memory of past TV shows that only lasted a single season. Other tests deliberately incorporate people or events that were extremely well-known at the time but have since become less famous. Examples might include Hale-Bopp (1996), Costa Concordia (2012), Ever Given (2021), and why we all argued over a two-tone dress (2015). (By the way, Eyjafjallajökull is an Icelandic volcano that caused the cancellation of 100,000 flights in April 2010.)

Concussion and retrograde amnesia: Head trauma (concussion) is probably the most frequent cause of brief retrograde amnesias (Figure 17.9). Indeed, some definitions of concussion require a period of memory loss. Other acute symptoms of concussion include feeling dazed, poor concentration, and blurred vision. A loss of consciousness may also happen. Following a concussion there is typically a brief, near-complete retrograde amnesia for those events just preceding the accident, which may be accompanied by a more diffuse disturbance of memory for earlier events. Contact sport is, unsurprisingly, a frequent cause of concussion.

Concerns about concussions have been heighted by advances in brain imaging. Diffusion MRI reveals how concussions not only bruise the brain but also cause previously unsuspected levels of white matter damage. Worryingly, studies of concussion in American Football players show that white matters changes can persist for months, long after the concussion has apparently resolved. Such findings amplify concerns over repeat concussions and the protocols that allow concussed players to return to games. At present (2024), there is no minimum time set by the NFL (American Football), although the median is reported to be nine days. For English Rugby Union, a 14-day period of relative rest is required, if symptom free, followed by a gradual return to play. I anticipate stricter protocols in future.

American Football has also helped us to understand what happens at the time of a concussion. In 1973, Steve Lynch and Phillip Yarnell patiently waited at the sidelines until a player was 'dinged'. The researchers would then rush to the groggy player and, as soon as possible, try to assess his memory. Surprisingly, when asked immediately after the hit, the players could often recall the events just before the collision, such as the last play. But within a few minutes, substantial forgetting occurred, and the memory was lost, suggesting

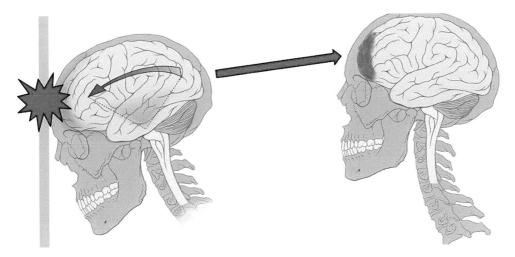

Figure 17.9 Head trauma and concussion. On impact the brain continues moving, striking the skull, resulting in bruising and damage to nerve tracts.

a failure of consolidation. Building on their findings, Lynch and Yarnell concluded that when assessing mild concussions on the field, tests of immediate memory, including digit recall, simple arithmetic, and reverse spelling are likely to be insensitive. World Rugby now recommends asking questions such as Where are you playing? Which half is it now? Who scored last in this game? What team did you play in the previous match? Relevant information that should have been consolidated.

Concussions do not just happen in sport. Two young Italian men received mild head traumas as a result of separate car crashes. Neither lost consciousness but both suffered retrograde amnesias that resolved over the following months (Stracciari et al., 1994). In both cases they displayed a selective loss of autobiographical memories, including forgetting their girlfriends from the past few months. One girlfriend only evoked a vague sense of familiarity even though her name had been recently tattooed on his arm. Both men recognised their homes but initially had difficulty in remembering where things were normally placed. They also both forgot their recent vacations. In contrast, skills, such as cycling and driving, seemed unaffected. In both men, the loss of past information was not confined to episodic memory as it also extended to autobiographical factual memory. Furthermore, in both cases, more recent memories were the most vulnerable. Over time, both men also showed a gradual recovery of memory, although some memories never returned.

The recovery of memory after head trauma often follows a similar sequence. There is initially a variable period of confusion, after which old memories start to return. More recent memories are often particularly stubborn, with some close to the time of the accident never returning. This gradual return of previously inaccessible memories can take place over a period of many months. As many memories were not completely lost, this recovery presumably reflects a gradual reinstatement of the relevant retrieval mechanisms.

In patients coming out of a coma the most common sequence of memory recovery begins with personal knowledge about who they are, followed by where they are, and finally when it is. This sequence of person, place, and then time is seen whether the closed head injury is mild or severe. An intriguing feature is that when patients are first asked to give the current date they typically gave one that is pushed back in time, in some cases by many years. This temporal disorientation then diminishes over the following days and weeks.

Retrograde amnesia after permanent brain injury: There is appreciable overlap between those brain sites that cause retrograde amnesia when damaged and those that cause anterograde amnesia, though the list is not identical. For example, tissue loss in either the medial temporal lobe or in the medial thalamus (diencephalon) can result in retrograde amnesia. Consequently, both anterograde and retrograde amnesias often co-occur in these cases. However, extensive frontal lobe pathology can also cause retrograde amnesia while largely sparing new learning.

A feature of retrograde amnesia is that the more extensive the frontal, temporal, or diencephalic pathology, the greater the loss of past memories. For example, patients with tissue loss largely restricted to the hippocampus have a less severe retrograde amnesia than those individuals where the pathology extends to include temporal lobe cortex. As seen in Clive Wearing, for some unfortunate individuals the memory loss can be extremely severe. This occurs when there is combined damage across multiple brain areas.

In October 1981, at the age of 30, K.C. crashed his motorbike, causing substantial head injuries leading to a dense, permanent retrograde amnesia accompanied by anterograde amnesia. K.C. suffered bilateral brain damage that included the hippocampus, an array of related diencephalic sites, along with parts of his left cortex (Rosenbaum et al., 2005). Decades later, K.C. still showed the same absence of both new and old episodic memories, so that personal experiences only exist in the present, disappearing as soon as his thoughts are distracted. His memories for episodic events from before his accident are essentially non-existent. Even when prompted, K.C. could not recall important incidents from his life such as the circumstances surrounding the drowning of his brother, crashing a dune buggy he had built, or the derailment near his house of a train carrying lethal chemicals that required thousands of people in the area to evacuate their homes.

Despite being unable to remember any personal episodes, K.C. could provide factual information such as the names of schools attended, names of classmates from photographs, details of the motorbikes he owned, and how to change a flat tyre. He remembered how to play chess but could not recall any individual games. Remarkably, his store of semantic facts from the first 30 years of his life seemed similar to that of many of his age mates, despite losing all personal episodes. In this way K.C shows a striking contrast between lost episodic memory and spared factual knowledge. In doing so, K.C. helped to highlight how episodic memory is a distinct entity within long-term memory.

The amnesic Korsakoff's syndrome often causes a dense retrograde amnesia. Given the association of Korsakoff 's disease with alcoholism it is tempting to suppose that the failure to recall past memories is due to excessive alcohol consumption throughout that period. In other words, the apparent retrograde amnesia is in reality a prolonged period of failed new learning that finally reaches a crisis point, so that much of the past doesn't exist.

At least in one case we know that this explanation is incorrect. The eminent academic P.Z. published his autobiography. Later P.Z. was diagnosed with alcoholic Korsakoff's disease and showed a severe retrograde amnesia for the same personal events that he had recorded in his autobiography. Clearly those events had been learnt, only to be later lost with the arrival of his amnesia. This means that his retrograde amnesia was a genuine failure to retrieve memories that had once been acquired. By assessing past memories recorded in his book, it became clear that his oldest memories were the most likely to have survived while his more recent memories were the most likely to be lost, an example of Ribot's law.

Ribot's law: Any discussion of retrograde amnesia must include Ribot's Law (1881). Théodule Ribot observed that in many cases of retrograde amnesia, older memories were more likely to be preserved than more recent ones (Figure 17.10). Put simply, last in, first out. This was the pattern seen in the academic P.Z. who suffered a near-complete loss of memory for events from the most recent decade but, thereafter, a slowly improving pattern of memory preservation for events going back in time over four decades. A similar greater resilience for older memories has been repeatedly found in other cases with Korsakoff's disease and following various disorders afflicting the temporal lobes. This same profile can also be seen in Alzheimer's disease, in which, the more recent past is the most vulnerable.

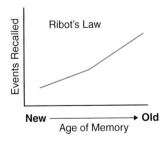

Figure 17.10 Older memories can be more resilient than newer memories following brain injury.

Explaining Ribot's law is integral to the much bigger challenge of identifying where and how memories are stored in the brain – one of the holy grails of neuroscience. Any viable model of episodic memory storage and retrieval needs to explain why older memories can show greater resilience. I will compare two leading models of memory storage and retrieval, which provide very different explanations for Ribot's law. Both models remain highly influential as it has proved difficult to dismiss either.

Consolidation and retrieval – the Consolidation Model: Probably the best-known explanation of Ribot's law is the 'Consolidation Model'. This model supposes that memories are initially created in the hippocampus, but over days, months, and years they are transferred and consolidated in the cortex, creating a more durable representation that slowly becomes independent of the hippocampus (Squire et al., 2001). As this transfer to the cortex only happens gradually, full memory resilience takes time. Only once the memory is fully incorporated across the cortex does it become independent of the hippocampus and maximally resilient to insult.

Initial support for this model came from descriptions of what happens to old memories after hippocampal damage. The Consolidation Model predicts that, in this circumstance, remote memories will be preserved (as they are now cortical) while more recent memories remain increasingly vulnerable (as they still partially rely on the hippocampus). A further prediction is that with additional cortical damage the retrograde amnesia will go back further and further in time.

The famous hippocampal amnesic H.M. was thought to provide especially strong support for the Consolidation Model. Descriptions of H.M. initially concluded that his memory for childhood events before his surgery was largely preserved. He was, for example, able to recognise faces of people in the news from before his surgery. Initial assessments estimated that his retrograde amnesia only stretched back three years before his surgery. The implication was that his older memories had become independent of the hippocampus after three years, and so survived the removal of that structure.

However, later assessments increased the extent of H.M.'s remote memory loss to eleven years, leaving him with spared autobiographical memories up to the age of 16. The picture became increasingly confused when H.M. was re-assessed in his 70s. His childhood memories were seen as lacking specific episodes that had unique time and place attributes. The implication is that the loss of hippocampal tissue had affected all past episodic memories. There does, however, remain the concern that H.M.'s age at the time of testing may have played a part. Furthermore, Scoville removed far more than just the hippocampus from H.M. Either way, the evidence from H.M. is not as definitive as once believed.

Stronger evidence for the Consolidation Model comes from those amnesics with more hippocampal-centred pathology who show a temporally graded retrograde amnesia for more recent memories, alongside preserved older memories. For example, when adults with hippocampal damage were given an Autobiographical Interview they showed a restricted retrograde amnesia going back a year. In those cases with additional medial temporal cortical damage, the amnesia reached back another ten years as cortical contributions to the storage of past memory were assumed to became increasingly significant (Kirwan et al., 2008). However, in some instances a 'flat' retrograde amnesia is seen. This term refers to how the degree of memory loss does not diminish going back in time (so does not resemble Ribot's curve). Proponents of the Consolidation Model argue that this flat gradient reflects increasing cortical loss beyond the medial temporal lobe.

Some amnesic cases, however, do not match the predictions of the Consolidation Model. For example, patients with more discrete hippocampal pathology can show a flat profile of autobiographical memory loss that stretches back to childhood. As a consequence, there is no temporal gradient (Yonelinas et al., 2019). This flat profile is inconsistent with the Consolidation Model, which predicts that older memories will be increasingly preserved as they become independent from the hippocampus. A further problem with the Consolidation Model is that it struggles to explain why it might variably take months, years, or even decades for a memory representation to finally become independent of the hippocampus. Why, for example, should it take many years for memories to clear the hippocampus in one amnesic, but only one year in another, similar case? (Kirwan et al., 2008).

Consolidation and retrieval – the Multiple Trace Theory: These limitations take us to the second model of memory consolidation, the 'Multiple Trace Theory'. This model again attempts to explain Ribot's law. Like the Consolidation Model, there is a critical interplay between the hippocampus and cortex for memory storage and retrieval, but there the similarities end.

The core difference between the models is that in the Multiple Trace Theory the hippocampus *always* remains vital for past episodic memories. In other words, past recollections rely on the hippocampus, no matter how old (Moscovitch et al., 2016). This reliance means that when re-visiting a past memory the hippocampus is activated to ensure that the episode contains the appropriate contextual features, but this same activation may cause the hippocampus to create a duplicate trace.

This duplication process has already been described within the phenomenon of 're-consolidation'. The assumption is that when an episodic memory is retrieved it may enter a fragile, malleable state. Consequently, following retrieval, the memory may be subtly altered and then consolidated again, in other words, 're-consolidated' (Figure 4.5). In the Multiple Trace Theory, this re-consolidation process standardly occurs, yet the original memory still persists. Consequently, repeated retrieval leads to the creation of increasing numbers of hippocampal – cortical traces for the same event ('multiple traces'). Having more versions of the same memory creates greater resilience. At the same time, the model argues that the cortical component of the memory trace is sufficient to provide gist-like memories in the absence of the hippocampus. Such memories would including semantic autobiographical facts, such as the name of the school attended. In contrast, the hippocampus remains necessary for past episodic memories that contain rich contextual information, such as detailing individual events within that school.

Perhaps the clearest prediction from the Multiple Trace Theory is that complete loss of the hippocampus will leave a flat profile of retrograde amnesia for past episodic memories, meaning that there will be no temporal gradient. This prediction follows because the hippocampus is thought to remain vital for the activation and retrieval of all episodic memories, irrespective of their age. Instead, only gist or semantic-like memories will persist in the absence of a hippocampus as such memories remain available in the cortex.

Just this pattern was seen in patient K.C. who, as you may recall, suffered bilateral hippocampal damage following a motorcycle accident. His loss of personal episodic memories was essentially complete, stretching back through his entire life, in other words he suffered a 'flat' retrograde amnesia. He did, however, retain some factual knowledge about his life, consistent with the idea that cortical representations are sufficient for this level of semantic autobiographic information.

An analysis of multiple patients concluded that, for personal events, most cases with selective hippocampal pathology show a flat temporal profile of retrograde amnesia (Yonelinas et al., 2019). As explained, this pattern is inconsistent with the Consolidation Model. Further support for the Multiple Trace model comes from how fMRI studies frequently show hippocampal activation at episodic memory retrieval, irrespective of whether the memory is recent or remote. Both sets of evidence point to hippocampal involvement persisting throughout the life-history of an episodic memory, and not being lost once the cortex takes responsibility. While adjudicating between these two models remains tricky, the tide of recent evidence favours the Multiple Trace Theory.

Storage and retrieval: This debate between these two consolidation models takes us to the long-standing issue of whether chronic retrograde amnesias reflect a storage failure or a retrieval failure. The Consolidation Model presumes that hippocampal damage results in a greater loss of recent memories as their storage still depends on the hippocampus. Consequently, as its name suggests, the Consolidation Model emphasises the importance of storage loss in retrograde amnesia. The Multiple Trace Theory differs as it highlights the significance of memory reactivation via the hippocampus, so incorporating retrieval mechanisms along with storage. The likelihood is that retrograde amnesias can arise from a loss of retrieval mechanisms, a loss of storage, or a combination of the two. These multiple causes help to make sense of the variety of pathologies associated with retrograde amnesia.

The idea that retrograde amnesia is predominantly a failure of retrieval helps to explain those cases suffering prefrontal cortex damage. In these patients, performance on executive tasks that depend on the prefrontal cortex can predict the ability to recall remote memories. Furthermore, brain activity studies reveal that when initiating episodic memory recall, the brain enters a 'retrieval mode' state that is partly generated within prefrontal cortex. This retrieval state predicts better subsequent recall. These findings reinforce the belief that prefrontal cortex helps to guide retrieval searches by acting back upon the temporal lobe, including the hippocampus. This interpretation fits with how the similarities between frontal lobe retrograde amnesias and temporal lobe retrograde amnesias outweigh any dissimilarities.

The surprising case of developmental amnesia

Until 1997 no one had thought to find out what happens to children who suffer the same brain pathology as that causing anterograde amnesia in adults. Is the amnesic syndrome the same in children? What happens as these children grow up? A group led by Faraneh Vargha-Khadem in London asked these very questions. What they discovered surprised everyone.

Sadly, some babies and some children suffer a brief period of oxygen loss (hypoxia). Any resulting brain damage often includes the hippocampus. Following from studies of adult anterograde amnesia caused by hypoxia, the expectation was that these children would show very obvious problems with memory, in particular, with episodic memory.

Another safe prediction was that these children would struggle badly at school where new learning is at a premium. A lot of childhood learning is factual, requiring semantic memory. But to acquire factual knowledge, it is usually assumed that we amass and integrate similar episodic experiences that share core facts. Those constant components may then create semantic memories, which typically lack context. For example, I know that the quagga is an extinct form of zebra. That knowledge was acquired over a series of individual episodes, leaving a core of factual quagga information that is context-free. Consequently, episodic memory should be a vital stepping stone to making semantic memories.

The first description of 'developmental amnesia' in 1997 focussed on three individuals (Elward & Vargha-Khadem, 2018). The three had suffered bilateral hippocampal damage at birth, or at the ages of four or nine. When initially tested, they were all teenagers. As might be expected, all three suffered a pronounced anterograde amnesia for the day-to-day episodes in their life. As a result, they could not navigate familiar surroundings, remember where belongings were placed, anticipate appointments, or describe the events of each day.

The utterly astonishing discovery was that all three teenagers attended mainstream schools and acquired levels of speech, language, literacy, and factual knowledge within the average to low range. Almost all of their factual learning occurred after the onset of the brain pathology that severely impaired their episodic memory. While their parents felt that none of the children could be left alone because of their memory problems, they each successfully progressed through school.

The first such patient to be thoroughly tested in 1997 was 'Jon'. He suffered hypoxia in the first few weeks of life. Astonishingly, Jon was able to describe historic events such as the assassination of the Archduke Ferdinand, which precipitated the World War I. He was also aware of current affairs, such as the handover of Hong Kong to China, though he was unaware of how he knew this information. Formal testing showed that Jon's verbal I.Q. was an impressive 114, which is above the average I.Q. of 100. At the same time, Jon struggled to recall new experiences. For example, when visiting London, he failed to recall that he had just walked up 171 steps when the lift in the underground station had failed. Instead, he said that he had taken the lift, as would be normal.

The severity of the anterograde amnesia in this syndrome is highlighted by a survey of developmental amnesic cases (Elward & Vargha-Khadem, 2018). The 18 cases displayed a 30-point drop between their I.Q. (mean 95, 'normal range') and their Memory Quotient (MQ, mean 61, 'exceptionally low range'). Performance on I.Q. tests draws heavily on semantic knowledge, which was largely spared. Yet, these same developmental amnesics all showed severe losses of episodic memory.

Case K.A. presents another fascinating example of developmental amnesia (Jonin et al., 2018). He suffered hypoxia at birth, but at age three had acquired normal language and motor abilities. As a child he showed clear difficulties in remembering instructions and struggled at school. As an adult, K.A. had a 44-point difference between his preserved I.Q. and devastated Memory Quotient. Because of his memory problems he cannot live independently. Yet, astonishingly, he has an impressive store of general knowledge. Indeed, for some factual tasks, such as identifying famous faces, he can outperform normal subjects.

An early observation on Jon was that, unlike recall, his performance on tests of recognition memory was relatively spared. This pattern has since been replicated in larger groups of developmental amnesics, revealing how their recognition memory is supported by preserved feelings of familiarity. Like Jon, the developmental amnesic K.A., also showed relatively spared recognition memory. While K.A. could readily recognise familiar stimuli, he was poor at remembering their location, again indicating a reliance on feelings of familiarity to solve recognition problems.

How do developmental amnesics acquire new factual information? Immediately following the first description of this condition, the uppermost question was how is it possible to effectively establish semantic memories when episodic memory is lacking? Most adult-onset amnesics, such as H.M. struggle to acquire new semantic knowledge, such as words or phrases that entered the vocabulary after the onset of their learning difficulties. Modern-day examples of such words might include terms like 'gaslighting', 'cryptocurrency', and 'oat milk'. Although some studies have described limited new semantic learning in adults with anterograde amnesia, this is never close to the impressive scale seen in developmental amnesia. While adult-onset cases of hypoxic amnesia show difficulties with recalling or recognising those famous news events that occurred after the start of their amnesia, developmental amnesics can be good at these same tasks.

One potential explanation for the spared learning in developmental amnesia is that the hippocampal pathology in this syndrome is unusually restricted. The spared hippocampal tissue might then be sufficient for some learning to proceed. This explanation, however, seems most unlikely. The extent of hippocampal shrinkage in cases of developmental amnesia is comparable to that seen in adult-onset hypoxic amnesics. Furthermore, a large survey revealed that the typical pathology in developmental amnesia extends beyond the hippocampus to involve diencephalic structures including the mammillary bodies and parts of the thalamus, those same areas most implicated in diencephalic amnesia. A lack of pathology does not seem to be the explanation.

These findings bring us back to the question of how these children acquire so much semantic knowledge. One key component to the success of developmental amnesics in acquiring semantic knowledge seems to be repetition. Another is the use of cues to help discriminate the correct response from incorrect alternatives (Elward & Vargha-Khadem, 2018). Even so, these strategies do not fully explain the impressive semantic learning that is seen in developmental amnesia but not in adult-onset amnesia. The assumption is that the immature brain has more flexibility in how it acquires some classes of information. The sparing of familiarity information may also add to these capabilities.

Another surprising feature of developmental amnesia is the extended period of early years associated with this syndrome. Hippocampal pathology that occurs between the time of birth all the way to the onset of puberty, is associated with a loss of episodic memory that contrasts with the effective acquisition of semantic knowledge. In other words, the developmental amnesic syndrome is not restricted to those who experience hippocampal pathology just around the time of birth. It is thought that across childhood there is an enhanced ability to flexibly use temporal lobe structures, making it possible to acquire semantic knowledge, despite hippocampal pathology. This explanation accords with the realisation that the temporal lobes take many years to mature fully. For example, recent measurements indicate that the medial temporal lobes, which include the hippocampus, take about a decade to reach their peak volume.

Transient global amnesia

For Trip Gabriel, a 61-year-old political journalist, the 27th June 2015 was "*the day that went missing*". Trip Gabriel was a keen sailor. On that day in 2015 he was racing his boat off Long Island Sound in miserable weather. The amnesic episode, probably triggered by cold water, left him alert and able to control and manoeuvre his boat, yet he could not recall completing two races or sharing a beer afterwards (Gabriel, 2017). He found that could not locate his car and did not know where he was or where he lived. His inability to get home led to his wife calling and realising something was very wrong. She helped him drive home and then took him to the hospital. His MRI brain scan appeared normal. About nine hours after the start of the episode he began to interact more normally. His first memory of the episode was of being inside the MRI machine. His amnesic state finally resolved about 23 hours after its onset.

Transient Global Amnesia is a rare clinical condition in which there is a rapid onset of a severe anterograde amnesia. Although there need not be a loss of personal identify, these individuals can appear disoriented and will often repeatedly ask the same questions, such as 'Why am I here?' 'What time is it?' or 'How did I get here?' Unfortunately, the answers are almost immediately forgotten because of the dense anterograde amnesia.

In reality, the term 'global' is misleading as procedural skills, such as a driving a car, are retained. Fortunately, as the name suggests, Transient Global Amnesia is typically brief, lasting a few hours and usually no more than 24 h. Recovery thereafter is normally complete, although the events during the episode are lost. In a small minority of cases, a further episode of Transient Global Amnesia can occur.

Transient Global Amnesia is more often seen in those over 50, with about 75% of episodes being in people aged between 50 and 70. The condition is often preceded by a precipitating event such as emotional distress, cold water immersion, strenuous physical exercise, sexual intercourse, or pain. There is also a weak association with suffering from migraine. During the episode the person may seem restless or confused but remains alert and retains speech, along with preserved motor and sensory functions. In addition to the anterograde amnesia, there is often a degree of retrograde amnesia. One patient during a transient global amnesic episode discovered she did not know the date or the year, where she was, or how long she had been there. Family events were vaguely remembered, though she recognised her husband's voice on the phone. This form of amnesia is not caused by head trauma, epilepsy, or localised stroke. Instead, brain imaging studies point to transient disruptions of hippocampal blood flow. Thankfully, this rare condition lives up to its name in that it is truly transient and does not leave persistent memory problems.

Psychogenic amnesia

The term psychogenic amnesia describes the loss of personal memories when there is no clear evidence of brain damage. The loss of past autobiographical memories can be confined to a particular event or may extend over long periods, even years. There may also be variable periods of anterograde amnesia affecting the learning of new personal events after the onset of the amnesia. Consistent with other amnesias, short-term memory and implicit memory are only rarely affected.

Instances of psychogenic amnesia (sometimes known as dissociative amnesia) are often thought to be provoked by extreme adversity. Precipitating events include severe stress such as marital break-up, bereavement, financial crises, war-related traumas, depression, and suicidal thoughts. Nevertheless, as extreme stress is not guaranteed to cause psychogenic amnesia, other individual factors must play an important role.

Extreme trauma and amnesia: It is hard to conceive of more extreme adversity than enduring a World War II concentration camp. Willem Wagenaar and Jop Groeneweg compared the testimonies of survivors from Camp Erika taken between 1943–1947 and again, 40-years later, between 1984–1987. The question was whether the intense, painful emotions would increase memory preservation or whether they would create periods of apparent amnesia.

In general, many concentration camp experiences were well-retained, suggesting that the heightened emotions had boosted memory. At the same time, details of traumatic incidents were sometimes forgotten. These forgotten experiences included being maltreated, the names and appearance of their torturers, and being a witness to murder. This mixed picture highlights how intense emotions can have opposing actions on memory retention, strengthening some and weakening others. Nevertheless, in spite of their terrible sufferings, the survivors did not have amnesias for lengthy periods of their ordeal.

A separate study interviewed 20 Auschwitz survivors (Kuch & Cox, 1992). Despite living for over a month in an extermination camp with the constant threat of death, surrounded by extreme atrocities, only two (10%) displayed psychogenic amnesia. Meanwhile, over 80% of the same 20 survivors endured intrusive recollections and recurrent nightmares. Even lower rates of psychogenic amnesia (~4%) were seen in those concentration camp survivors who were less directly exposed to the same atrocities.

Interviews of Dutch survivors of Japanese/Indonesian concentration camps revealed a similar pattern (Merckelbach et al., 2003). Psychogenic amnesia was evident in only one of the 29 survivors, while flashbacks and nightmares were common. Many of the survivors felt that their most adverse war memories were more permanent than their neutral childhood memories.

Together, these three studies of concentration camp victims show that even the most horrific circumstances need not guarantee a psychogenic amnesia, indeed the frequency was relatively low. In other words, while severe mental stress is associated with psychogenic amnesia, it is often not sufficient to induce the state.

Fugue states: Psychogenic amnesias come in different forms. Helpfully, they have been categorised into four types (Harrison et al., 2017). Probably the most famous type of psychogenic amnesia is the 'fugue'.

On the 3rd December 1926, a world famous writer discovered that her husband was having an affair and wanted a divorce. In a distressed state, she drove off, almost resulting in a serious crash. She then disappeared, feared dead. Despite many thousands of people searching, the lady was not found for 11 days. She was finally identified hundreds of miles away in a Harrogate hotel where she had registered under a different surname (taking the surname of her husband's lover). The lost celebrity was Agatha Christie (Figure 17.11). While we will never know what really happened during those 11 days, the precipitating events, and the lack of any description for that period are consistent with a fugue state. (Appropriately, the French word 'fugue' means to run away.) In the case of Agathe Christie, most contemporary newspapers believed that her disappearance was planned, but many features of those 11 days are consistent with a genuine fugue.

As seen in the case of Agatha Christie, during a fugue state there is a sudden loss of personal identity. The fugue, which is often associated with a period of wandering, can last from a few hours up to several days. During the fugue state there is a severe and uniform loss of memories for personal autobiographical facts and events dating back across one's lifetime. After recovery, there is typically a dense amnesia covering the period of the fugue. A psychogenic fugue may sound very similar to a Transient Global Amnesia but differs because, in a fugue, repetitive questioning is rare but personal identity is usually forgotten, while in Transient Global Amnesia the opposite pattern is characteristic.

Because of their sudden onset and the lack of obvious brain injury, there is a natural concern over whether fugue states are genuine or whether they are fabricated. As far as could be ascertained a genuine fugue was diagnosed in a young man, P.N. The last thing P.N. recalled was walking at night in downtown Toronto in a state of shock and depression after his grandfather's funeral (Schacter et al., 1982). During the fugue he could not remember his name, address, or almost any other information about himself though, on questioning, he could give the names of local baseball and hockey teams. His ability to identify famous faces also indicated some preserved semantic knowledge. The next evening his amnesia began to clear so that he could recall his grandfather's death and the recent funeral. Over the next few days his amnesia continued to clear so that aspects of his personal past that had been inaccessible now returned, but he remained unable remember what happened immediately after his night-time walk in Toronto.

MRS. CHRISTIE FOUND AT· HARROGATE

Dramatic Re-union With Husband in Famous Hydro.

"HER MEMORY GONE"

How Missing Novelist· Spent Time While Police and Public Looked for Her

Mrs. Christie, the missing inventor of detective stories, was traced last night to the Hydro, Harrogate, by her husband, Colonel Christie.

In an interview after a dramatic meeting between the pair, Colonel Christie told the DAILY HERALD that his wife had suffered from the " most complete loss of memory." She did not even recognise him, he added.

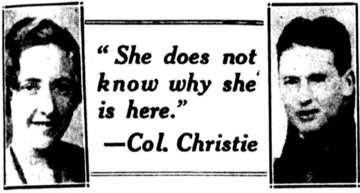

" *She does not know why she is here.*"

—*Col. Christie*

Mrs. Christie   **Col. Christie**

Figure 17.11 Contemporary newspaper report of Agatha Christie's disappearance and later discovery.

Other psychogenic amnesias: Other types of psychogenic amnesias have been given the following rather awkward labels: fugue-to-focal retrograde amnesia, psychogenic focal retrograde amnesia following a minor neurological episode, and patients with gaps in their memories (Harrison et al., 2017). As we have just seen with P.N., the pure fugue state shows an abrupt absence of autobiographical memory, including a loss of personal identity, often accompanied by a period of wandering. The term 'fugue-to-focal retrograde amnesia' is given when, in addition to the acute fugue episode, there remains after recovery, a period of dense retrograde amnesia for events predating the fugue episode.

In the third category, 'psychogenic focal retrograde amnesia following a minor neurological episode', there are holes in part of the person's past. In other words, there are islands of preserved past memories alongside apparently lost periods. This condition is often associated with a minor neurological event, but one unlikely on its own to cause the amnesic state. Unlike fugues, the incomplete retrograde amnesia can persist for many weeks or even years. However, having relatively intact new learning means that the person can re-learn who they are and their history.

The fourth and final category, 'gaps in their memory' refers to people who suffer discrete periods of memory loss, associated with enhanced stress, as in PTSD. The periods of memory loss range from hours to several weeks. Unlike a fugue state, there is not a loss of all earlier memories, so wandering and loss of identity are rare.

While these attempts to classify psychogenic amnesia offer a valuable framework, individual cases can defy simple classification. One such example is A.T. During a period of severe marital stress and probable depression, A.T. suffered a psychogenic amnesia during March 1990. After delivering her children at school on the 6th March she recalled nothing until finding herself seven days later in a London Underground station and seeking help from the police. Over the following year A.T. complained of a loss of new autobiographical memories. Careful analyses revealed that while the seven-day period constituted a real psychogenic fugue, the subsequent anterograde amnesic period was, in part, simulated. This mixture of genuine amnesia and part fabrication underlines the complexity of these conditions.

What causes psychogenic amnesia? Various explanations have been offered for the loss of memory in psychogenic amnesias. In one leading model, emotional traumas promote the release of stress-related hormones (glucocorticoids) creating what has been called an 'amnestic block syndrome'. The hormones cause a breakdown in communication between the frontal and temporal lobes, disrupting memory retrieval.

There are, however, potential problems with this account. One problem is that emotionally charged events are often *better* remembered than neutral experiences. The underlying mechanism for this memory enhancement also involves the release of glucocorticoids, which stimulate noradrenaline to act upon the amygdala and influence the hippocampus. Consequently, the 'amnesic block' explanation seems to invoke mechanisms that would normally improve, not remove, memories. A related problem comes from the survivors of concentration camps. The expectation would be of much higher rates of psychogenic amnesia than often observed given the likely levels of glucocorticoids provoked by the constant threat to life. For this hormone-based explanation to hold, we need to know a lot more about when and how this mechanism can boost or block memory.

A different explanation centres on how the combination of a severe precipitating crisis, depressed mood, or any past neurological insult, such as a minor head injury, might cause frontal lobe executive mechanisms to inhibit autobiographical memory retrieval. This account is, in part, an extension of the phenomenon called 'motivated-forgetting' (see Chapter 6, *Why do we forget*). Motivated-forgetting refers to our ability to suppress the memory of some information when instructed or when desired. Brain activation studies suggest that motivated-forgetting is brought about by actions of the prefrontal cortex on the medial temporal lobe, including the hippocampus. Problems with this explanation include how motivated-forgetting in the laboratory often has only limited effects, quite unlike a dense psychogenic amnesia. It also has to be appreciated that, for ethical reasons, laboratory studies on motivated forgetting lack the degree of ecological validity needed to determine any role in real-life, trauma-induced memory loss.

Faking amnesia

It may come as a surprise to discover that many people deliberately pretend to be amnesic. There are two main categories of people who might choose to simulate amnesia. The first consists of those people claiming financial compensation in the aftermath of an accident. The second is those accused of a crime who claim to have a blackout for the critical period. Ironically, it is peoples' confusion over the true nature of amnesia that has often made it possible to identify those simulating memory loss. For that we can thank the misrepresentation of amnesia in the media.

Despite the enormous clinical burden of traumatic brain injury to medical services, it has been estimated that nearly 40% of those receiving evaluations following mild head injury may be feigning some symptoms. Memory loss is a frequent component of the 'post-concussion syndrome', which is often associated with traffic accidents. This syndrome has been the mainstay of many dubious compensation claims. The cynic might note that in countries where litigations based on 'post-concussion syndrome' have been abolished, the condition has largely been cured.

Identifying simulated amnesia: Tests for malingering tap into the tendency of those feigning amnesia to exaggerate their cognitive difficulties. This exaggeration is captured in both formal tests of memory and self-report measures. There are, however, two cautions. One is that people with dementia might, at first glance, resemble those who are malingerers, although dementias have a much wider impact on cognition that is backed up by MRI differences. The second caution is that depression can adversely affect memory, along with other aspects of cognition.

When trying to distinguish real from simulated *anterograde* amnesia, a favoured approach is to give forced-choice tests of recognition memory. Imagine I show you 50 pictures, followed by 50 pairs of pictures, each pair comprising one of the previous pictures next to a novel picture. Your task is to identify the now-familiar pictures. As there is one correct and one incorrect choice, a chance score is 25 (50%). People simulating anterograde amnesia are likely to exaggerate their 'amnesia' by performing at or even less than chance. Interpreting chance recognition scores can, however, be tricky as some genuine amnesics may perform close to chance. For this reason, only below chance scores provide compelling evidence for malingering.

Also, in most amnesias, short-term memory is preserved yet this is often not appreciated by would-be feigners. Consequently, people malingering may give abnormally low scores on tests such as digit span. In the 'coin-in-the-hand' task the experimenter shows their open palms, one of which contains a coin. The potential malingerer then closes their eyes, counts back from ten, and then points to the hand that had contained the coin. Despite the apparent degree of memory challenge, confirmed organic amnesics perform well on this short-term memory task. In contrast, suspected malingerers and those asked to simulate amnesia often drop to near-chance levels.

The distraction/no distraction test has a similar rationale. Subjects read three words printed on a card, and 20 seconds later are given a semantic cue to one of the three words. People simulating amnesia perform far worse at recalling the target word than true amnesics, reflecting the misguided belief that true amnesics could not overcome this brief delay. Other variants of this task apply the same logic; take a simple memory task but dress it up so that it appears more demanding. This facade tempts the malingerer to perform at abnormally low levels, not realising that brief memory spans can still be bridged by those with genuine amnesia. A complementary approach involves training people on an implicit memory skill that true amnesics can learn and retain unaffected. One example would be learning to draw when looking in a mirror. Those simulating amnesia are prone to believe that the skill will not be acquired or will be rapidly forgotten, causing them to underperform.

Testing for real or simulated *retrograde* amnesia brings new challenges. One problem is that retrograde amnesia involves a loss of autobiographical memories, yet we may not know what memories the person had before the onset of amnesia. Nevertheless, those who simulate tend to exaggerate the loss of highly salient personal semantic memories such as the names of schools attended and the names of close friends. The Dead or Alive test has also been used with some success, probably because malingerers are unsure how true amnesics would react. Lastly, because claims of memory loss based around head trauma would normally reflect organic injury, structural and functional brain imaging can have an important role. The development of imaging methods to measure the status of the brain's numerous white matter pathways creates an additional way to test for any abnormalities.

Crime Motivated Amnesia: Determining whether a claim of amnesia for a committed crime is true or false brings a different set of challenges. Here, there is no expectation of brain pathology, unless the perpetrator received a head injury during the crime. Furthermore, the memory loss is for a particular episode in time so there need be no chronic effects on cognition. The reasons for feigning amnesia also differ. Faking amnesia may help to diminish responsibility, avoid questions about others involved in the crime, or even suggest incompetence to stand trial.

At the start of the Nuremberg Trials in 1946, Rudolf Hess claimed to have no memory for his Nazi atrocities, but later admitted he was feigning amnesia. (Jean Delay, who we met in the earlier section on the neurological basis of anterograde amnesia, was one of the psychiatrists charged with examining Hess.) Hess spent the rest of his life in Spandau Prison, until he committed suicide in 1987. More 'successfully', General Augusto Pinochet repeatedly avoided having to defend himself in court from multiple allegations of his involvement in the death and torture of thousands of civilians when he was head of the military in Chile from 1973–1990. The decision that he was mentally unfit to stand trial drew much criticism from clinical experts given the lack of objective evidence.

It is important to clarify whether having no memory of a crime you committed is a true defence. The answer is nearly always no. If the memory loss was caused, for example, by alcohol, you remain responsible as you are expected to know the risks of excessive alcohol (or any other drugs). The legal situation is different if the alcohol (or drug) consumption was unwitting or forced. In addition, there may be some mitigation if the defendant can show that because of the intoxication he or she could not form the relevant criminal intent.

A different defence is that of 'automatism'. Here, the defence needs to show that the criminal action was involuntary and beyond any conscious control. Such actions are deemed to be 'automatic'. However, if the automatic state is knowingly self-induced, for example because of taking illicit drugs or not taking prescribed medication, the person must demonstrate that they could not possibly have anticipated the consequences. Someone with type 1 diabetes who is struggling to regulate their glucose levels could be legally liable for a car crash caused by a hypoglycaemic episode. Sadly, fatal car crashes have resulted from this tragic combination of events. (In the U.K. it is a legal requirement for type 1 diabetics to check their blood glucose no more than two hours before driving, and to then check every two hours if on a long journey.)

Some defences based on automatic behaviour have led to acquittals. In 2009, Brian Thomas from Wales was acquitted of murdering his wife who he strangled while he dreamt. Brian Thomas suffered chronically from night terrors, and it was decided that his murderous actions were automatic. In a more controversial case from 2001, a man in the Netherlands said he had no memory of killing his wife. He strangled her after she threatened to accuse him of sexually abusing their daughter. Following her accusations, all he claimed to remember was that 'his ears started to sing and the light went out in his eyes'. His next memory was of his wife's body in the backyard and his hands loosely around her neck. The court experts recommended that had suffered an acute dissociative reaction and had been unable to control his behaviour, though no one had tested his memory profile. He was acquitted in the belief that the murder had been an automatic action so that it was out of his control.

A slightly different situation arises when the crime is seen as a form of temporary insanity that results from extreme provocation. In the U.K. there is a 'loss of control' defence. As a consequence, the killing of a spouse might be exonerated if it had been provoked by a lengthy period of violent abuse, occurred during a state of intense commotion, and was not pre-meditated. Famously, France had a special defence for '*crime passionnel*', but this was phased out in the 1970s. It is, however, still used as a defence in some counties, including Portugal.

To get an idea of how many people who commit a serious crime also report no memory of that same crime, a survey was conducted of those sentenced to life imprisonment in England and Wales in 1994 (Pyszora et al., 2003). Around a third claimed amnesia for the crime. This proportion is consistent with other surveys of murder and manslaughter, which give rates of claimed amnesia of between 25% and 40%. Of those sentenced to life imprisonment in 1994, claims of amnesia were strongly associated with a history of alcohol abuse, psychiatric disorder, and crimes of passion.

Three years after their convictions, only ~3% admitted that their 'amnesia' was feigned (Pyszora et al., 2003). Furthermore, those claiming amnesia were just as likely to plead guilty as those who were not amnesic. Together, these factors were seen as consistent with the criminals experiencing a genuine loss of memory. However, these same 'amnesic' cases were also more likely to claim provocation, as well as diminished responsibility, or lack of intent because they were intoxicated. These additional claims suggest that they might be trying to use their supposed amnesia for their benefit.

It is often thought that most of these amnesias are promoted by intense emotion, resulting in an affective dissociative state, also called a 'red-out' (to distinguish it from a 'black-out'out). A red-out is a form a psychogenic amnesia, with potential causes including the 'amnestic block syndrome', described above. Such explanations have, however, been challenged given that many extremely emotional events are well-remembered; so why should this specific situation encourage amnesia? Other concerns are that in a fifth of those cases claiming amnesia there was evidence that the crime was premeditated.

When excessive drinking is involved, a different explanation for crime-related amnesia is that the memory loss stems from an alcoholic blackout (see below *Losing Memory: Drug Induced Amnesia*). Even so, measures of alcoholic intake show that this explanation still leaves many other cases of crime-related amnesia unexplained. A further explanation is that the memory loss reflects state-dependency (Figure 7.2). This term means that the physiological and emotional states of the perpetrator were so abnormal at the time of the crime that normal retrieval cues are unable to reinstate that same extreme condition and help bring back the lost memories. However, attempts to demonstrate state-dependent memory loss in criminal cases have been unsuccessful.

Other clues come from the repeated finding that criminals who claim amnesia tend to be older, suggesting a greater experience of the legal system. One possible reason is that claims of amnesia increase the likelihood of examination by a psychiatrist or neurologist which, in turn, might lead to a diagnosis of a condition such as epilepsy, sleep disorder, or schizophrenia. These same conditions could then be used to suggest diminished responsibility.

While only ~3% later admitted to feigning amnesia in the study of those imprisoned for life in 1994, many believe that the proportion is far higher. One concern is that crime-related amnesia is sometimes a deliberate strategy when faced with overwhelming evidence. Consequently, a potential 'red-out' should be investigated rather than accepted. In an analysis of violent crimes, testing for malingering helped to distinguish those cases in which a genuine red-out seemed most plausible and those where it was more dubious. To assist in this difficult task, 'symptom-validity testing' was introduced. This method involves creating 12 or more questions about the specific crime, each followed by two equally plausible answers, only one of which is correct. The rationale is that the perpetrator with genuine memory loss will perform at or around chance, while the malingerer will be tempted to score below chance.

An obvious concern is that better-informed, well-coached malingerers may prove extremely difficult to detect. By searching the internet (or reading this book), people should become better prepared. To combat this problem, neuropsychologists are increasingly encouraged to use multiple methods to detect feigned memory loss. This is also one of the reasons why the promise of fMRI lie detection is so attractive. The assumption is that it would be difficult to mask the extra work the brain has to do when simulating memory loss, so coaching will be of little avail.

As early as 2006, two companies began offering fMRI-based lie detection services for reducing insurance fraud. The method assumes that we have different brain activity patterns when deliberately lying and when telling the truth. In particular, that lying is more effortful and may result in slower responses. Partial support comes from finding that activity changes associated with deliberate deception are most often located in parts of prefrontal cortex, as well as the inferior parietal lobule and anterior insula. But there is considerable variation from study to study. No single region consistently signals the presence of lying. This means that there was no reliable way of identifying deliberate deception in an individual person.

In a recent review of fMRI experiments, deliberate lying was compared against incorrect memories, in other words, unintentional lying. A range of brain areas may help to distinguish these two classes of false memories. Nevertheless, it was still not possible to find a brain activity measure that would reliably detect deliberate lying in a given individual. Even so, we are getting closer to the time when fMRI evidence will be routinely used in court. We already know from simulated experiments that jurors are likely to find MRI evidence persuasive. There is a need to proceed with the utmost caution and care.

Drug induced amnesia

It is all too easy to disrupt memory with drugs. The focus here is on those few drugs that can produce an almost complete absence of memory. Many other drugs have milder state-dependent effects on memory recall (Figure 7.2). (State-dependency occurs when a drug alters your physiological or emotional state, making it harder to subsequently recall information when not in that state.)

Alcoholic blackouts: The acute alcoholic blackout is almost a rite-of-passage in some cultures. It is estimated that of those who consume alcohol, between a third and a half of college students experience a blackout. A blackout is not the same as passing out.

A blackout occurs when you have no explicit memory for a past intoxicated period, despite remaining conscious throughout. Consequently, the episodic memories for that period are lost.

During an alcoholic blackout, while access to semantic information is reduced, people are able to interact and carry on conversations, even though those same experiences will later be lost from memory. The resulting blackout can be complete for a specific period ('en bloc'), with a precise moment of onset, or it may be partial ('fragmentary'). 'En bloc' memory loss is usually permanent, so that trying to jog your memory with cues does not help. For example, drinking alcohol to regain lost memories by combatting state-dependent effects does not appear to lessen an 'en bloc' blackout.

Blackouts do not happen every time someone is drunk. They are closely associated with a rapid rise of blood alcohol. Consequently, speedy drinking on an empty stomach, especially when consuming spirits, is commonly associated with a blackout. Related risk factors include a history of binge drinking, previous blackouts, and prior head injuries. For some, there may be a genetic predisposition to suffering blackouts. In general, women are more susceptible to alcoholic blackouts and show a slower recovery from the impact of alcohol on cognition. This greater sensitivity may reflect sex differences in the transfer and clearance of alcohol.

Unsurprisingly, alcoholics are prone to blackouts, especially those who drink spirits. The behaviour of alcoholics when intoxicated can, however, appear very similar whether or not they are experiencing a blackout period. The preserved ability to converse and interact helps to explain some of the most alarming aspects of blackouts. A sizeable minority of alcoholics describe coming out of a blackout and finding themselves in a place with no recollection of how they got there. In a survey of 100 alcoholics by Donald Goodwin, three reported blackouts lasting longer than 48 hours. Astonishingly, one man reported a blackout lasting five days. His last memory was of sitting in a bar in St Louis on a Monday, only to 'awake' with a mild hangover in a hotel in Las Vegas on the following Saturday. He was so alarmed by what had happened that he abstained from drinking for two years.

Alcohol disrupts most brain functions, but it can be especially harmful to memory. It is a non-specific drug that affects many neurotransmitters, including the major excitatory and inhibitory systems in the brain, which respectively involve glutamate and GABA receptors. Not surprisingly, alcohol has multiple effects on memory. Alcohol directly disrupts working memory, episodic memory, and semantic knowledge (a warning to pub quizzers). It also has indirect effects, including a loss of attention. Its more direct actions are on those neuroplastic process that help to form and consolidate memories. These disruptive actions are dose-dependent. As alcohol levels rise, plasticity within key brain areas such as the hippocampus becomes increasingly vulnerable. One consequence is the failure to link and store ongoing events with their appropriate contextual signals, i.e., with the where? and when? hallmarks of episodic memory. To make matters worse, alcohol disrupts sleep, which further impairs memory consolidation.

In researching for this book, I came across some extraordinary studies, but a study published in the esteemed journal Nature may take some beating. Insights into what occurs during a blackout were obtained by recruiting men who were willing and able to drink a pint of spirits in a few hours (Goodwin et al., 1970). The volunteers drank between 16 and 18 ounces of 86 proof bourbon in four hours, during which time they received both immediate and delayed memory tests. These tests included showing the drinkers scenes from an erotic movie every 30 minutes and then asking the increasingly drunk subjects to describe the content of that film two minutes and then 30 minutes later. (The authors claimed that the 30 minutes retention period taxed short-term memory, which is simply wrong.) Despite the alcohol, the volunteers demonstrated reasonably effective immediate memory, but those who could not recall details of the erotic film after 30 minutes were those who suffered blackouts. One message is that blackouts do not reflect a failure to maintain the most recent memories, rather a failure of further encoding, consolidation, and later retrieval. A second message is that ethical approval was very different in 1970.

Benzodiazepines and memory: Many years ago, I travelled to Sunderland to have a wisdom tooth removed. Before the extraction, I hopefully asked if they would use a general anaesthetic. The dentist said 'no', and that is about the last thing I remember until after the procedure finished. A week later I returned for a check-up and I took the opportunity to challenge the dentist by saying that he had misled me over not using a general anaesthetic, as I had no memories of the extraction. He replied with the ominous words 'Oh, we remember you'. He then explained that prior to the extraction I had asked what drugs they were giving me. The dentist answered, saying that it was a benzodiazepine. During the procedure I apparently kept his assistants amused by insisting on telling them all about the amnestic properties of benzodiazepines and their actions on the brain.

Apart from my embarrassment, I learnt two important lessons. First, some drugs, in addition to alcohol, can have such a strong amnestic action that they leave a complete blackout. Second, during that amnesic period you can remain cogent, hold a conversation, and act in ways that might appear quite normal. Incidentally, the hugely successful 2009 film 'The Hangover' used this same device. Three friends wake up in Las Vegas with no memory of the previous night and what happened to their fourth friend. They also wake up to discover a tiger in the bathroom and a baby in the closet. Retracing their steps, the trio discover they were drugged with Rohypnol, a benzodiazepine.

Benzodiazepines are a class of drugs with many clinical uses, including the treatment of anxiety, sleep disorders, and epilepsy. Well-known examples include Librium (Chlordiazepoxide) and Valium (Diazepam). Benzodiazepines are depressants that promote an inhibitory neurotransmitter called GABA, encouraging sedation. High doses of benzodiazepines can have amnestic and dissociative properties. (Dissociative means causing a feeling of detachment between yourself and your environment.) These same properties make them an attractive pre-medication for medical or dental procedures as patients cannot recall what may be an unpleasant experience, such as having a wisdom tooth removed.

All benzodiazepines can cause an anterograde amnesia. Different benzodiazepines vary, however, in their speed of onset and duration. Although their sedative actions may contribute, this is not the main reason for the resultant memory loss. While short-term memory tasks are relatively unaffected by benzodiazepines, new long-term memory tasks at even modest delays are impaired. Some benzodiazepines can also have mild effects on implicit memory.

The principal action of benzodiazepines is to disrupt consolidation into long-term memory, while having only modest state-dependent effects. The degree of memory impairment is related to task difficulty, so that recall is more affected than recognition, verbal tasks are more affected than visual tasks, and lengthier retention delays are increasingly sensitive. Benzodiazepines do not affect the retrieval of information acquired prior to their administration, allowing me to explain the actions of benzodiazepines to my Sunderland dentist. This pattern of findings suggests that the benzodiazepine-induced blackout is a failure of memory consolidation.

Benzodiazepines, most notably Flunitrazepam, have sadly acquired a reputation as date rape drugs. (The term 'date rape' is a misnomer as it can convey the false impression that it is not as serious as other forms of rape.) Flunitrazepam, better known as Rohypnol (also roofies, forget-me pills), is similar in action to Valium but far more potent. It is quick acting but long-lasting, remaining in the blood stream for up to 60 hours. Furthermore, Rohypnol is colourless, odourless, and flavourless, making it easy to administer without knowledge. When consumed at higher doses it causes memory loss, lack of motor control, and unconsciousness. Aside from alcohol, it is the drug most implicated in date rape. According to the BBC, U.K. police forces received almost 5000 reports of drink and needle spiking over the course of 2022. Sadly, it remains necessary to take precautions when out socialising.

Other amnestic drugs: The drug scopolamine is also known as hyoscine. The drug achieved notoriety as it was used by Dr Crippen to murder his wife Cora. It is also one of the active ingredients of henbane, a plant associated with witchcraft and death. Scopolamine acts by blocking one of the brain's major neurotransmitters, acetyl choline. The drug principally affects the initial acquisition of information, having far less effect on subsequent retrieval. The elderly seem to be particularly sensitive to the amnestic effects of scopolamine.

The power of scopolamine is conveyed by one of its more chilling names, 'Devil's Breath'. In a formal demonstration of the amnesic properties of scopolamine, the drug was compared with Diazepam, a benzodiazepine (Ghoneim & Mewaldt, 1975). Healthy students were given 128 words to learn after an injection of either scopolamine, diazepam, or saline. Scopolamine led to the poorest delayed recall (a mean of only six words), compared with 13 words for Diazepam, and 45 words for the saline control condition. Despite have such a powerful effect on subsequent recollection, scopolamine had little effect on recognition memory. Because of its actions on acetyl choline, it also causes a dry mouth, pupil dilation, sweating, and sedation. Sadly, scopolamine is another of the drugs associated with date rape. In a curious twist, scopolamine was also thought to be a potential truth serum (see *T is for Truth Serums*).

A further class of drugs that can cause amnesia consists of those chemicals that block the synthesis of proteins in the brain. It is believed by many that the formation of long-term memories involves structural alterations in the brain, a process that requires the production and transport of new proteins. Anisomysin, which is also an antibiotic, is a protein synthesis inhibitor. In animals, inhibiting protein synthesis with anisomysin during or immediately after an experience can induce an amnesia for that event. This amnestic effect has been demonstrated in a wide range of animals including goldfish, day-old chicks, pigeons, and mice. While it is natural to assume that the principal actions of such drugs are on memory consolidation, there is some evidence that they also affect the ability to produce memory tags that assist retrieval.

One fascinating clinical application of protein synthesis blockers is in trying to eradicate traumatic memories. The phenomenon of re-consolidation describes how a memory can enter a labile state when recalled, so that it might be modified (see Chapter 4, *How accurate and durable are our adult memories?*). By simultaneously administering an amnestic drug such as anisomysin, it might be possible to remove the traumatic memory that the sufferer had brought to mind. Initial studies with animals show that this memory extinction procedure is feasible. Naturally, there is great interest in how this method might be adapted for conditions such as Post-Traumatic Stress Disorder where intrusive, traumatic memories play such an important role in maintaining the condition.

18   Losing memory

Alzheimer's disease and other dementias

> It seems that when you have cancer you are a brave battler against the disease, but when you have Alzheimer's you are an old fart. That's how people see you. It makes you feel quite alone.
>
> Terry Pratchett (2008)

The belated appreciation of dementing diseases

In 2007 the best-selling author Terry Pratchett was diagnosed with a rare form of Alzheimer's disease. He sadly died in 2015, but not before reminding us how our attitude to dementia can only improve. The quote also highlights how fame provides no protection from this disease. Notable people who reportedly had Alzheimer's disease include Rita Heyworth, Ronald Reagan, Rosa Parks, Harold Wilson, James Stewart, Margaret Thatcher … (the list goes on and on). It is worth adding that Ronald Reagan greatly promoted research into Alzheimer's disease, both before and after his diagnosis.

The concept of dementia has a long history. The word was present in the medical community by the 18th century (the word dementia comes from the Latin for being without a mind). It is, however, an umbrella term that applies to numerous neurodegenerative conditions. About one person in 14 over the age of 65 has a form of dementia, with the proportion rapidly rising with advancing age. It is also worth repeating some truly frightening global numbers from the Introduction – around 57 million people currently have dementia, a number thought to rise to around 152 million by 2050. Approximately, two thirds of these cases will have Alzheimer's disease, that is around 100 million people by 2050. This vast number is, in reality, an underestimate as Alzheimer's disease is no longer just seen as a late-in-life medical syndrome, rather its pathology builds silently for decades before cognitive impairments become detectable.

We are now so familiar with the term Alzheimer's disease that it is hard to believe that the medical community took a long time to embrace this diagnosis. Up until the 1960s, 'senile dementia', as it was then called, was largely seen as a problem with the delivery of blood to the brain. Indeed, for some forms of dementia, vascular problems are the principal cause, but this is not the case for Alzheimer's disease. In a landmark study from 1968, based on the post-mortem study of brains in Newcastle, it was possible to establish that the neuropathology described by Alzheimer was the main cause of dementia in later life, and not vascular pathology.

DOI: 10.4324/9781003537649-18

Alzheimer's disease

It was at the beginning of the 1900's when Alois Alzheimer (with whom I share a birthday) made the breakthrough of linking a form of dementia with a particular pattern of brain pathology. On 26th November 1901, he met a 51-year-old woman named Auguste Deter in a Frankfurt asylum (Figure 18.1). He was struck by her strange behaviour, which included worsening memory and speech, as well as emotional outbursts. Auguste Deter died in 1906. After studying her brain microscopically, Alzheimer saw the cerebral 'plaques', 'tangles', and brain shrinkage that we now know classically accompany this disease. Soon, thereafter, Alzheimer described his observations at the 1906 Tübingen meeting of the Southwest German Psychiatrists. The audience, however, seemed uninterested, asking no questions. It is thought that the attendees were impatient for the following talk, which concerned compulsive masturbation. Alzheimer's disease was formally named in 1910, but it was not until the 1970s that it started to become clear that this disease is the commonest form of dementia, posing an unimaginable medical burden.

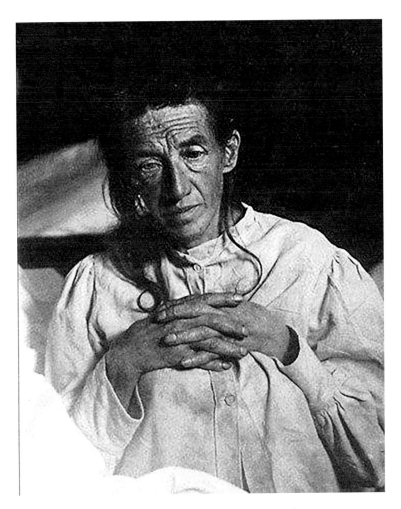

Figure 18.1 Auguste Deter. The first described case of Alzheimer's disease.

Sadly, some people develop Alzheimer's disease before the age of 65, a condition originally called presenile dementia. That term is often now replaced with early-onset or young-onset dementia. For those over 65, the term late-onset Alzheimer's disease (LOAD) is typically used. Early-onset dementia often has a stronger genetic component than late-onset. Given Auguste Deter's age, she clearly would have qualified as suffering from early-onset dementia. Amazingly, Auguste Deter's original medical records were discovered in 1996, records that include verbatim questions and answers between Alois and Auguste.

There is so much that could be written about Alzheimer's disease, but I will just concentrate on those issues with the most practical importance. The first issue concerns how Alzheimer's disease is diagnosed, including why memory loss is so often an early symptom of this disease. The second issue considers those factors that increase or decrease our vulnerability to this terrible condition. While a few novel medications exist that seem to slow down the cognitive decline in Alzheimer's disease, there is none that can stop, or even reverse, the condition. For this reason, those modifiable lifestyle behaviours that can hold back the onset of Alzheimer's disease remain of special significance. Their significance was further underlined by the realisation that Alzheimer's disease has a long, hidden incubation period.

The diagnosis of Alzheimer's disease: In 1990, Ernest Saunders was found guilty of fraud in the headline making 'Guinness Trial'. In 1991, he successfully appealed on the grounds that he was suffering from Alzheimer's disease. Evidence included his inability to repeat more than three numbers backwards, his misidentification of Gerald Ford as the American President, and apparently becoming lost when visiting a consultant. The diagnosis was accepted and his sentence much reduced. Subsequent events, when Ernest Saunders returned to full work, showed that he was either the only person on the planet to make a complete recovery from this incurable neurodegenerative disease or the diagnosis of Alzheimer's disease was wrong. The latter is almost certainly the correct conclusion.

The cautionary tale of Ernest Saunders highlights how difficult it can be to diagnose Alzheimer's disease with any confidence. Many illnesses cause a loss of cognitive abilities. Just one of many examples not related to dementia is depression. Consequently, it is vital not to jump to any conclusions when an elderly person is struggling with their memory. Despite the introduction of increasingly-sophisticated brain scanning methods, the diagnosis of Alzheimer's disease still remains a challenge.

The first diagnostic step involves a cognitive assessment. Favoured tests are the Mini-Mental State Examination (MMSE) and the MoCA (Montreal Cognitive Assessment). The MMSE has proved especially popular. A cut-off score of 24, i.e., 23 or less, is usually seen as an indicator of dementia, but this cut-off needs to be adjusted for some groups. It may, for example, be raised for highly educated individuals. Other adjustments include focussing on those MMSE subtests that assess temporal orientation, delayed recall, attention/concentration, and copying geometric drawings, as they can be the most sensitive. Even so, as a stand-alone test the MMSE remains only a moderate predictor of dementia, highlighting the value of additional tests. Examples include the Five-Word Test, which measures initial and delayed recall.

The problem is that many conditions, including other dementias, disrupt cognition. At present, the only reliable way to confirm Alzheimer's disease is by measuring a series of biological markers ('biomarkers'). This task requires specialised equipment. One biomarker for Alzheimer's disease is raised levels of a brain protein called beta amyloid (β amyloid or $A\beta$), which can be measured from cerebrospinal fluid (CSF) or by specialised brain scans using Positron Emission Tomography (PET). The β amyloid protein forms distinctive clumps, called 'plaques', that increasingly accumulate between neurons (Figure 18.2 left). It is these same plaques that Alois Alzheimer first described in 1906 from looking at Auguste Deter's post-mortem brain.

Other changes in Alzheimer's disease include excessive tissue degeneration, which causes brain shrinkage (Figure 18.3). This shrinkage, which is visible from MRI scans, is not uniform across the brain. One of the most vulnerable regions is the temporal lobe. In addition, the brains of those with Alzheimer's disease contains increased levels of a protein called Tau, again measurable from cerebrospinal fluid. Tau protein forms what are called neurofibrillary tangles, which develop inside neurons (Figure 18.2 right). Many now believe that Tau is a key agent in promoting the disease. A further change in those with Alzheimer's disease is a reduction in energy consumption by the brain.

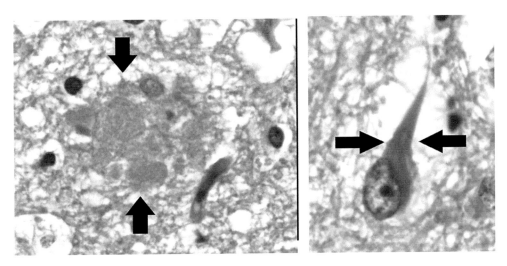

Figure 18.2 Amyloid plaque (left) and neurofibrillary tangle (right), diagnostic features of Alzheimer's disease.

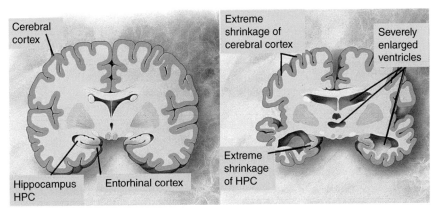

Figure 18.3 Gross pathological changes in Alzheimer's disease (right). Shrinkage of cerebral cortex and hippocampus, enlargement of ventricles (as subcortical sites shrink), alongside increased plaques and tangles.

Given the complexity and cost of measuring these various biomarkers, which rely on specialised brain scans or CSF taken from lumbar punctures, only a small proportion of people receive a confirmed diagnosis. Consequently, there is a huge demand for a simple blood test that will diagnose Alzheimer's disease. In recent years, rapid advances have been made in measuring both β amyloid and Tau levels from blood. While we are at the dawn of their roll-out, we will need to correlate any data from biomarkers with clinical signs and symptoms to reach an accurate diagnosis. Such tests will also need to diagnose the disease at its early stages, as this is when any treatment will be most effective. At the same time, it is vital to ensure that targeted, new treatments are only given to those with the disease. There are currently many attempts to create and validate a blood test for Alzheimer's disease, and recent results are highly promising.

Prodromal Alzheimer's disease: The word prodromal describes the incubation period prior to the development of the full disease symptoms. Our understanding of Alzheimer's disease has been transformed with the discovery that is has a very long prodromal phase, lasting decades. This means that there is a lengthy period with largely hidden neurological and cognitive changes that precede the overt stages of the disease. This discovery has profound implications because medical treatments should be given as early as possible in the course of the disease, which might be years before normal diagnosis. There are also beneficial lifestyle changes that could be put in place decades before any external hint of the disease.

It is now believed that Alzheimer's disease might begin 25-30 years before any obvious symptoms. For many, this would be when in their forties and early fifties. The very start of this disease begins with a pre-clinical 'at-risk' stage during which there is increased accumulation of Tau and β amyloid, but no discernible symptoms. Subsequently, some at-risk preclinical candidates will start to develop subtle cognitive difficulties. This initial prodromal stage, which can last many years, is barely discernible to others.

As these cognitive problems slowly increase, the person is likely to be diagnosed with the common condition called Mild Cognitive Impairment (MCI). Sadly, for many, Mild Cognitive Impairment represents a stage towards Alzheimer's disease, though for others the condition remains stable. Mild Cognitive Impairment is found in 10-20% of those aged over 65. Up to around one half of those with Mild Cognitive Impairment will develop Alzheimer's disease over the following five or ten years. Its most typical symptoms are a loss of episodic memory and prospective memory, forgetting what you just did in the past and forgetting what you should do in the future. Mild Cognitive Impairment can also affect language and decision-making. Depending on the most marked cognitive changes, this condition has been subdivided into amnestic Mild Cognitive Impairment and non-amnestic Mild Cognitive Impairment. The second group are at greater risk of other types of dementia, including dementia with Lewy bodies.

The key difference between amnestic Mild Cognitive Impairment and Alzheimer's disease is that daily living activities remain possible with Mild Cognitive Impairment, and sufferers do not usually require additional support, even though there is a decline in cognition beyond that expected for the person's age and education. While MMSE scores consistent with Mild Cognitive Impairment usually range from 23 to 27, this test can be insensitive. In practice, the MoCA (Montreal Cognitive Assessment) is often a better test of Mild Cognitive Impairment. While neuroimaging can help rule out other disorders, it is likely to be advances in the use of blood biomarkers combined with cognitive testing that will prove particularly helpful when identifying those most likely to develop Alzheimer's disease. As already noted, these biomarkers include blood plasma levels of Tau proteins and the ratio of different forms of Aβ (Aβ42/Aβ40). For cognition, it is best to take regular tests to see if the condition is stable or deteriorating. A continuing decline in episodic memory is most often seen in those Mild Cognitive Impairment patients who progress to Alzheimer disease. Also, as will be described below, genetic screening for the *APOE* ε4 allele helps to identify those with Mild Cognitive Impairment who are most likely to deteriorate and develop Alzheimer's disease.

Because of its frequency and indeterminant status, a legitimate concern is how Mild Cognitive Impairment affects quality of life. One practical issue is whether the condition impairs driving skills, which are often critical for maintaining independence. Experiments show that Mild Cognitive Impairment does affect a variety of driving skills, leaving sufferers at the same level as poorer drivers who are cognitively normal. In addition, Mild Cognitive Impairment often impacts spatial memory, affecting navigation. Clearly there is a need for increased vigilance among family members, especially as this condition often progresses. With continuing cognitive decline, driving skills deteriorate further. For example, tests using driving simulators show that those with mild Alzheimer's disease are more likely to react wrongly when there is a potential collision.

Memory loss and the progression of Alzheimer's disease: It is worth considering why memory, and in particular episodic memory, is so often an early victim of Alzheimer's disease. Post-mortem analyses, along with non-invasive brain imaging studies, have tracked the temporal progression of the pathology in this disease from three key perspectives. As you might predict, these are the patterns of brain shrinkage, the accumulation of β amyloid plaques, and the build-up of Tau protein tangles.

There is agreement that the cortical areas in the temporal lobe next to the hippocampus – including the entorhinal cortex – are often the first to be affected by Alzheimer's disease. Soon thereafter, the hippocampus is affected (Figure 18.3). Given this pattern of pathology it should be no surprise that memory, and in particular episodic memory, is so vulnerable. In addition to the hippocampus, other key sites for episodic memory are also affected in the early stages of this progressive disease, these sites include the retrosplenial cortex and anterior thalamus. This same network of brain structures is also crucial for spatial processing, helping to explain why becoming disoriented and feeling lost are often early symptoms.

Working memory is also affected in the early stages of Alzheimer's disease. Dual, rather than single, task performance is especially vulnerable. For this reason, the central executive is thought to be more susceptible than some other components of working memory. Meanwhile, there is a common belief that memories from childhood and one's youth are better protected from the disease. Formal tests do, indeed, show that in Alzheimer's disease both episodic and factual autobiographic information from ages 10–30 are more likely to be spared, in contrast to similar classes of memory from more recent decades, which are increasingly lost.

As the disease progresses, semantic (factual) knowledge is increasingly lost. This breakdown in the organisation and structure of factual information occurs as the neurodegeneration reaches those cortical areas believed to store semantic representations. This same break-down results in naming problems, including difficulties in 'fluency'. Here, the term 'fluency' describes the ability to spontaneously provide words when given a particular prompt. Examples include thinking up words beginning with a particular letter (phonemic fluency) or words that belong to a particular category, such as naming animals (semantic fluency). Semantic fluency appears to be especially vulnerable as Alzheimer's disease progresses. By the later stages of the disease there can be widespread language loss. In contrast, Alzheimer's disease relatively spares implicit memory.

Combatting Alzheimer's disease: The 64,000-dollar question is whether there is a cure for this disease. When reflecting on the desperate need for a cure, the author Terry Pratchett wryly observed, "*A cure? I would gnaw a dead mole if there was any science behind it*". At present, we do not have a cure despite some encouraging advances. The next best thing is to identify those biological and lifestyle factors that might ward off this terrible disease. Most important are those factors that can be modified, so that we can make a difference to our future health. Sadly, the largest risk factor for Alzheimer's disease is increasing age, something that cannot be modified.

Fortunately, not all 80-year-olds have dementia, highlighting why we should identify the risk factors associated with different dementias, including Alzheimer's disease. In this quest, researchers have produced an ever-growing list of modifiable and non-modifiable risk factors. However, identifying factors associated with dementia is only the first half of the challenge. The second half is to separate those factors that directly promote Alzheimer's disease from those that are merely associated but have no direct clinical significance. In other words, separating causation from correlation. It is known that across the 12 months of the year there is a striking correlation between U.S. ice cream sales and U.S. shark attacks, both reaching a peak in the summer, but obviously one does not cause the other. One way to help resolve this problem is to set up and analyse longitudinal studies.

One of the most informative, long-term studies into dementia began in 1986 with over six hundred American nuns who were members of the School Sisters of Notre Dame. David Snowdon, the instigator of the now-famous 'Nun Study', realised that convent life offered a unique opportunity to study dementia in a uniform community where everyone shares core aspects of their lives, while also being protected from unpredictable, external elements (Snowdon, 2002). [I once flew into Newark airport where the well-informed U.S. immigration officer decided to check the occupation stated on my passport (Neuropsychologist) by asking me what I thought of the Nun Study.]

On admission to the convent, when aged 19–21 years old, each sister completes an autobiography just before they take their vows. Astonishingly, aspects of these autobiographies, including the degree of positive content and the density and sophistication of the ideas expressed, predicted greater resilience against Alzheimer's disease many decades later. The associations between higher education levels and higher I.Q. with delayed dementia onset in the nuns has since been repeated many times in other studies. Related to this same finding, type of occupation, mentally stimulating leisure activities, and size of social network, all appear to affect the risk of developing clinical dementia. Consequently, experts recommend staying mentally and socially active throughout life. The likely explanation is that more stimulating and demanding activities are associated with creating greater cognitive 'reserve', meaning that one can function effectively for longer during the early stages of dementia.

The Nun Study also found that those sisters who took daily exercise were more likely to retain their cognitive abilities with aging. This preventive effect has since been seen in numerous studies, where both strength exercise and cardiorespiratory exercise can help to prevent cognitive decline. This relationship makes sense as exercise promotes vascular health and can promote the creation of new neurons (neurogenesis) within the hippocampus. However, studies looking at the potential benefits of exercise on those already with Alzheimer's disease have reported a mixed pattern of results. The beneficial impact of exercise appears to be greatest before obvious symptoms emerge, diminishing as the disease takes hold.

One popular idea is that taking 10,000 steps (four or five miles) each day should be a target for healthier living. In fact, the World Health Organisation is far less ambitious, with targets that include a total of at least 150 minutes of moderate-intensity aerobic exercise across the week. (10,000 steps a day would equate to something like 700 minutes across a week, nearly five times the WHO target.) A recent study of nearly 80,000 individuals in the U.K. over a seven-year period found that a more modest 3800 steps per day was associated with a reduced risk of dementia by around 25% (del Pozo Cruz et al., 2022). But the apparent benefits do increase with further walking. The optimal amount seemed to be close to the magic 10,000 steps a day, which was associated with a dementia risk reduction of 50% over the study period. Speed of walking also appears to matter as brisk walking was better than slow strolling.

Rather more surprising associations from the Nun Study include how smaller head circumference and suffering more tooth loss are associated with an increased likelihood of eventually suffering Alzheimer's disease. Perhaps less surprising is that previously suffering a stroke can hasten the onset of dementia.

Related to this last finding is the fact that brain trauma increases the risk of a wide range of dementias. This risk was first recorded almost a century ago, when it was realised that many boxers became 'punch drunk'. About a fifth of professional boxers develop this form of dementia. This link explains why there is mounting concern over the long-term effects of those sports that increase head-to-head contact or head-to-ball contact, such as American football, soccer, ice-hockey, and rugby. Chronic traumatic encephalopathy (CTE) is the name given to trauma-related dementia, which is closely related to Alzheimer's disease. Alarm bells include the finding that a sport-related concussion is far more disruptive to the brain's white matter than had previously been suspected, a discovery only made possible by the development of new forms of brain imaging.

In 2020, the Lancet medical journal highlighted 12 potentially modifiable factors that contribute to an increased risk of dementia. The twelve were: less education, hypertension, hearing loss, cigarette smoking, obesity, depression, physical inactivity, diabetes, low social contact, excessive alcohol consumption, traumatic brain injury, and air pollution. Together, these same modifiable risk factors account for around 40% of worldwide dementias.

The important message is that about 40% of dementias can be delayed or even prevented. To test this message, it has been necessary to turn to animal studies, where it is possible to separate correlation from causation. For example, age-related hippocampal changes in rodents can be counteracted by increasing physical activity, reducing calory intake, and enriching the animal's environment. Another important message from these studies is that we should improve our lifestyles not in later life, but much earlier.

It should come as no surprise that the list of lifestyle factors that might combat the development of Alzheimer's disease and other dementias is exactly the same of those for successful aging and super-aging. One prominent member on both lists, which might seem surprising, is hearing loss. In fact, the degree of association between age-related hearing loss and dementia, including Alzheimer's disease, makes it one of the highest risk factors that is easily diagnosed and capable of remedy (with hearing aids). There are a number of ways by which hearing loss might advance the onset of dementia, such as through decreased social interaction or the depletion of cognitive reserve. Another predictive factor for Alzheimer's disease is sleep-disturbance. To complicate matters, Alzheimer's disease is known to decreases sleep-quality. This is unfortunate as disrupted sleep will have negative effects on memory consolidation, making matters only worse.

Women show higher rates of Alzheimer's disease than men. One reason is that women tend to live longer. Hormones may also play a part, as earlier menopause is associated with increased risk of Alzheimer's disease. Consequently, oestrogen is thought to have a protective effect. Some, but not all, studies show that hormone replacement therapy can have a preventive action. These mixed results may reflect the individual genetic make-up of participants, so that only some women can benefit.

You may have read that a modest amount of alcohol can protect against Alzheimer's disease. Indeed, some, but not all, meta-analyses implied that light drinking, especially of red wine, can delay Alzheimer's disease. In contrast, excessive consumption consistently increases the risk. Unsurprisingly, the apparent protective effects of modest alcohol intake caused much debate, partly because of the many confounding factors that could render this association misleading. Indeed, more sophisticated analyses now reveal that even modest alcohol consumption is probably associated with an earlier onset of Alzheimer's disease. The advice is that those who abstain should not begin alcohol consumption to improve 'cognitive health', while those who do drink should reduce consumption given the overall harmful effects of alcohol.

Biological risk factors: Up to now, the focus has been on risk factors that stem from our lifestyle and, hence, are potentially modifiable. In contrast, those genetic factors that increase or decrease the risk of Alzheimer's disease cannot be changed by lifestyle. These genetic factors can, however, provide unique insights into the molecular causes of this disease, insights that have stimulated ideas for possible treatments. They can also help to identify those at highest risk of suffering Alzheimer's disease, should one wish to know.

The initial genetic breakthroughs came from studying families with unusually high levels of early-onset Alzheimer's disease. A common feature of these families is that they have gene variants that increase the amount of β amyloid in the brain (one of the biomarkers for Alzheimer's disease). These gene mutations include those that directly affect the gene on chromosome 21 that helps to produce β amyloid. This association with β amyloid levels also helps to explain why people with Down's syndrome are so prone to Alzheimer pathology in later life. In Down's syndrome there is an extra copy ('trisomy') of chromosome 21, the same chromosome that contains the gene that produces the β amyloid protein. The extra copy causes heightened levels of β amyloid. This same link with β amyloid also helps to explain why mutations of genes called Presenilin 1 (on chromosome 14) and Presenilin 2 (on chromosome 1) are also associated with early-onset Alzheimer's disease. These mutations both increase β amyloid within the brain.

Unsurprisingly, emerging potential treatments have targeted the β amyloid pathway using immunotherapy. So far, the clinical results have been modest but encouraging. The U.S. Food and Drug Administration (FDA) recently approved some anti-β amyloid monoclonal antibodies (Donanemab and Lecanemab) for mild Alzheimer's disease. While the drugs can reduce levels of β amyloid in the brain, the important question is whether they can slow down or even stop the decline in cognitive symptoms. Recent clinical trials of Lecanemab and Donanemab point to a slowing down of around 25% in the loss of cognition in those with early Alzheimer's disease, though some patients show no apparent benefits. In other words, memory and other cognitive abilities continue to decline but, in some cases, at a slightly slower rate. Clearly this is not a cure.

Some clinicians believe that amyloid is the wrong target. Instead, Tau protein should be the target of future treatments. This belief springs from how levels of Tau protein often correlate better with cognitive decline than β amyloid. Consequently, there is enormous interest in developing methods to remove Tau protein from the brain. While animal studies using Tau immunotherapy look encouraging, it is only after human trials that will we know if this approach is helpful. Clinical trials are currently underway, but because they have to track disease progression over many years we have yet to discover their outcomes. Many predict that we will eventually need a cocktail of drugs that attack both β amyloid and Tau.

Others believe that this is still only part of the puzzle, and other factors, such as neuroinflammation, will also need to addressed before any early treatment will prove effective.

For some of us, the version of a gene that we all carry called Apolipoprotein E (*APOE*) is of considerable significance. Apolipoprotein E, which supports fat transport and tissue repair, can occur in three different variants (three alleles). The form *APOE* ε2 is protective against Alzheimer's disease, *APOE* ε3 is neutral, while *APOE* ε4 increases β amyloid levels and vulnerability to the disease. This means that people with Mild Cognitive Impairment who carry the *APOE* ε4 allele are more likely to progress to Alzheimer's disease. This *APOE* ε4 risk is found for both early and late onset Alzheimer's disease.

The numbers of people with the *APOE* ε4 allele varies with ethnicity, but around 15–20% of the population have a single copy. Thankfully, only about 2–5% of the population carry two copies of *APOE* ε4. While a single copy of *APOE* ε4 increases the risk of Alzheimer's disease by two to three times, those with two copies roughly have a tenfold increased risk. As the *APOE* ε4 allele can be identified by genetic screening, there is the potential to encourage carriers to adopt those lifestyle behaviours that might delay Alzheimer's disease. At the same time, such genetic screening brings an array of ethical concerns.

In more recent years, the search has extended to find other gene variants associated with late-onset Alzheimer's disease, as this condition is far more common than the early-onset variant. We now know that a large number of gene variants are associated with the more frequent late-onset form, but for each gene variant this association is weak. Consequently, none of the individual gene variants is sufficient to cause Alzheimer's disease on its own, limiting their value as part of a screening test or as the starting point for a radical new therapy. This leaves *APOE* ε4 as the best genetic predictor for late-onset Alzheimer's disease.

Other dementias

The prominence of Alzheimer's disease has overshadowed the many other forms of dementia. These other types of dementia are very varied in nature. Not all, for example, are dominated by memory problems. I have selected three, principally because together they make up the large majority of dementia cases beyond those with Alzheimer's disease. All of these dementias are progressive, in other words the symptoms become more and more pronounced as the person gradually deteriorates. Sadly, some people suffer a mixed pattern of two different types of dementia.

Lewy body dementia: Imagine suddenly hallucinating that an army is marching up your lawn. This is an example of the bizarre visual hallucinations that are associated with Lewy Body dementia. Other symptoms include having violent dreams. About 15% of dementia cases have Lewy Body disease, which is often divided into two closely related disorders. These two conditions are called 'dementia with Lewy bodies' and 'Parkinson's disease dementia'. The two disorders are grouped together because they share a common pathological feature, namely protein deposits called Lewy bodies.

These protein deposits were first described by Frederick (Fritz) Lewy when he worked in Alois Alzheimer's laboratory in Munich. He described 'Lewy' bodies in Parkinson's disease in 1912 (Figure 18.4), yet ten years later he seems to have almost completely forgotten these protein clumps, overlooking their enormous clinical significance. The reason for this neglect remains unknown, yet he must have been very close to making the critical link between these bodies, Parkinson's disease, and dementia. It was fifty years later that John Woodard connected Lewy bodies with a form of dementia, although the term 'Lewy body disease' only became established after 1980.

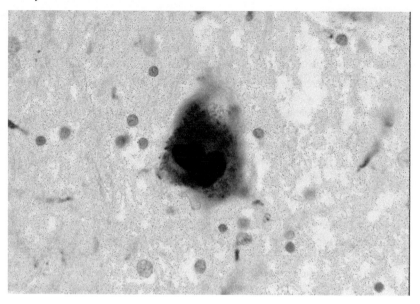

Figure 18.4 Two overlapping stained neurons containing Lewy bodies, formed by the protein alpha-synuclein.

In addition to its well-known motor effects, people with Parkinsons' disease are at a considerable risk of developing dementia as it afflicts around a half of all sufferers over the age of 65. In Parkinson's disease dementia, the classic motor symptoms, such as a resting tremor, problems with initiating movement, and a changed style of walking, precede the decline in cognition. Typical cognitive symptoms include problems with attention, executive functions such as planning, visuospatial function, and free recall. Patients can also show a lack of drive, while visual hallucinations may occur.

Dementia with Lewy bodies has a similar cognitive profile to Parkinson's disease dementia, but it is not preceded by a lengthy period of Parkinson's disease. There is a 'one-year rule'. If the dementia occurs at least one year after established Parkinson's disease, it is diagnosed as 'Parkinson's disease dementia'. If, however, the dementia precedes, or occurs at the same time, or within a year of the onset of Parkinsonism, it is regarded as 'dementia with Lewy bodies'.

The symptoms of dementia with Lewy bodies typically fluctuate and can include sudden periods of Parkinsonism as well as visual hallucinations. These hallucinations, which often appear early in the course of the disease, typically involve people, animals, objects, and landscapes. Examples include a small boy in the bedroom shouting fire, a line of nuns waiting to cross the road, rats and mice running along the skirting board, and a collection of buses and lorries.

Here is just one example

Every night I would see a man and a young child standing in the corner of the room staring at me… it was really queer. They would move but not come any closer to me and didn't say anything…they both had on old fashioned clothing, like Victorian style with cloaks on.

(Collerton & Perry, 2011)

The concentration of Lewy bodies in temporal lobe structures such as the amygdala, inferior temporal cortex, and parahippocampal region is associated with these well-formed, complex hallucinations. In general, visuospatial functions are more affected in dementia with Lewy bodies than in Parkinson's disease dementia, possibly reflecting greater parietal cortex abnormalities in the former condition.

A curious aspect of Lewy Body disease is the presence of 'rapid-eye-movement sleep behaviour disorder', which can precede the full syndrome. Here the patient may dream of being attacked by a person or by an animal. The sufferer then acts out their dreams by shouting, screaming, and waving their limbs, including punching, and kicking. Drugs that raise levels of the neurotransmitter acetyl choline are often prescribed for dementia with Lewy bodies as they might slow down the cognitive deterioration, meanwhile L-Dopa is given for the Parkinsonism.

Vascular dementia: This disease is responsible for around 10–15% of dementias. The study of vascular dementia is complicated by the presence of multiple subtypes, although most are associated with brain infarcts. (An infarct is the term given to the local death of brain tissue as a result of the loss of blood reaching that area.) Inevitably, age is a risk factor for vascular dementia, but other factors include having had a prior stroke and depression. As with Alzheimer's disease, further risk factors are those that increase the likelihood of circulation problems, such as smoking, obesity, diabetes, heart disease, high blood pressure, and raised cholesterol levels.

Because the pattern of pathology in vascular dementia is varied, so are the cognitive changes. While there are frequent impairments in attention and executive functions, long-term memory loss need not be a prominent feature. For this reason, tests such as the MMSE (Mini-Mental State Examination) can be insensitive, though the attentional measures from the MoCA (Montreal Cognitive Assessment) might be informative. Diagnosis is typically dependent on using brain scans to show infarcts and related white matter damage. Drug treatments for vascular dementia have largely proved disappointing, with the emphasis being placed on lifestyle changes that may reduce future stroke risk and slow progression.

Frontotemporal dementia: The announcement in 2022 that the Hollywood actor Bruce Willis had been diagnosed with frontotemporal dementia suddenly brought this form of dementia into the spotlight. The label is used for a group of degenerative conditions in which the brain pathology centres on the frontal lobes ('fronto') and the temporal lobes ('temporal'). Frontotemporal dementia is relatively rare, causing less than 5% of dementias. It is, however, relatively more frequent in those under 65, and can appear in people as young as 45. As yet, there are no effective treatments.

Frontotemporal dementia was first described as long ago as 1892 by Arnold Pick, a Czech psychiatrist. This led to the subsequent adoption of the name 'Pick's disease' in 1922. As different variants emerged, this name was dropped. The classification of this form of dementia has undergone a lot of recent changes. The current terminology is awkward as the different variants have been given long, complex titles, often making them difficult to remember.

The 'behavioural variant of frontotemporal dementia', which largely reflects frontal lobe degeneration is associated with executive deficits, along with personality changes. Behavioural changes often include a lack of inhibition or apathy. The disinhibition can lead to impulsive or reckless behaviour, even criminal actions.

The 'non-fluent variant - primary progressive aphasia', is characterised by a gradual deterioration in speech, grammar, and word output. While language functions continue to decline, there need not be the same obvious loss of episodic memory as seen in Alzheimer's disease.

Meanwhile, the 'semantic variant - primary progressive aphasia' describes a gradually increasing aphasia accompanied by a loss in the meaning of objects and words. (The term aphasia is used for language disorders that block effective communication.) Early on in the course of this variant it is the naming or understanding of relatively unusual or atypical objects that is most affected, but as the disease progresses even common nouns lose their meaning. For this reason, it is more commonly known at semantic dementia.

Semantic dementia – a subtype of frontotemporal dementia: If I ask you 'what is a violin?', you will know the answer. For someone with semantic dementia (also 'semantic variant - primary progressive aphasia') this question gradually becomes impossible to answer. For various reasons, semantic dementia has attracted considerable attention from neuropsychologists.

One reason is that semantic dementia has reinforced the conceptual division between semantic memory and episodic memory. Repeated studies show how the loss of semantic knowledge in this condition far outstrips that of episodic memory. For this reason, memory for recent day-to-day events can remain relatively normal, in stark contrast to what happens in Alzheimer's disease where episodic memory loss is often the principal symptom. In semantic dementia, the front of the temporal lobes, especially the left temporal lobe, is most afflicted, with the severity of the semantic impairment being directly related to the total loss of anterior temporal lobe tissue. While the hippocampus is not at the core of the pathology it is often disrupted, making the relative preservation of episodic memory in this condition somewhat perplexing.

A further curious feature of semantic dementia is that there can be a better recall of recent autobiographical memories compared with those from the distant past. This is the reverse pattern to that often seen in people with Alzheimer's disease, where older memories are often the best protected (Ribot's law). One interpretation of the reversed Ribot's law in semantic dementia is that the functioning hippocampus benefits more recent memories, while the loss of temporal cortex hastens the demise of old memories.

Semantic dementia has also influenced our understanding about how concepts are stored and organised by the brain. While patients with this condition can repeat even long complicated names, such as 'hippopotamus' or 'chrysanthemum', their definitions are sketchy and lack detail. For example, when asked 'What is a hippopotamus?' a patient might reply 'A big animal'. Difficulties with naming people extends to not knowing why their name or face is famous or in what circumstances are they known.

In the early stages of the disease, naming errors may reflect semantically related items, so that a drawing of a zebra is called a 'giraffe'. But, as the disease progresses, the person may refer to more familiar members of the same category, such as a 'horse', before naming develops into something even more generic, e.g., a zebra simply becomes an 'animal'. Eventually, the patient will state that they do not know what the drawing represents.

The ability to name or describe an item is strongly affected by familiarity. The names of less common items are the first to be lost as the disease progresses. This pattern explains why patients are better at identifying everyday home objects such as knives and cups, while struggling with less familiar things such as corkscrews or thermometers. A similar pattern is found for 'typicality'. Patients struggle to name or comprehend items that are not obviously typical of their group. This effect is seen both for objects (naming a seahorse, which is of course a fish despite its appearance), as well as the spelling of words ('blud' for blood) or generating irregular verbs ('drinked' rather than drank).

The pattern of deficits in semantic dementia has been one the principal sources of evidence for the 'hub and spoke' model of semantic knowledge (Patterson & Ralph, 2016). The notion is that cortex in the anterior part of the temporal lobe contains the abstract essence of a concept, for example, the concept of a magpie. This representation is the 'hub'. Two-way associations (spokes) link the hub with modality specific areas in the brain that provide the various elements of a 'magpie', such as its size, movement, colour, sound, name, and behaviour.

A characteristic feature of semantic dementia is that the break-down of semantic knowledge is broad, affecting different concepts, be they concrete, abstract, living, or human-made. Furthermore, the semantic deficits remain, irrespective of how conceptual knowledge is probed. Consequently, cues to a target item, be they a picture, spoken word, written word, environmental sound, taste, or touch all begin to fail. These features support the idea that essentially all semantic knowledge is stored in a similar manner, and that storage involves a web of related information from areas that are themselves more dedicated to specific modalities. In semantic dementia, the anterior temporal lobe damage gradually destroys the hub so that the multiple spokes are all affected and rendered useless. Objects that are typical for their class or are highly familiar can be relatively preserved as they contain richer, more plentiful links, making them more available and more resistant to tissue loss.

19 An alphabet of memory curiosities

A Aphantasia: People who lack imagery

> Implacable November weather. As much mud in the streets, as if the waters had but newly retired from the face of the earth, and it would not be wonderful to meet a Megalosaurus, forty feet or so, waddling like an elephantine lizard up Holborn-hill.
>
> *Bleak House*, Charles Dickens (1853)

Great writers, like Charles Dickens, employ striking visual imagery that ignites the mind. His opening paragraph to Bleak House paints London in an unforgettable manner, setting the tone for the book. Most of us take imagery for granted, but this is not true for everyone. Consider the following two questions. Is a strawberry darker or lighter red than a cherry? Does a kangaroo or pig have a longer tail in comparison to their body? These are just two questions designed to test visual imagery.

The Vividness of Visual Imagery Questionnaire asks people to imagine a series of scenarios. For example, 'picture a rising sun in a hazy sky'. What do you see in your mind? These images are then self-rated.

1 No image at all, you only 'know' that you are thinking of the object.
2 Dim and vague; flat.
3 Moderately clear and lively.
4 Clear and lively.
5 Perfectly clear and lively as real seeing.

Such questions reveal a surprising degree of variability in our ability to employ imagery. This individual variation has long been suspected. In the 1880s Sir Francis Galton tested people's power of visual imagery by asking them to recollect and describe the image of their breakfast table that morning. Some people, including Galton's cousin Charles Darwin, displayed impressive imagery. The ability to create unusually vivid mental images, almost as though you are seeing in real-life, is called 'hyperphantasia'. The mnemonist 'S' demonstrated hyperphantasia, as does the savant artist Stephen Wiltshire who draws cityscapes from memory.

But what if you are unable to form visual images? People who seemingly lack mental imagery have 'aphantasia'. Estimates suggest that between 1% and 3% of the population have congenital aphantasia, in other words, they lack from birth what most of us would call 'our mind's eye'. This condition, which may be a little commoner in women, often runs in families. In addition to vision, congenital aphantasia often extends to other senses, reducing

DOI: 10.4324/9781003537649-19

auditory, tactile, gustatory, and olfactory imagery. Curiously, most people with aphantasia can have visual dreams, although they are more likely to have non-visual dreams. One fascinating consequence is that people lacking imagery are less likely to sweat when listening to very scary stories.

Surprisingly, people with aphantasia perform normally on many memory tests. Imagery would seem intrinsic to visual working memory, yet people with aphantasia often show apparently normal visual working memory. In order to compensate for their loss of visual imagery, people with aphantasia seem to pick out key characteristics of an item to create a verbal label. This label is retained for use within working memory. This recoding, which has been refined over a lifetime, often appears to be automatic, helping to explain the effectiveness of this strategy. Spatial working memory also seems to be largely unaffected in aphantasia, as a coordinate system is employed instead of mentally placing items in space. Despite having effective recognition memories, nearly half of the people with aphantasia do have problems with face recognition.

Autobiographical memory is, however, different. Individuals with aphantasia often have poor autobiographical memory, with fewer sensory details, resulting in less vivid memories. They can recall memories but fail to picture them. Likewise, imagined future scenarios lack the normal degree of detail. Consequently, aphantasia is associated with a diminished ability to re-experience the past and simulate the future. These findings remind us how visual imagery is an important element in the reconstruction of episodic details for both past retrieval and future planning. Presumably for the same reasons, some people with aphantasia describe themselves as 'living in the present'. As a result, aphantasia may limit intrusions from past emotional memories, be they good or bad.

It would be rash to assume that aphantasia is a handicap. People with aphantasia may tend to have higher I.Q. scores than those with hyperphantasia. It is thought that people with aphantasia are more likely to work in mathematical, computational, or scientific professions. Examples of notable people thought to have aphantasia include the neuropsychologist Oliver Sacks, one of the lead decoders of the human genome Craig Ventnor, and Blake Ross, the co-creator of Mozilla Firefox. Meanwhile, those with elevated object imagery (hyperphantasia) may incline towards the visual arts.

B Bilingualism: Does it aid memory?

Dwyieithrwydd: Ydy e'n cynorthwyo'r cof?

Approximately half of the world's population speak two or more languages fluently. Being bilingual could have two opposing effects on cognitive capacity. If aspects of cognition, such as memory, have finite resources, then filling part of the system with a second language will reduce capacity elsewhere. On the other hand, if being bilingual promotes and strengthens valuable mental skills, these acquired abilities may spill over to have wider benefits for cognition.

The second account is correct. Being fluent in two languages can boost aspects of cognition, including memory. This is good news for my country of Wales. (The subtitle for this section is in Welsh.)

One focus has been on working memory. There is a small, but real, capacity increase for those who are bilingual. This benefit can be seen in both adults and children. A popular explanation is that being bilingual produces constant mental juggling created by the two competing languages. This competition occurs because a word in one language can activate its counterpart word in the second language. For example, the phrase 'good morning' would activate the Welsh equivalent 'bore da' (Figure 19.1). This duplication creates the need to control the competition between the two languages. This constant demand strengthens our cognitive control processes. These same control processes are critical for the effective use of the central executive within working memory.

What of episodic memory? Numerous studies now show that being bilingual can boost episodic memory in both children and adults. This enhancement is found for those fluent in a variety of language pairs, so it is not specific to certain language combinations. The benefits to episodic memory might again arise from enhanced cognitive control, but there are probably additional reasons. Being bilingual is likely to increase depth of encoding and help to create multiple representations. Both actions would then aid subsequent storage and recall. Support for this explanation comes from how episodic memory is further enhanced when the memory task explicitly involves switching between languages, such as translating text. This enhancement is to be expected because translating involves more mental effort and more elaboration, leading to deeper processing.

Chapter 3 of this book introduced the Lothian Birth Cohort. Briefly, all Scottish children born in 1936 were given a variety of intelligence tests when 11 years old. Many decades later, almost 1000 were traced and re-assessed. Those who had learnt a second language after the age of 11 subsequently achieved better cognitive scores than would have been predicted from their childhood I.Q. In other words, learning a second language helped to combat the effects of cognitive aging in a way that was independent of childhood I.Q. These benefits were found for both those who acquired a second language in early life and for those who learnt a second language in later life. As these beneficial effects seemed greatest for those with low childhood scores on tests of cognition, the conclusion is that being bilingual aided cognition rather than *vice versa*.

If mastering two languages is good, what happens if you are proficient in even more languages? Current evidence indicates that people who can speak three or more than languages have better episodic recall than those who are bilingual. One possible reason is that being proficient in multiple languages further boosts cognitive control, which in turn benefits episodic memory. That same study found that middle-aged multilinguals outperformed bilinguals on the Mini-Mental State Examination (MMSE). This finding is relevant as the MMSE is widely used to screen for evidence of dementia.

The good news for half of the world's population is that being bilingual protects against a range of dementias, including Alzheimer's disease. It has been estimated that being fluently bilingual throughout life delays the onset of dementia by around four years.

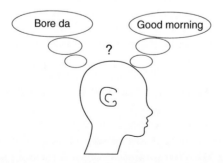

Figure 19.1 The cognitive control demands of being bilingual.

The likely explanation is that bilingual people have more cognitive reserve with which to combat neurodegenerative disorders. Again, one key element is the refinement of cognitive control which, in turn, supports memory and executive tasks. The latter effect may be especially valuable as age-related declines in cognition are often most evident for executive tasks that involve the switching and inhibiting of attention, along with the transfer and updating of information. The long-term benefits of acquiring a second language in adulthood still occur, but they are typically smaller than a lifetime of being bilingual.

C Computerised brain training: Does it work?

You may hear that memory, like a muscle, can be improved with exercise. So regular mental work-outs must be good for memory. Such logic has fuelled the claim that computerised 'brain-trainers', with their targeted mental exercises, improve memory. One common target is working memory, providing a potential route to wider improvements in cognition.

There is little doubt that repeatedly tackling the same cognitive challenge will strengthen performance on that task. Solving the daily sudoku will improve performance on subsequent sudokus. The critical question is whether these narrow improvements generalise to benefit other cognitive skills. (Will doing the sudoku help you solve the cryptic crossword?) Put another way, does brain-training a particular task cause wider cognitive benefits that make a genuine difference to real-life memory problems?

This issue has proved to be highly contentious, with scientist seemingly lined up on both sides of the divide. To complicate matters, brain-training has become big business, with many vested interests. As a warning, in 2016 the U.S. Federal Trade Commission charged one commercial provider of brain-trainers with "deceptive advertising".

As you might anticipate, there are mixed claims over the key issue of whether brain-training can improve those cognitive skills not directly being 'trained'. The problem is that we currently lack rigorous evidence as to whether these methods can improve everyday tasks, whether any benefits are persistent, whether this form of training works for everyone, or how many weeks, months, or years of training you might need. The reason for all of this uncertainty is that many studies fail to conform to best scientific practice. The inclusion of weaker studies only increases the apparent confusion over whether brain-training really works.

One generous approach has been to examine the peer-reviewed intervention studies cited on the websites of leading brain-training companies (Simons et al., 2016). We might expect these studies to be the most supportive of the technique. Unsurprisingly, there was good evidence that brain-training improves performance on the specific tasks being trained. There was, however, less evidence for improved performance on closely related tasks. Most importantly, there was little evidence that brain-training enhances performance on distantly related tasks or assists everyday cognitive performance. Overall, the analysis highlighted the lack of compelling evidence that cognitive brain-training produces lasting benefits for a wide range of real-world cognitive challenges.

A very similar conclusion was reached from a series of studies that assessed whether commercially-available brain training can assist older adults, including those with Mild Cognitive Impairment. Evidence was found for a modest transfer to tasks similar to those in the training programmes. This transfer was seen for both healthy participants and those with Mild Cognitive Impairment. There was, however, no convincing evidence for helpful transfer to a wider range of cognitive problems.

Further scepticism over the value of brain-training comes from an online survey that questioned over 1000 adults who had used a variety of computerised 'brain trainers'

(Stojanoski et al., 2021). After giving multiple tests of attention, reasoning, working memory, and planning, the researchers found no relationship with cognitive performance and current brain training or duration of training, which ranged from two weeks to five years.

Overviews of brain-training programmes for children and adolescents reach much the same conclusion. Many studies into the issue are poorly designed. Even so, the consensus is that there can be 'near-transfer' effects (benefits for similar tasks), while long-term benefits for less-related tasks ('far-transfer') seem largely absent. Once again, the conclusion is that commercial Brain Training Programmes are not as effective as first expected or as apparently promised in their advertisements.

In the absence of better experimental studies, there is little reason to believe that commercial brain-training products have beneficial effects that spill over to make a real difference to day-to-day memory problems. Nevertheless, it remains the case that cognitively stimulating leisure activities are associated with increased cognitive reserve, which, for instance, help to stave off the effects of aging. Here, a useful contrast can be made between commercial brain training and being bilingual. Language learning is a form of brain-training with benefits for memory that transfer across different domains. Critical differences include how the cognitive demands of being multilingual are incessant, extend over a lifetime, and impact on something as fundamental as how we represent written and spoken words.

D Duplicates, delusions, and familiarity disorders

In the sleepy town of Mill Valley, in California, an invasion is happening. People are being replaced with perfect physical duplicates that share the same knowledge and memories but are devoid of emotion or feeling. The real humans are extinguished. This terrifying picture, which comes from *The Body Snatchers* by Jack Finney (1954), was subsequently turned into a number of films, including *The Invasion of the Body Snatchers* (1978). Weird as this scenario seems, it is not dissimilar to the delusion held by those rare people suffering from the Capgras delusion.

The Capgras delusion refers to the belief that a close friend, spouse, parent, or other close family member has been replaced by an imposter. In one of the first descriptions of this delusion, the sufferer not only believed that her family and neighbours had been replaced by doubles, but the doubles had repeatedly been replaced by yet more doubles. The strength this delusion can be so powerful that the sufferer can, in extreme circumstances, consider killing the 'imposter'. Clearly, the Capgras delusion is very distressing. There may, for example, be the belief that you are sleeping with someone other than your spouse.

While most often seen in schizophrenia, the Capgras delusion can also accompany some dementias. It can also occur in people with limited psychiatric history. The student Y.Y., on returning home from university after a stressful period, which included a brief stay in hospital, locked herself in the family house. When her father rang the doorbell, Y.Y. called the police because "there was an impostor outside the house who was picking the lock and pretending to be her father" (Brighetti et al., 2007). For the next two months, Y.Y. failed to acknowledge close family members (mother, father, uncle, paternal grandparents, maternal grandfather) but she correctly identified her other relatives, including her aunts, and could also identify friends and schoolmates. While the delusion waned over months, it persisted for her father, such that she maintained that her mother and the impostor had killed him to start a new life together.

Explanations for this delusion centre around the idea that identity recognition is preserved but there is a disconnect between identification and the familiar feelings normally evoked by that person. These lost feeling include aspects of emotional and autonomic arousal. As a result, your gut feeling is wrong around this familiar person, so you come to the logical, but false, conclusion that they have been replaced. This explanation helps to explain why the delusion only happens for very close family members and friends. For the same reason it can apply to pets, including dogs and cats.

There are other bizarre delusions than can arise when familiarity gone wrong. In the Fregoli syndrome the sufferer believes that different people are just a single individual in disguise. This rare syndrome was named after the Italian actor Leopoldo Fregoli (1867–1936), who was famous for quick character changes while on stage. Indeed, he was so quick that there were rumours that there must be more than one Fregoli. To add to the distress of those with the Fregoli syndrome, the sufferer often believes that that they are being persecuted by these disguised imposters. For this reason, the Fregoli syndrome is often accompanied by threats to the misidentified person. Like the Capgras delusion, this is a misidentification syndrome and like the Capgras delusion, it is most often seen in psychotic patients or those with neurodegenerative diseases.

E Exercise: Is it worth it?

On the 2nd October 2004, 13 runners went for a timed five-kilometre run in Bushy Park, London. There were no prizes, just the pleasure of participating in a free, social event. The event was repeated over the following weeks. Twenty years later, the weekly ParkRun takes place at 2000 different locations in more than 20 countries, with over nine million participants who can run, walk, or push a pram. There is an enormous appetite for exercise, which is good for your body and your brain (Figure 19.2).

Both aerobic exercise (such as walking, jogging, swimming, cycling), and anaerobic exercise (such as weights, jumping, sprinting) can boost mood and brain well-being. For the lucky few, there is a post-run 'high'. This mood lift is often thought to be linked to the release of endorphins, the brain's own opioids. Both aerobic and anaerobic exercise can increase β-endorphin release, although this release is more strongly associated with anaerobic exercise. Nevertheless, there is some question over whether endorphins cause the post-run 'high', as some believe it is due to the release of endocannabinoids, substances produced by the body that resemble cannabis. To complicate matters, exercise can also affect a wide range of the brain's major neurotransmitters, including 5-HT, GABA, dopamine, and acetylcholine, in ways that can benefit mood in both the short and long-term.

Exercise is good for brain health in many ways. It helps to reduce neuroinflammation, neurotoxicity, and neurodegeneration. One consequence is that physical exercise helps to maintain the structural integrity of our brain's white matter as we age. Exercise also benefits grey matter. The hippocampus remains the centre of much research, partly because of its importance for memory but also because exercise increases the production of new hippocampal neurons. It is thought that the release of BDNF (brain-derived neurotrophic factor) is a key promotor of hippocampal neurogenesis associated with exercise. Other hippocampal benefits following exercise include greater neuronal resistance to stress, along with increased dendritic length and neuronal spine density. Aerobic exercise is also associated with relatively larger hippocampal volumes. This 'gain' may partly reflect how exercise can slow down the loss of hippocampal volume associated with normal aging.

Another site under the spotlight is the prefrontal cortex. Long-term exercise is often associated with benefits to functions such attention, task switching, and working memory,

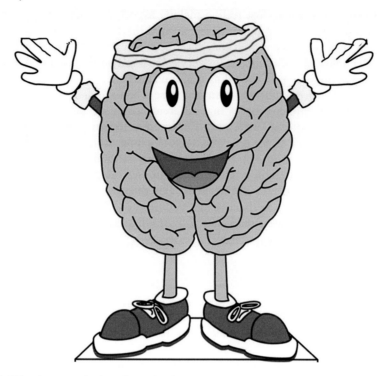

Figure 19.2 Why does exercise benefit the brain?

Source: Illustration, Lorraine Woods.

functions that involve the prefrontal cortex. Remarkably, even a single bout of exercise can assist prefrontal cognitive functions, in addition to enhancing mood and reducing stress. One possible explanation is that once exercise stops, there is a circulatory rebound causing greater than normal blood supply to areas such as prefrontal cortex.

If you cast your mind back to the Nun Study you may recall that those nuns who took daily exercise showed greater resistance to the onset of dementia. This is not surprising as one of many actions of physical exercise is on reducing neuronal inflammation, helping the prevention of various neurodegenerative diseases, including Alzheimer's and Parkinson's disease. Related benefits of long-term exercise include increased cerebral blood flow, as well as reduced blood pressure and heart rate. We know, for example, from the U.K. Biobank that a resting heart rate of 80 or over predicts an increased risk of dementia in older adults, along with greater hippocampal atrophy and a loss of white matter integrity. Exercise is a natural way to reduce resting heart rate.

So how much exercise should we take? An extensive review concluded that walking about 4000 steps per day can reduce the risk of dementia but taking nearer 10,000 steps is even better. The World Health Organisation (WHO) recommends that people aged 18–64, should do at least 150–300 minutes of moderate-intensity physical activity (such as brisk walking) per week. In addition, they should engage in muscle strengthening activities (such as weights, squats, sit-ups) at least two days a week. If you are over 65 you should also include exercises to help your balance. However, it is all-too-easy to sound evangelical when it comes to promoting exercise, and we need to remember that it is a real struggle for many. Surely the loudest support at Parkrun should go to those at the back, not those at the front.

F Food preferences and learnt taste aversions

There is a life-changing form of learning that about half of the population acquire. I am referring to a conditioned taste aversion. This term describes the persistent, deep dislike of a taste or smell that had previously been associated with an illness. Powerful taste aversions can form even when we are confident that something else was responsible for the illness. In a famous example, the psychologist Martin Seligman acquired an aversion to Sauce Bearnaise, despite being convinced that flu, rather than the sauce, had made him ill. This phenomenon is also highly selective, as the learning is closely linked to feeling nauseous rather than with other symptoms of illness.

Now might be the time to admit that I have a conditioned taste aversion to whisky (Figure 19.3). Surveys of college students find that over half report at least one aversion, often for an alcoholic drink. My overdose of whisky let to an aversion that has lasted over

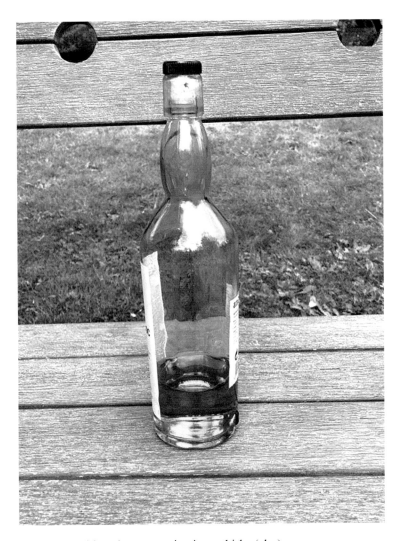

Figure 19.3 My own conditioned taste aversion is to whisky (alas).

four decades. Modest, titrated doses of single malts over the intervening years have thankfully helped to diminish this aversion.

My self-treatment highlights how 'extinction', the subsequent consuming of the aversive food or drink with no bad after-effects helps to reduce learnt aversions. However, when that extinction happens in a place different to where the taste aversion was acquired, the learnt aversion can be partly re-instated by going back to original learning location. I have to confess I have avoided returning to the pub in Oxford where my disastrous experience occurred, but my prediction is that I would again find it very hard to enjoy their whisky.

There are a number of features that, together, make conditioned taste aversions unique. As already indicated, the learnt aversion is typically very long lasting, sometimes persisting for a lifetime. This same aversion can be acquired after just a single-taste illness-episode. Furthermore, the taste and the illness may happen hours apart, yet the learning remains powerful. Normally a time-lag will stop aversive conditioning. Lastly, the aversion is focussed on the taste and smell of the food or drink, while its visual appearance is often far less disliked even though it is a salient part of any food or drink consumption. Given these characteristics, it is thought that we have specialised neural systems for acquiring conditioned taste aversions.

There are good biological reasons for this heightened form of learning. Humans are omnivorous, allowing us to exploit an astonishing array of environments. But this versatility brings risks. How do we know what is safe to eat? One solution is to acquire our food preferences by imitating those around us. This strategy is normally safe and effective, and so it should not be surprising that observational learning is one of key ways that children acquire food preferences. Consequently, children and parents have similar food likes and dislikes. Our sensitivity to the likes and dislikes of others also explains why, when in a restaurant, someone expresses their dislike of a meal (or drink) we have also ordered, our pleasure is often diminished.

Novel foods pose a special challenge. We cannot afford to ignore them as they might prove to be highly nutritious, but there is also a risk that they might prove to be poisonous. Our solution is to be 'neophobic'. This means that we are wary of new tastes, only consuming a small amount on first exposure. This strategy reduces the likelihood of serious illness. The same neophobic strategy is shown by rats, who are also omnivorous and can also acquire conditioned taste aversions. Rats have a further trick. They can detect novel food odours on the breath of other rats, using that second-hand familiarity to reduce the neophobia for that particular food.

A related feature, shared by rats and humans, is that novel foods and drinks induce the most intense learnt aversions. This again makes biological sense as a familiar food will have previously been consumed without subsequent sickness. It also means that we are most likely to acquire an aversion to just the novel food in the buffet, should we fall ill. For the same reason, learnt aversions to alcoholic drinks are often to novel distinctive tastes, such as unusual cocktails.

Moving to a clinical setting, conditioned taste aversions may contribute to the dislike of food seen during some cancer treatments. Both chemotherapy and radiotherapy can induce nausea, creating conditions for taste aversion learning. These aversions are directed at foods consumed shortly before these nausea-inducing treatments. An ingenious solution is to offer a novel foodstuff, between the familiar foods and the chemotherapy. As might be predicted, the aversion becomes associated with the 'scapegoat' novel food, helping to protect familiar tastes.

The power of acquired taste aversions has also been used in wildlife management. Here, animals receive bait deliberately laced with non-lethal levels of poison so that they will form a long-lasting aversion to that particular type of food. Examples include giving poisoned meat to coyotes and wolves to reduce livestock predation. Other instances involve racoons and egg predation. The procedure is not without problems. One limitation is that it often presumes that the learnt aversion will generalise to similar foods, thereby creating wider protection. This generalisation cannot be guaranteed. Over decades the practice has been much refined, but there is still a need to identify those contexts and those species for which it is most effective.

Up to now I have largely focussed on acquired aversions, but we can also acquire food preferences. Many of our food preferences are the consequence of observational learning combined with early exposure, which can even happen before birth (see Chapter 2 *From before birth to adolescence*). The early experience of a wide variety of foods further helps to create a broad palate of pleasant flavours. As a result, familiarity, along with sweetness, almost completely accounts for the taste preferences of children aged between two and three.

Studies with rats show how recovery from illness can sometimes create new food preferences. For example, thiamine-deficient rats will learn to prefer those foodstuffs containing the missing B1 vitamin. (If you recall, thiamine deficiency is the principal cause of the amnesic Korsakoff's disease.) However, this 'medicine effect' probably only accounts for a very small proportion of human food preferences.

We begin life with an innate tendency to reject bitter tastes. This dislike of bitter tastes probably originates from the need to avoid consuming plant-based poisons, such as alkaloids. Their bitter taste helps the plant from being eaten and helps us to avoid ingesting their poison. Happily, this innate distrust of bitter tastes can be overcome with associative learning, such as pairing the bitter taste with a liked taste or a high energy nutrient. Coffee is bitter, so most coffee drinkers begin by adding sugar, which they may later remove and yet still enjoy the bitter taste. Another bitter substance is quinine, yet when added to carbonated water and repeatedly combined with gin, it can become surprisingly pleasurable.

Our subjective 'liking' of a taste is moderated by exposure. For example, when encouraged to sample different amounts of unfamiliar tropical fruit drinks, people stated a preference for those drinks they had sampled more often. As with many things, greater familiarity is associated with greater liking. This hedonic reaction is often described as the 'mere exposure effect'. But it is also easy to overdo things. Repeating the same, familiar taste over a mealtime will often cause 'sensory-specific satiety'. This term refers to how the subjective pleasure associated with the taste of a food declines across the course of a meal as we continue to consume that same food. Changing to a different food can then re-instate our pleasure. This is one of the reasons why it is so easy to overindulge at buffets and why there is always 'room' for a dessert. Rather alarmingly, we eat up to 50% more when offered a variety of foods.

G The 'generation effect', the Aha! moment, and memory

The 'generation effect' describes how self-generated information is remembered better than information that you have read or heard. The effect still works if you generate an error, as long as that error is corrected.

To begin, try and generate the only common English word that begins ONI. A word that you self-generate is likely to be better remembered than a word you merely read. Now imagine you are given a list of single words and asked to generate the missing word that has the opposite meaning, e.g., Higher – L.... For comparison, you are also asked to read pairs of opposite words that are provided, e.g., Smooth – Rough. The self-generated word 'lower' is more likely to be subsequently recalled than the word 'rough'. Other ways to self-generate words include producing rhymes and solving anagrams, as well as completing words from their initial letters. (The word in the first sentence is, of course, onion.) If, you have ever tackled a 'Wordle' problem you will know that you have to generate a specific five-letter word by a process of elimination. There is a clear prediction that Wordle solutions will be well remembered as they are self-generated.

The generation effect is especially powerful for recognition memory, but it is also consistently found for cued recall and free recall. Likewise, it is found for both intentional learning, where subjects know they will later be tested, and incidental learning in which the memory test is unexpected. While the overall memory benefit for self-generation can sometimes appear modest, its effectiveness may increase with longer retention delays, highlighting its practical potential.

Intuitively, we might suppose that this memory advantage reflects the greater mental effort required for self-generation. Surprisingly, an extensive meta-analysis failed to support this idea as there appeared to be no difference in the size of the generation effect when comparing tasks of low difficulty and high difficulty. A clearer difference is, however, seen when comparing the generation of real words with tasks involving generating non-words. This same difference suggests that activating our word lexicon contributes to the generation effect. The resulting factors that influence the generation effect appear to arise from two related processes – interrogation of the features of the target item and enhanced processing of the relationships between the cue words and target words.

The generation effect is not confined to the psychology laboratory. In the classroom, self-generation improves the learning of new information when compared with simply reading that same information. For example, the generation effect is used to help second-language learning, where trying to come up with the desired word is encouraged. Another example is when students were asked to generate their own mnemonics for terms used in neurophysiology. Subsequent recall of those same terms was superior when using personal mnemonics rather than ones provided by the instructor.

An obvious hazard is that self-generation in the classroom will inevitably produce some errors, which might disrupt memory. However, if feedback is provided to correct these errors, the benefit of self-generation is preserved. As the industrialist and engineer Henry Ford astutely observed *"The only real mistake is the one from which we learn nothing."*

Guess the meaning of the word 'skep'. Don't worry if you do not know, just make a guess. The likelihood is that you will get it wrong. I can now tell you that it is a kind of basket. This combination of self-generated error and corrected feedback still results in better memory for the meaning of 'skep' than just reading its meaning. In other words, the benefits of self-generation and error feedback extend to information that is completely novel. Intriguingly, students subjectively feel that error-generation is ineffective, even though their objective scores confirm that it is better than merely reading the correct information.

"The haystack was important because the cloth ripped." This ambiguous phrase is now quite famous within cognitive psychology. Memory for this sentence was tested when the critical cue word ('parachute') was embedded within the phrase '… because the parachute cloth ripped'. Recall was, however, much better when the same cue word 'parachute' was only given after the conclusion of the sentence and after a delay. The delay helped to create an 'Aha!' moment associated with the sudden, self-generated insight into what the sentence really means.

Self-generated experiences associated with an 'Aha!' moment are remembered better than those lacking a sense of self-discovery. Examples of the kinds of problems used to deliberately create an Aha! moment include working out how a magic trick is done and solving a riddle. For example, *What runs, but never walks. Murmurs, but never talks. Has a bed, but never sleeps. And has a mouth, but never eats?* As already explained, self-generation helps memory, but the Aha! moment has an added emotional element of pleasure that further enhances memory. (The answer to the riddle is at the end of the next section.)

H Hypnosis, memory, and the law

Chapter 4, *How accurate and durable are our adult memories?* considered the value of hypnosis and described why recollections made under hypnosis are prone to error. This unease led the U.S. Department of Justice to highlight concerns over its practice in legal cases. Their Archives state that *"The information obtained from a person while in a hypnotic trance cannot be assumed to be accurate."* Nevertheless, they also state that *"in certain limited cases, the use of forensic hypnosis can be an aid in the investigative process"*. Worryingly, of the 17 U.S. States that currently allow hypnotically induced testimony, ten have active capital punishment laws.

Moving to the U.K., the Code for Crown Prosecutors issues very clear warnings about the use of hypnosis. There is the stark statement that *"Any confession obtained by hypnosis is likely to be ruled inadmissible under sections 76 or 78 Police and Criminal Evidence Act 1984."* Furthermore, *"Under no circumstances should suspects or persons who may be implicated in the commission of an offence be hypnotised."* The same document urges extreme caution when considering the hypnosis of witnesses and that such testimony should only be used in exceptional circumstances. The advice highlights how such memories are prone to confabulation (making up missing information) and cueing (where something suggested or imagined becomes fixed in the mind of the subject). (It is a river.)

I Illusions of learning and illuminating text

I have in front of me a second-hand copy of a textbook on memory. I strongly suspect the previous owner was a student as on many pages there are passages highlighted in yellow. Illuminating text in this way is very popular (Figure 19.4). The question is whether this is a useful memory aid or just a memory illusion. The answer is yes and no. Reaching this conclusion takes us to a number of memory illusions.

A recent meta-analysis involving 36 studies, the first dating as far back as 1938, found that text-highlighting by students can help with subsequent tests of memory but not with tests of comprehension (Ponce et al., 2022). Any beneficial effects of highlighting on memory were boosted by complementary approaches such as note taking or constructing a memory map. However, the benefits of text-highlighting were marginal for less experienced learners, pointing to the need for training in what to highlight.

High-quality highlighting by the instructor helps both memory and comprehension while, unsurprisingly, inappropriate highlighting hinders learning. Helpful instruction includes how to pick out the main ideas from among the supporting ideas and how best to use the overall structure of the text. The benefits of highlighting are presumed to arise from the 'generation effect' allied to the push for deeper, semantic processing, along with promoting salience for the key content.

Before rushing out to buy more highlighter pens it is important to appreciate the opposite view – that highlighting or underlining text, which you then re-read, is one of worst learning strategies. For one thing, too much highlighting is counter-productive as it becomes

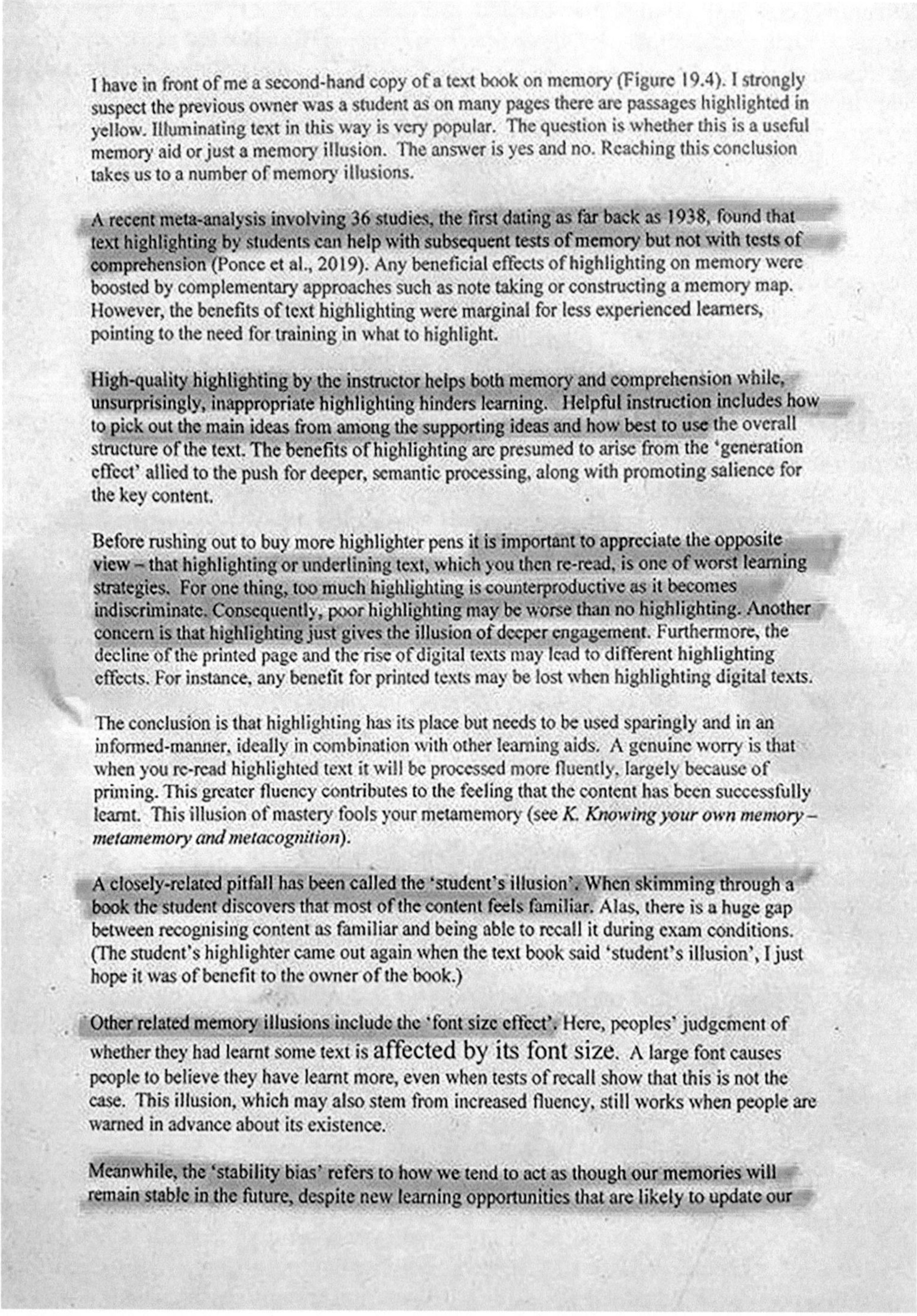

I have in front of me a second-hand copy of a text book on memory (Figure 19.4). I strongly suspect the previous owner was a student as on many pages there are passages highlighted in yellow. Illuminating text in this way is very popular. The question is whether this is a useful memory aid or just a memory illusion. The answer is yes and no. Reaching this conclusion takes us to a number of memory illusions.

A recent meta-analysis involving 36 studies, the first dating as far back as 1938, found that text highlighting by students can help with subsequent tests of memory but not with tests of comprehension (Ponce et al., 2019). Any beneficial effects of highlighting on memory were boosted by complementary approaches such as note taking or constructing a memory map. However, the benefits of text highlighting were marginal for less experienced learners, pointing to the need for training in what to highlight.

High-quality highlighting by the instructor helps both memory and comprehension while, unsurprisingly, inappropriate highlighting hinders learning. Helpful instruction includes how to pick out the main ideas from among the supporting ideas and how best to use the overall structure of the text. The benefits of highlighting are presumed to arise from the 'generation effect' allied to the push for deeper, semantic processing, along with promoting salience for the key content.

Before rushing out to buy more highlighter pens it is important to appreciate the opposite view – that highlighting or underlining text, which you then re-read, is one of worst learning strategies. For one thing, too much highlighting is counterproductive as it becomes indiscriminate. Consequently, poor highlighting may be worse than no highlighting. Another concern is that highlighting just gives the illusion of deeper engagement. Furthermore, the decline of the printed page and the rise of digital texts may lead to different highlighting effects. For instance, any benefit for printed texts may be lost when highlighting digital texts.

The conclusion is that highlighting has its place but needs to be used sparingly and in an informed-manner, ideally in combination with other learning aids. A genuine worry is that when you re-read highlighted text it will be processed more fluently, largely because of priming. This greater fluency contributes to the feeling that the content has been successfully learnt. This illusion of mastery fools your metamemory (see *K. Knowing your own memory – metamemory and metacognition*).

A closely-related pitfall has been called the 'student's illusion'. When skimming through a book the student discovers that most of the content feels familiar. Alas, there is a huge gap between recognising content as familiar and being able to recall it during exam conditions. (The student's highlighter came out again when the text book said 'student's illusion', I just hope it was of benefit to the owner of the book.)

Other related memory illusions include the 'font size effect'. Here, peoples' judgement of whether they had learnt some text is affected by its font size. A large font causes people to believe they have learnt more, even when tests of recall show that this is not the case. This illusion, which may also stem from increased fluency, still works when people are warned in advance about its existence.

Meanwhile, the 'stability bias' refers to how we tend to act as though our memories will remain stable in the future, despite new learning opportunities that are likely to update our

Figure 19.4 Highlighted passage from memory book.

indiscriminate. Consequently, poor highlighting may be worse than no highlighting. Another concern is that highlighting just gives the illusion of deeper engagement. Furthermore, the decline of the printed page and the rise of digital texts may lead to different highlighting effects. For instance, any benefit for printed texts may be lost when highlighting digital texts.

The conclusion is that highlighting has its place but needs to be used sparingly and in an informed manner, ideally in combination with other learning aids. A genuine worry is that when you re-read highlighted text it will be processed more fluently, largely because of priming. This greater fluency contributes to the feeling that the content has been success-fully learnt. This illusion of mastery fools your metamemory (see *K. Knowing your own memory – metamemory and metacognition*).

A closely-related pitfall has been called the 'student's illusion'. When skimming through a book the student discovers that most of the content feels familiar. Alas, there is a huge gap between recognising content as familiar and being able to recall it during exam condi-tions. (The student's highlighter came out again when the text book said 'student's illusion', I just hope it was of benefit to the owner of the book.)

Other related memory illusions include the 'font size effect'. Here, peoples' judgement of whether they had learnt some text is affected by its font size. A large font causes people to believe they have learnt more, even when tests of recall show that this is not the case. This illusion, which may also stem from increased fluency, still works when people are warned in advance about its existence.

Meanwhile, the 'stability bias' refers to how we tend to act as though our memories will remain stable in the future, despite new learning opportunities that are likely to update our thinking. Finally, the 'underconfidence-with-practice effect' describes how we often under-estimate the memory benefits of multiple study-test cycles. Like several illusions, this last effect stems from poor metamemory, which is discussed later.

J Jennifer Aniston neurons

It's fair to say that the neuroscientific world was stunned in 2005 by the description of 'Jennifer Aniston neurons'. The 'grandmother cell', once discredited, was suddenly back in the spotlight. The notion of a grandmother cell arose from the debate over how our brains store information and concepts. The hypothetical grandmother cell is only activated when a person sees, hears, or otherwise discriminates their grandmother. In one extreme version, we contain a single grandmother cell (or just handful), and these are the only ones that encode that specific concept.

As a prelude to the surgical removal of brain tissue responsible for intractable epilepsy, a patient may have recording electrodes implanted to confirm the source of the seizures. This procedure creates the unique opportunity to measure the activity of individual neu-rons in awake people. From this start point, Rodrigo Quiroga and his colleagues published a set of findings that set the neuroscientific world alight. They found neurons in the medial parts of the temporal lobe that responded in a highly selective way to specific stimuli. One such stimulus was Jennifer Aniston (Quiroga et al., 2005).

Rodrigo Quiroga described a neuron in the hippocampus that consistently increased its activity whenever the patient was shown a photograph of the 'Friends' star, Jennifer Aniston. That same neuron showed little or no reaction to other photographs, which also included other famous people. It did, however, react to Lisa Kudrow, a co-star in 'Friends'. The only Jennifer Aniston photo the neuron did not react to was when she was pictured with Brad Pitt (whom she subsequently divorced).

Another hippocampal neuron in a different patient responded selectively to photographs of Halle Berry, as well as the name of the same film star. While the neuron responded to Halle Berry dressed as Catwoman, it did not react to other people dressed as Catwoman. Other neurons have been found that selectively and consistently responded to Julia Roberts, Kobe Bryant, Diego Maradona, Mother Teresa, Luke Skywalker, as well as the Sydney Opera House and the Tower of Pisa. These various identity neurons were located in the hippocampus or in the adjacent parahippocampal cortex.

Identity neurons appear to encode an abstract representation of the concept triggered by the stimulus. This explanation fits with how these same cells may respond to the written name of the person or hearing that same name. For this reason, they have also been called 'concept cells'. It is probably a mistake, however, to imagine that a given cell only responds to just one individual. Indeed, cells have been found that respond to two different basketball players, while the Luke Skywalker cell also responded to Yoda from 'Star Wars'.

The impression that these neurons somehow captured the abstract representation of a specific entity resurrected the concept of the 'grandmother cell'. As explained, this hypothetical cell is only activated when a person sees, hears, or otherwise discriminates their grandmother. This is an immediately attractive idea as it seems to explain our exceptional ability to identify the same entity from different perspectives or different cues. This idea, raised in the 1960s, was, however, rapidly dismissed at the time. The proposal suffers from the obvious problem that if our grandmother cell were to die, then the concept of our grandmother would also disappear.

While a Jennifer Anniston neuron is highly reminiscent of a grandmother cell, there is no reason to believe that the cell is unique, rather it is one of many that share those attributes. Indeed, if only one neuron out of the many millions in the medial temporal lobe represented Jennifer Anniston, the scientists would never have discovered that specific match.

Given these facts, it has been estimated that of the 10^9 neurons in the medial temporal lobe, around 10^6 (one million) are involved in the representation of a given concept, such as Jennifer Aniston or Halle Berry. At the same time, each of one of these 10^6 medial temporal neurons might encode up to a few dozen of the 10,000–30,000 things a person can recognise. These representations may form the building blocks of our explicit knowledge base.

K Knowing your own memory: Metacognition and metamemory

The term 'metacognition' describes our understanding of our own cognitive processes. It is not always accurate. One obvious example is that 65% of Americans believe that they possess above average intelligence (Heck et al., 2018). I might add that the bias to believe that you are above average intelligence is more exaggerated in men rather than women. Within metacognition is the ability to monitor your own memory capabilities, this is called 'metamemory'.

When considering metamemory it is difficult not to begin with a famous statement made by Donald Rumsfeld in 2002 concerning the Iraq war. He said *"as we know, there are known knowns; there are things we know we know. We also know there are known unknowns; that is to say we know there are some things we do not know. But there are also unknown unknowns— the ones we don't know we don't know."* His statement captures the essence of metamemory and some of its limitations.

Imagine you are watching a TV quiz, and the contestant is asked 'What is a jerboa? You may realise that you have no idea as to the answer correct – *"the known unknowns"*. On the other hand, you might think you know the answer – *"the known knowns"*. You may also be able to also judge how confident you would be of getting it right if you had to choose from various options. [A jerboa is: a) a type of drinking vessel, b) a type of rough cloak, c) a small desert animal, or d) the leading feather on a wing.] Metamemory is pushed to the very limits in TV programmes such as 'Make Me a Millionaire' where participants will gamble huge sums of money based on the strength of their belief that they know the correct answer.

The cognitive process at the heart of metamemory is not the memory itself, rather, the awareness of the memory. This awareness helps us to track our learning and stop us from wasting time on something we have already acquired. It also helps us to predict those future memory tasks that will be easy and those that will be challenging. For example, Willem Wagenaar's famous five-year diary study showed that he was good at predicting his subsequent ability to remember an event several years later, though he tended to be overconfident. This same predictive ability helps us to decide when to offload those memory tasks that we think will prove too demanding by, for example, making notes on our phones or writing down lists.

A familiar aspect of metamemory is the 'feeling of knowing'. This is the cognitive sense that we know that we know something, even if it cannot be retrieved. One frequent consequence is the 'tip-of-the-tongue' effect. Not only do we know that the memory exists, but we can also often describe some of its attributes such as the first letter or the number of syllables, along with how confident we are in our ability to eventually retrieve the target word. To generate the effect, you might wish to try and remember the name of the disillusioned weatherman in the film 'Groundhog Day'.

Returning to the question of 'what is a jerboa?', when people cannot recall the answer, they are still better than chance at judging whether they will correctly pick out the correct answer from among false answers that they have yet to see. In other words, they know whether a memory has previously been established. However, many people are overconfident in their judgements of knowing. This overconfidence persists even when given the opportunity to bet against the experimenter for real money. (A jerboa is a small desert animal.) This same bias has been termed the 'overconfidence effect', the tendency to have an unreasonable confidence in one's own answers. This same bias is often present in those who think they have a particularly good sense of direction. Likewise, it is this overconfidence effect that helps to explain why 65% of Americans think they are above average intelligence and why 85% of American drivers think they are better than average drivers.

Students are prone to overconfidence when predicting future exam results. In one study, students took no less than 13 exams in an introductory course on educational psychology (Foster et al., 2017). Not only were many students overconfident, but their overconfidence did not decline across the multiple exams. Furthermore, their predictions were often unrelated to their prior exam scores. It is clear that many students underuse past performance, despite its value in making more accurate future predictions. Even after receiving feedback, those people who tended to be overconfident often persisted with this bias.

Rather alarmingly, overconfidence is also seen among investors as their memories are positively skewed. They tend to recall their money returns as being better than they really were and are more likely to remember winning, rather than losing, stocks. As you might guess, the overconfidence bias, along with the gambler's fallacy, are important cognitive props for pathological gamblers. (The gamblers fallacy concerns the likelihood of random events, and the misguided belief that it is affected by the outcome of past events. If successive coin tosses land on heads nine times in a row, the likelihood of a tail on the tenth toss still remains at 50%.)

Another area of practical concern is the relationship between confidence and accuracy for eye-witness testimony. The ability to detect whether one's memory is real is thought to depend, in part, on reality-monitoring, as real memories are presumed to contain more contextual, sensory, and semantic detail, as well as feeling more plausible. In addition, our knowledge of how memory works can add to that information. For example, a memory that readily comes to mind with little effort would be perceived as being stronger and more likely to be accurate. Consequently, we are more confident about memories that feel easier to retrieve. In practice, this is often a good rule of thumb. When participants watched a film of a staged crime, incorrect memories appeared more effortful and were rated as less confident. However, as you increase retention delays, both accuracy and confidence judgments decrease. Worryingly, the confidence–accuracy relationship also deteriorates over time so that those remaining high confidence responses start to contain relatively more errors.

L L learners: Spaced versus massed practice

Knowing the right thing to do is often easy, putting it into practice can be surprisingly difficult. It is very likely that you have been told that it is better to space out learning rather than cramming it all at the last moment. Yet, massed (or block) training is often more convenient and can lead to quick gains. Consequently, it often feels effective. Indeed, for those of us who procrastinate, massed learning it is often an inevitability. So, it is worth considering whether spaced learning, also called distributed practice, is as good as it is claimed to be.

Before going further, it is helpful to appreciate that when psychologists compare spaced with massed learning they focus on performance after the same total time spent learning. It is almost inevitable that massed training will initially race ahead if performance is simply judged against the interval from the start gun.

As 'L' is the sign for learner drivers I will first consider different training strategies for passing the driving test (Figure 19.5). The strategy we adopt matters as it will affect your finances, the likelihood of passing, and your resulting safety. Much of the current advice on the internet is for learners to take frequent block (massed) lessons in order to pass the test quicker, claiming that this is also beneficial for your brain (not true) and bank balance. There seems to be a concerted push for intensive courses, which include lessons that last from two up to five hours.

The RAC (Royal Automobile Club) appears to support this idea as its current website states that "*Intensive courses (otherwise known as the poorly named 'crash course') will give you the best chance of passing your driving test in the shortest amount of time.*" As you will spot, this advice is misleading. If by 'the shortest amount of time' the RAC is referring to the date from your first lesson then this is very likely to be true. If by 'the shortest amount of time' the RAC is referring to total lesson hours (and total cost), then they will be wrong if spaced learning is more effective.

Although Learner drivers do not appear to have been systematically studied, it is possible to predict the winner with some confidence. For other perceptual-motor skills, the findings are remarkably consistent. Spaced training is far more effective. This is true for mirror-drawing, for learning medical procedures, for the many sports that have been tested, for music-making, for the skill components of computer games, and much more.

In one famous study, British Post Office sorters were trained to type (Baddeley & Longman, 1978). Four different training regimes were compared. The best rate of learning was in those sorters receiving one hour of training each day (spaced condition), while the worst was in those receiving two two-hour sessions each day (massed condition).

Figure 19.5 L is for learner.

The spaced training meant that far fewer total hours of training were needed to reach the same level of typing proficiency (55 hours versus 80 hours). In addition, the spaced training led to much better retention of those new typing skills after the completion of training. Improved retention is an added bonus associated with spaced learning, and one that is repeatedly observed.

While we do not appear to have objective data for driving lessons, there is every reason to believe that it is just like other perceptual-motor skills. Not only should spaced learning be more efficient regarding total lesson-hours, but spaced training is likely to ensure better subsequent retention, which must be a good thing given the gravity of getting things wrong. Nevertheless, more condensed training is popular for various reasons. Along with the sense of rapid gains, there is the greater ability to predict when to book a test.

An opportunity exists to determine the best training regime by the use of driving simulators. We already know from driving simulators that making errors, followed by correction, is more valuable than errorless driving. It is thought that responding to errors helps with the transfer of skills and reduces misplaced self-confidence. In other words, getting it wrong can help – but preferably not on a hazardous road.

Sticking with Learner drivers for the moment, there is understandable interest in the number of lessons that give you the best chance of passing your test. This number will be much affected by the training regime (massed versus spaced), by the on-road demands of the driving test in that country, as well as their supervision rules, which vary enormously from country to country. In the U.K., the RAC along with the Driving Standards Agency recommend about 45 hours of professional lessons as well as 20 hours of supervised practice before taking your test.

Some countries demand a minimum number of hours of driving experience, which may have to include professionally supervised instruction. However, these rules vary enormously both across and within countries. For example, three states in Australia, including New South Wales, require 120 hours of supervised driving prior to taking a road test. Western Australia only requires 50 hours. In the U.K. there is currently no requirement, so that the minimum is zero hours before taking a test.

Beware of overconfidence. There is repeated evidence that crash risk initially *increases* as the hours of practice rise prior to obtaining a licence. At first sight, this correlation makes little sense, but part of the explanation concerns overconfidence – the illusion of mastery. The good news is that there must be an inverted U-shaped curve so that as practice hours continue to increase, crash rates start to decline. Studies of novice drivers in Sweden showed that those who took advantage of an extended period of supervised driving had far fewer crashes after passing their test. A practice effect can also be seen in the much-repeated finding that the risk of a car crash falls dramatically over the first year of licensed driving, starting from a worryingly high rate. These same statistics help to explain why states like New South Wales have opted for 120 hours of supervised training.

Returning to spaced versus massed practice, it is time to consider verbal learning. "*What European nation consumes the most spicy Mexican food?*" This was a trivia question used in one of the most ambitious studies of massed versus spaced learning (Cepeda et al., 2008). Over 1350 individuals were asked to learn 32 obscure trivia facts. (The surprising answer was Norway when measured by percentage of population). Each individual had an initial study session, followed by a second learning session, followed by retention test. Different gaps between these learning sessions (either 0, 1, 2, 7, 21, or 105 days) were given to different subjects, along with varying the subsequent interval before the retention test (7–350 days). The final results were clear. Spaced learning (one day or more between the first and second session) was consistently superior to re-learning just three minutes after initial learning ('massed').

All of the spaced learning conditions outperformed the massed condition. Increasing the interval between the first and second study initially improved performance but reached a tipping point so that performance began to slip back when the interval between the two learning sessions was as long as 105 days. However, these longer spacings were effective when the participants had to retain that information for a long time. This meant that there was no single spacing between the first and second learning session that was optimal, as that depended on how long you wished to retain that information. Or as the authors put it "*if you want to know the optimal distribution of your study time, you need to decide how long you wish to remember something*" (Cepeda et al., 2008).

Similar effects are seen when people learn a second language. Once again, spaced learning is superior to massed learning. Although, shorter spacing can be as effective as longer spacing when tested immediately, longer spacing was superior when retesting comes after a longer delay. This spaced training benefit for later retention was, for instance, seen when second language learning was tested as long as eight years after initial learning.

Again and again, spaced practice produces better learning and better retention over time. Although the disadvantages of cramming are less severe for information to be examined immediately, a later unexpected test will catch out those who crammed, as their forgetting will have been faster. It is, therefore, surprising that when given a choice, students typically opt for block (massed) learning. This preference probably reflects its familiarity, the sense of speedy acquisition, along with the illusion of mastery, as well as the fear of making more errors with longer intervals between learning sessions. In reality, making errors, followed by correction, is more helpful. This is one of the reasons why trying to retrieve information in the form a test before restudy can add to the effectiveness of spaced learning.

From the students' perspective, spacing might appear wasteful as it leaves blank intervals. But spaced learning can be embedded into other tasks. For example, by interleaving related but different problems, information spacing becomes time-effective. It may be easiest to understand this 'interleaving' by considering how to acquire sports-related skills. Rather than continually repeat the same action within a training session, different but related skills are mixed together. For tennis training this means combining shorter blocks of different facets of the game, rather than spending the session on just one, such as serving.

A similar interleaving benefit is seen when people learnt to identify the artists responsible for paintings they had not previously seen. Intermingling the paintings of the various artists was more effective than giving a block of one artist's paintings followed by a block of another artist. Further examples of the benefits of interleaved training include such diverse topics as maths learning and training nurses to distinguish different stethoscope sounds. Again, participants often thought that massed trials were more effective than spaced, interleaved trials. In reality, the opposite result was seen.

Finally, it is worth considering why spaced learning works. One intuitive explanation is that learners pay less attention to subsequent presentations of the same material when they are close together in time (massed). Reasons for paying less attention include the learner's misguided belief that the material is now known well enough to ignore. Support for this idea comes from comparisons of the study time given in massed or spaced conditions, where massed trials can lead to less inspection time when the same material re-appears.

An additional explanation centres on what is called 'encoding variability'. It is argued that by increasing the spacing between learning trials, you increase the likelihood that the target item is encoded in association with a wider array of other information. This encoding variability then provides more routes to retrieval. Other explanations are that spaced trials allow more cognitive rehearsals or independent reactivations, thereby aiding cumulative consolidation, and so increasing the persistence of the memory. Cramming is also likely to induce fatigue, as well as boredom.

There are also neuroscientific explanations for the benefits of spaced learning. These accounts typically centre on the idea that the intervals between massed trials are too short to take advantage of those neural consolidation processes that enable the summation of the same memory traces over successive trials. One such explanation is that massed training can saturate key plasticity mechanisms, so dampening the cumulative effect of two trials when they closely follow each other. Such accounts often centre around the idea of an unresponsive ('refractory') period so that the plasticity mechanisms for the same memory trace cannot be repeatedly recruited if they are too close together in time. A spaced trial can allow this refractory period to disappear. Another suggestion is that plastic mechanisms can be primed so that a second stimulus, at a suitable interval, can best promote neural changes that underly learning, such as dendritic spine growth. As is clear, there are both cognitive and neural explanations for the superiority of spaced learning. It is unlikely that just one explanation is sufficient to explain all the benefits of spaced learning.

M Mozart, music, and memory

There is a beguiling idea that playing certain classical music to our children (it has to be classical, of course) will somehow promote intellectual growth. Because of the music used in the original studies, this claim has been called the Mozart effect. In that study from 1993 by Frances Rauscher, it was reported that those college students who listened to Mozart's Sonata for Two Pianos in D Major (K448) for ten minutes showed a temporary improvement when performing certain spatial tests taken from the Stanford-Binet I.Q. test. These tests included the Paper Cutting and Folding Task, which involves mentally opening a folded piece of paper with cut sections and deciding its unfolded appearance.

In the original study the spatial benefit did not persist beyond the 10-15-minute test session. However, the same authors next reported that after hearing ten minutes of Mozart's Sonata K448, students performed better on the same Paper Cutting and Folding Task when tested on the following day, but not thereafter. The rationale given for selecting Mozart was that because he was composing at the age of four he may have exploited 'the inherent repertoire of spatial-temporal firing patterns in the cortex' (Rauscher et al., 1995). (This is the kind of neurobabble that should set alarm bells ringing).

From these transient, selective effects, the Mozart effect was born. The notion that classical music can stimulate learning had a meteoric rise in popularity. The original studies received much media attention, despite it being clear that any enhancement of spatial reasoning was temporary. This same publicity often implied that listening to Mozart would improve intelligence. These claims inevitably attracted parents. They also attracted entrepreneurs who created a variety of products based on the Mozart effect for those with infants and young children. By 1998, the Governor of Georgia, Zell Miller, tried to raise State money so that every newborn child in Georgia should be given a cassette or compact disc of classical music to make them smarter. Belief in the Mozart effect has persisted. A 2020 survey of Australian teachers revealed that 71% believed that listening to classical music increases children's reasoning ability (Hughes et al., 2020).

The persistence in this belief is remarkable as the initial findings were greeted with much scepticism given their apparent transience and the frequent failure of many psychologists to repeat the Mozart effect. These follow-up studies included an attempt to copy in full the original 1993 study. This replication found no evidence for the Mozart effect. The resulting debate was played out in a single issue of 'Nature' in 1999.

An analysis that combined the results of many studies concluded that there was no effect on general intelligence or reasoning, but there might be a small, temporary effect on transforming visual images. In response, Rauscher emphasised that the improvements they reported were for spatial reasoning and they did not claim wider improvement in I.Q. A decade later, the Mozart effect was largely discredited by experts, featuring in '50 Great Myths of Popular Psychology' (Lilienfeld et al., 2009). Nevertheless, it has remained popular, not least among Australian teachers.

If any Mozart effect does exist, it probably results from increased arousal and heightened mood, effects that explain its transience. Consistent with this account are claims that enhancement of the spatial paper folding task is linked to the tempo and mode of a Mozart sonata. Superior performance on the spatial task may be seen when the tempo of the music is speeded up or when played in a Major rather than Minor mode.

In summary, the 'Mozart effect' is capricious, transient, very restricted in nature, and often not present at all. In keeping with this conclusion, a review of nearly 40 studies by Jakob Pietschnig entitled 'Mozart effect–Shmozart effect: A meta-analysis', found little evidence for an enhancing Mozart-based effect. Quite rightly, such reviews have reasonably asked whether children's spatial skills might be better served through appropriate direct practice rather than indirectly through music, the latter having no reliable effects.

Talk of the 'Mozart effect' did not, however, die, instead it evolved. Do violin lessons help you to understand quantum physics? You may have come across the many claims that childhood music lessons can improve I.Q. The reality is that children with a higher I.Q. are more likely to take music lessons and more likely to persist, though not necessarily become 'real musicians'. In other words, the association between music lessons and higher I.Q. is correct, but it is not the music lessons that are boosting I.Q. Likewise, a recent major meta-analysis concluded that music training has no impact on academic achievement or on people's non-music cognitive skills (Sala & Gobet, 2020).

N Neuromyths in education: Eight seductive ideas

By adding the right prefix, you can enhance the apparent scientific legitimacy of almost any term. The word 'Neuro' has suffered terribly in this regard. A glance at the internet comes up with neuroenergy, neurogum, neuroteaching, neurotraining, neurowellness, and many more. Given that any experience will have a neural correlate, you can put 'neuro' in front of anything and claim legitimacy – anyone for neurotennis?

For the letter N, eight neuromyths are considered. The first seven all come from a recent survey of Australian teachers (Hughes et al., 2020). All seven were endorsed by over half of the teachers (the percentages are included). A curious warning is that being more knowledgeable about the brain does not protect teachers from believing in neuromyths. The eighth is the neuromyth that we only use 10% of our brains. This famous claim is added as the story has a new twist.

i *Short bouts of motor co-ordination exercises can improve the integration of left and right hemispheric brain function (94%).*

The hint of plausibility in this idea comes from how the right cerebral cortex is more directly connected with the left side of your body. The opposite pattern holds for the left hemisphere which, therefore, is more directly connected with the right side of your body. Consequently, bouts of co-ordinated exercise might conceivably encourage the two hemispheres to get together.

This logic falls down as soon as you realise that the left and right cerebral cortices are directly interconnected by the corpus callosum and the anterior commissure, two huge brain tracts. The corpus callosum, which may contain ~200 million nerve fibres, ensures that sensorimotor information is constantly shared between the two hemispheres and needs no prompting or warming up. Brain activity studies show that a particularly strong pattern of integration is seen between the same cortical areas in the two opposing hemispheres. Their cross-talk continues through what are called 'resting states', when participants are lying still and asked not to think of anything in particular. In other words, no exercise is needed to encourage the two hemispheres to work together, which they have been doing all your life.

ii *Exercises that rehearse co-ordination of motor-perception skills can improve literacy skills (91%).*

This claim also sounds plausible. Motor-perceptual skills are integral to aspects of schooling, most obviously for writing. Furthermore, there are correlations between school children's motor skills with their levels of reading and mathematics. Possible explanations for a causal link include a greater ease of translating visual representations of concepts when able to use manual methods such as drawing letters, counting beads on a string, or sorting shapes into groups. Other possible reasons include how mastering a perceptual-motor skill might free up cognitive space for other tasks. At the same time, there are many reasons why such a correlation could exist without having any causal relationship as both might stem from more widespread aspects of neural maturation and health.

Brain Gym® (also educational kinesiology or Edu-K) is marketed worldwide as a physical programme that will improve a range of cognitive skills, including memory and literacy. Endorsing light exercise, drinking plenty of water, and taking regular breaks is fine, but the rest of the programme is pseudoscience. Perhaps as a result of the many stinging criticisms, the current official sites only make the vaguest comments about brain mechanisms. We are, for example, reminded that exercise is good for the brain. This is correct, but I would suggest outdoor recreation, going to a real gym, or brisk walking.

One of the 26 Brain Gym® exercises is called 'cross crawl'. Practitioners of Brain Gym® tells us that bringing together the left and right sides of our bodies will facilitate connections across our brain, thereby, enhancing whole brain thinking (see Neuromyth #1). Meanwhile, the Brain Gym® exercise optimistically called the 'brain button' involves massaging below your collarbone to activate your reticular activating system (which does exist) so the brain is awake for learning. Practitioners also recommend rubbing your ears ('the thinking cap') as this helps to improve short-term memory and listening ability. This is all nonsense with no scientific basis.

The reality is that well-designed studies have repeatedly failed to find evidence of improved academic learning due to Brain Gym® (Stephenson, 2009). Coming back to the specific neuromyth, research has failed to demonstrate that perceptual-motor training is an effective aid to literacy. The neuroscientific basis of these programmes has also been refuted. I was going to leave the last words to Ben Goldacre who wrote in his terrific book 'Bad Science' (2008) that *"Brain Gym® is so obviously, transparently foolish that nothing they could say could possibly justify the claims made on its behalf."* The bad news is that this neuromyth is still with us, with countless books, videos, and programmes.

iii   *Individuals learn better when they receive information in their preferred learning style (e.g., auditory, visual, kinaesthetic) (79%).*

It is safe to say that every student is unique, and individual differences will affect learning. A progression from this belief is the idea that individuals have their own optimal 'learning style'. This seductive concept has been applied all around the world. For example, in 2016, over 90% of Colorado State University instructors endorsed the idea of 'learning styles'. Furthermore, teaching based around this core belief has been applied across all ages, from kindergartens to universities, and beyond.

There are many different variants of 'learning styles', but a common theme is that learners should be categorised by their preferred sensory modality. In practice, the distinctions are typically between visual (V), auditory (A), or kinaesthetic (K). The student should then be mainly taught via their preferred modality which, in turn, benefits their individual learning. This means that visual learners should be shown diagrams, colourful pictures, videos, and related material that appeal to the eye to help them learn and retain information. Auditory learners should favour sounds, while kinaesthetic learners should move and physically react as part of their learning. The application of learning styles is not, however, cost-free. Its adoption consumes limited time and resources, such as when determining a student's supposed learning style and then adapting lessons to match that style.

It is true that children and adults will express preferences about how they like information presented to them. It is also true that multiple routes to the same memory can aid recall. The core question remains, however, does the learning styles method work?

An initial pair of meta-analyses provided apparent support for the learning styles approach. But those same analyses have since been much criticised. A major issue was that those early reviews were highly reliant on findings from dissertations that had not been subject to proper independent review and were essentially 'unpublished'. In other words, their data sampling was inappropriate. Other faults were identified in how the data were analysed and interpreted. Subsequent meta-analyses that corrected earlier shortcomings have repeatedly failed to find any consistent evidence that learning styles, as a teaching method, works. Such findings have led to the impassioned plea to "*stop propagating the learning styles myth*" (Kirschner, 2017). Nevertheless, recent surveys indicate that learning styles is still a staple of education practice, showing that this popular myth has yet to be effectively debunked.

iv   *Children are less attentive after consuming sugary drinks and/or snacks (75%).*

As described in the section *Smart drugs, supplements, and self-brain stimulation*, in the short-term, the opposite is often closer to the truth. That said, a dip in attention and arousal after a meal (post-prandial) is a real phenomenon. There are many different explanations for this all-too-frequent experience. Of practical concern is how schooling should be scheduled in the afternoon given this dip.

v   *Listening to classical music increases children's reasoning ability (71%).*

From reading the M entry (*Mozart effect – is it real?*) it should be apparent that this does not work.

vi   *A common sign of dyslexia is seeing letters backwards (66%).*

This idea dates back to the notion that letter reversal indicated problems with cerebral dominance that were associated with dyslexia. Consequently, interest focussed on whether readers switch letters such as p and q, as well as b and d (e.g., cob versus cod). While it is the case that poor readers will sometimes make letter sequence and reversal errors, the rate at which this occurs within total errors is often no different from that seen in good readers. For this reason, it is not diagnostic for dyslexia, although the idea has persisted. That said, there may be some dyslexic subgroups that do find left/right letter reversals particularly challenging.

vii   *Some of us are 'left-brained' and some are 'right-brained' and this helps explain differences in how we learn (56%).*

This myth stems from the false idea that some people predominantly use their left hemisphere, while others predominantly use their right hemisphere. This idea is at best a metaphor!! (I hate using exclamation marks but sometimes it feels necessary.) Yes, some people have better verbal skills than others, but it does not mark them out as being left-brained. Likewise, others may seem more creative, but they are not right-brained. Indeed, it would be impossible to be 'left-brained' or 'right-brained', however, hard you tried, and that includes learning to draw with your left hand, should you be right-handed. I mention this last example as the internet is full of bogus claims that this will enhance your creativity because it stimulates your right hemisphere.

It is true that the two hemispheres make slightly different contribution to cognition, most obviously for language. But, as already observed, there are something like 200 million nerve fibres in the corpus collosum, which is just one of the pathways that directly intercon-nect our two cerebral hemispheres. These interconnections ensure that we continually ben-efit from coordinated activity across these hemispheres. Furthermore, brain activity studies of visual creativity do not find a right hemisphere monopoly, instead both hemispheres are engaged. Likewise, language functions are not the preserve of the left hemisphere, as the right hemisphere makes many contributions. All cognition engages both hemispheres, so please never ever label someone as 'left-brained' or 'right-brained'.

viii   *We only use 10% of our brains (38%).*

The origins of this well-known claim can be traced back to the plausible claim that we do not harness our full mental potential. As far as anyone can tell, that infamous 10% figure was plucked out of the air, being used in 1929 in a self-help advertisement. Remarkably, the idea took seed and persisted in those who should, perhaps, know better. As mentioned in the introduction, a recent survey found that over a third of Australian school teachers still believe in the myth. Surveys in countries such as the U.K. and the Netherlands give similar results.

Neuroscientists refute this claim by pointing out that when brain activity is measured we do not encounter large areas of sleeping neurons. Neither do whole brain areas simply switch off, becoming silent. This evidence comes from neuronal recordings in animals, including those made in humans, along with measures from non-invasive brain imaging methods such as MRI. It is also clear that different parts of the brain support different functions, yet no function-less areas have been found. Other counter-evidence comes from estimates of how the brain consumes around 20% of the energy we utilise, so maintaining vast numbers of neurons that do nothing would make no biological sense.

As ever, there is the risk of overconfidence. Scrutiny of brain recording studies seems to reveal large numbers of neurons that appear silent, or have very low firing rates, or only fire to very specific stimuli. Even when state-of-the-art methods are used that should simulta-neously reveal almost all active neurons, large proportions of cortical neurons can appear largely unresponsive. These seemingly inactive cells have been described as 'dark neurons', with a nod to 'dark matter'. One reason is that, like dark matter, they may make up the majority of cortical neurons in the brain, with estimates of between 60% and 90%.

To explain their relative silence, it is thought that these neurons are held in an inhibited state, despite the energy costs to the brain. One speculation is that these silent circuits once supported functions in our evolutionary ancestors, functions that are no longer required. If correct, this implies that vast numbers of silent neurons have somehow eluded natural selection, given their energy costs. A different argument is that silent neurons are normally held inactive as otherwise the energy costs would simply be too great.

Another possibility that silent neurons create potential reserves for neural recovery and plasticity. Related, recent discoveries show how silent synapses, which are located at the ends of processes called filopodia, can be recruited into action. Their prior silence may mean less interference with previously acquired information, creating cleaner learning. For this same reason, they may have an important role in rapidly learning new information, by being able to start from a clean slate.

O Openness and the three Rs (reproducibility, robustness, and replicability)

Since the 2010s, both Psychology and Neuroscience have been in crisis. The source of that crisis stems from a simple question that sits at the heart of the scientific method. If I were to replicate a published finding, would I find the same result? If a key finding can be replicated then it may well be worthy of further study. But, if it cannot be replicated then it should be abandoned or at least questioned. (To paraphrase a cynical remark, the impact of a scientific study is measured by the time that it holds up progress in that field.)

Scientists have often been guilty of taking published findings on trust and not spending time on replications. The reasons are simple. Replicating another study takes time and money. Furthermore, copying someone else's ideas is unlikely to bring scientific prestige or enhance the prospects of further funding.

Well before the 2010s there were warning signs. Statisticians had long been concerned about the probability level that is standardly used in both Psychology and Neuroscience to determine whether an experimental change has occurred (is 'significant'). That probability is less than one in twenty (or below 5% by chance, or $p < 0.05$). In other words, if you repeat a study one hundred times, the 'significant' effect should only happen by chance less than five times. In other words, the experimental effect is far more likely to be real.

In a heroic study completed in 2015, the Open Science Collaboration replicated 100 psychology studies, a third of which centred on learning and memory. With the magic probability of $p < 0.05$ you might expect a successful replication well over 90% of the time. In reality it was around 40%. Put another way, less than half of the findings could be replicated. (For some psychology disciplines the replication level was less than 30%.) The only comfort was that those studies with the most statistical power and the largest effects were those most likely to be replicated.

The reasons for this replication failure are many but some have long been suspected. One major problem stems from publication bias, as journals are more likely to publish positive rather than negative findings. As a result, negative findings may gather dust as they go into the filing cabinet (hence the 'file drawer problem'). Other problems include a misplaced reliance on small sample sizes (giving low statistical power), along with an absence of any prior specification of planned data analyses. This last failure opens the door to what has been called 'P-Hacking', in which data are dredged through to find one 'significant' result, or subjects are added until the magical $p<0.05$ is reached (or the experiment stopped as soon as $p < 0.05$ is reached). All of these common practices create false pictures. I should add that while deliberate scientific fraud does occasionally occur, it is thankfully very rare.

In fixing this crisis, there is renewed emphasis on Openness and the 3Rs. Psychologists are increasingly expected to share all of their methods and all of their findings (not just the ones that were published). This culture of Openness also includes what is called 'pre-registration'. For this, the authors publish what they are going to do and how they will and will not interrogate the findings. Pre-registration helps to combat the hiding of negative results and P-Hacking.

The term 'Reproducibility' refers to the belief that if someone else analyses your data they will arrive at exactly the same results. Rather than being at 100%, reproducibility in Psychology is currently around 70% because of unavailable data or poor statistical analyses. 'Robustness' refers to whether the claimed findings are matched by complementary aspects of the data.

The importance of Replication has already been flagged, but this is not a straightforward goal. Once a finding seems well-established researchers may well be reluctant to try and publish a failed replication, feeling that they must have made a mistake. To complicate matters, an exact replication of a previous Psychology study is logically impossible, as all experiments are unique in some way. This challenge is made all the more demanding without full and open disclosure of methods and data.

Psychology, and Science in general, has had to take a long hard look at itself over the past decade. There is a call for greater openness, including the safeguard of pre-registration.

There is also a need for studies with more participants, greater statistical power, better statistical methods, and a willingness to publish 'failed' studies.

P Parrot learning: Learning by rote

Parrot learning means acquiring knowledge by repetition without necessarily understanding what it means. At school I was required to memorise the first 14 lines of Henry V's famous speech before the walls of Harfleur from Shakespeare's play. (I still have no idea why). The extraordinary thing is that I can still recite that speech, which begins '*Once more unto the breach, dear friends, once more…..*' My recitation stops abruptly at the 14th line, which is '*swill'd with the wild and wasteful ocean*', though I had no idea what many of the words meant.

I learnt these words by repetition, often called 'rote learning'. These thoughts prompted me to contact a classmate and ask him whether he also remembered the same 14 lines. Despite an interval of over 50 years, he did so. This anecdote highlights how repetitive learning can work, though in this case much aided by the rhythm and balance of the words. By contrast, my numerous failed attempts to learn the words of the Welsh National anthem painfully highlight the limitations of this approach. (More about that particular challenge to come.)

You might be surprised to discover that a playwright's contract often stipulates that an actor who deviates from the play's exact wording can be replaced. It is not sufficient to remember the gist, each word must be recalled. One of the greatest theatrical challenges is playing Hamlet. With around 30,000 words, Hamlet is Shakespeare's longest play. There are over 11,000 words for Hamlet himself. Given the enormity of the task and the need to get it absolutely right, it seems natural to assume that professional actors learn their parts by rote. As far as we know, this is not the case.

Actors may begin by learning the overall structure of a play, but this strategy is clearly not sufficient. As far as we know, actors unwittingly employ many of the same learning methods highlighted in this book. These memory aids include elaborative imagery and considering the same scene from the perspective of different characters, both of which employ deeper processing allied to imagery. In addition, the actor may break sections into chunks that reflect the steps in a speech, utilise mood congruency (trying to match your mood to that of the material), and identify those details that make a particular section unique. There are many similarities with the strategies used by mnemonists (see Chapter 9, *Superior memory for all: Mnemonics, memory, and imagery*). But that is not the end of the process. There is still the challenge of anticipating the mental and emotional interactions between the actors at every moment of the play.

You might also want to spare a thought for opera singers. They have to learn the musical notes along with the correct words, which are often in an unfamiliar language. Using an unfamiliar language reduces working memory capacity and removes the scaffolding provided by prior knowledge that, in turn, boosts long-term memory. Consequently, learning a song in a foreign language can prove daunting. John Redwood's famous inability to sing the National Anthem of Wales (*Hen Wlad Fy Nhadau*) when Welsh Secretary shows just how difficult this can be.

Even though rote learning often gets a bad press, it remains popular in East Asian education. There are understandable pleas for Western educationalist to be more sympathetic to these cultural differences. Advocates of learning methods within China stress how their methods are more than just rote learning, and that trained memorisation will lead to deeper understanding. It is also said that repetitive rote learning is an effective way to learn the Chinese language characters and the four-character Chinese idioms.

A common criticism of rote learning is that it is superficial, leading to inflexibility. Consequently, the learnt knowledge may struggle to transfer to novel problems. Like so many of my generation, I leant the multiplication tables by rote. Not the most enjoyable of experiences for teacher or pupil. The potential rigidity of rote learning can be seen when you consider the simple multiplication $4 \times 6 = 24$. In a hidden form, this same calculation pervades a host of mathematical problems that appear different yet require the same basic knowledge. Examples could include $4 \times 16 = 64$, $40 \times 60 = 240$, $0.4 \times 0.6 = 0.24$, $0.04 \times 0.06 = 0.0024$, $\frac{1}{4} \times \frac{1}{6} = \frac{1}{24}$, 40% of $60 = 24$, and many more. The good news is that, in addition to rote learning the multiplication tables, these same calculations can be learnt in many other ways, including visual aids, toys, finger multiplication, the abacus, Napier's bones, and a host of interactive games on the internet.

It seems only fair that the last word should go to parrots (Figure 19.6). Parrots can indeed be trained to acquire many tricks, seemingly without understanding their nature,

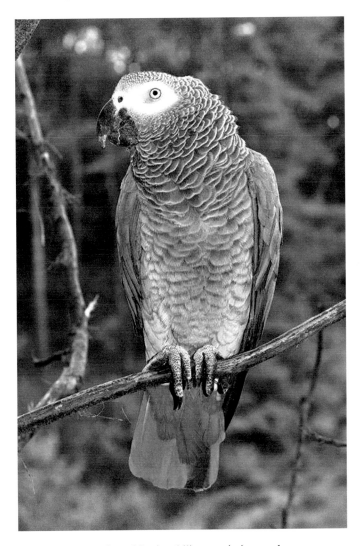

Figure 19.6 African grey parrot – famed for its ability to mimic speech.

hence 'parrot learning'. But I may be maligning parrots. A star of the parrot-world is surely the African grey parrot called Alex, who was trained for three decades by Irene Pepperberg. Alex astonished the world with his enormous vocabulary, its apparent flexibility, and his outward comprehension of complex ideas. He could recognise quantities up to six, name different colours and shapes, and seemingly grasp concepts such as bigger and smaller.

Alex learnt over 100 words. These were not restricted to specific exemplars. He could, for example, voice the word 'key' to sets of keys with quite different appearances. He also appeared to ask questions. Apparently his final words were '"You be good, I love you. See you tomorrow", with which he signed off every night. Unsurprisingly there has been much controversy over the nature of his accomplishments, whether they help to reveal the hidden depths of animal intelligence or whether they reflect little more than a highly complex form of discrimination learning. My advice is just to enjoy the many jaw-dropping videos of Alex on the internet.

QI Quite interesting and quite curious

The long-running BBC programme QI (which stands for 'Quite Interesting') derives its success from countless Aha! moments (see *The 'generation effect' and memory*) combined with how we are more engaged when interested, so furthering memory. The phrase 'curiosity-driven learning' captures this very notion. I personally find it quite interesting that the word 'curiouser' does not appear in my 'Oxford English Dictionary', despite being part of a well-known phrase made up by Lewis Carroll ("*Curiouser and curiouser!*" from 'Alice's Adventures in Wonderland'). A further, quite interesting fact is that the word 'quite' has different meanings in the U.K. and U.S. In the U.K. 'quite good' reflects modest approval, sometimes with a hint of disappointment. In the U.S., 'quite good' means extremely good. Getting these two forms wrong can prove quite embarrassing.

Both psychologists and educationalists have long been curious about the nature of curiosity. It is generally agreed that the word curiosity has two different connotations – having a general desire to seek new information or having the narrower goal of solving an uncertainty about a specific gap in one's knowledge (an 'information gap'). Advocates of the former meaning see curiosity as a personality trait, meaning that individuals vary in a relatively stable manner on this measure. Indeed, curiosity is regarded as a critical component of the 'Openness to Experience' trait, which is one of the 'Big Five' personality traits. Given that the derived trait of curiosity predicts better learning and academic success, there is much interest in how best to enhance this feeling of curiosity.

It is agreed that stimulating curiosity is central to effective education. The benefits to learning caused by high curiosity are long lasting and can be demonstrated weeks later. Increased curiosity is presumed to encourage deeper levels of processing and heightened motivation. But it is more than that because once you are 'curious', any incidental learning for adjacent information you have not explicitly been asked to learn, also improves.

Research into student learning also shows how the extent of an 'information gap' can matter. The term refers to the amount of missing information that is needed to solve a task or complete a problem. Those students with a large information gap found learning more difficult. This pattern was interpreted as reflecting low curiosity as the challenge to complete the 'gap' seemed too great. However, when individuals are close to resolving an information gap, their curiosity is increased, and their learning is better. A similar effect is seen when we suffer 'tip-of-the tongue'. Because we feel very close to the answer, a small information gap, we are even more driven to come up with the recalcitrant word.

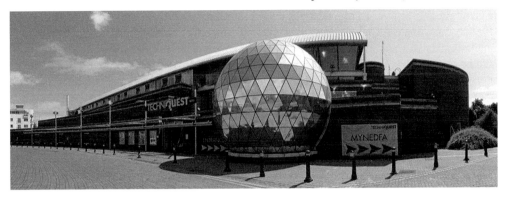

Figure 19.7 TECHNIQUEST, the hands-on science museum in Cardiff, designed to generate curiosity.

Given the importance of curiosity for education, it is useful to know how it might be increased. One approach is to complement traditional teaching with a series of tasks or puzzles that can only be solved by acquiring the target information. This approach also taps into the 'generation effect' (see *G for The 'Generation Effect', the Aha! moment, and memory*) as self-generated guesses are involved. Other applications include, when learning a second language, the provision of sentences with missing words for completion. It is also possible to approach this issue from the other end – namely, help students to identify the information gaps in their knowledge, which in turn may stimulate curiosity. The success of the many 'hands-on' science museums around the world (Figure 19.7) exemplify the enjoyment when curiosity and generation effects combine.

Additional educational methods include introducing a short, unpredictable delay before providing the feedback containing the correct answer. This delay-of-feedback effect seems to be most reliable when participants are curious to know the answer, which can help to create an Aha! moment. A similar trick of slightly delaying sought after information is repeatedly used on TV and radio Quiz Programmes. The anticipation that is created adds to the curiosity and the feeling of subsequent reward.

We are beginning to appreciate how a state of interest and curiosity provokes brain changes that encourage learning. Experiments using fMRI have compared brain activity when given trivia questions that are rated as being either of low or high curiosity. It appears that being curious increases activity in the neurotransmitter dopamine. One action of increased dopamine activity is to enhance hippocampal-dependent learning. This effect is thought to benefit not only specific information that we are curious about, but also accompanying information that we encounter while feeling curious. The link with dopamine takes us back to the idea that curiosity is often seen as a means to complete an information gap, which feels rewarding.

R Return trip effect

You are not alone in thinking that the outbound journey to a place often feels longer than the return trip, even though the distance remains the same. This illusion, called the 'return trip effect', can occur whether the trips are by bus, bike, or even when watching someone else make a journey on video. People also often spontaneously report the effect after walking there and back again. I recently experienced a variant of the return trip effect when, as part of an exhibition, I enjoyed back-to-back, identical Virtual Reality trips through a 'French countryside' that showed paintings by Vincent Van Gogh. The second time felt much quicker.

The intuitive explanation is that we add less new information to our memory on the return trip. On the outward trip, the surroundings are novel, grabbing our attention and inviting new learning. Changes in the environmental, our mood, and other contextual features increase our perception of past time. These changes are likely to be most marked at the start of a new journey. The return trip is familiar so there is less new information to learn. Consequently, when looking back, the return trip seems emptier and, hence, shorter in time.

This memory loading explanation, however attractive, is probably incomplete. The return trip effect persisted when cyclists returning to their start point used one of two routes. One group retraced the now-familiar outward route, but the other group took a novel return route. Both routes were the same distance. The memory loading explanation predicts that the return trip effect would only affect those retracing the original route. In fact, both groups showed the return trip effect, which shortened the apparent duration of both return journeys by about 20%.

To explain these surprising results, it was proposed that the return trip effect is caused by a violation of one's initial expectations of the journey (Van de Ven et al., 2011). We expect the outward journey to take less time than actually required, making it longer than anticipated. In contrast, the duration of the return trip feels appropriate as we have re-adjusted our expectations to make them more realistic. Both the expectation account and the memory loading explanation predict a loss of the return trip effect for frequent journeys.

A different explanation focusses on the roles of anticipation and arousal. There is much evidence that emotional arousal affects the perception of time, often making intervals seem longer. It is supposed that we are often more aroused on the outward journey as it is unfamiliar, and that increased arousal can result in time seeming to slow down, causing an overestimation when we look back. For a desired destination, the increase in arousal might come from a mixture of eagerness and the wish to not be late. Meanwhile, a destination perceived as unpleasant is likely to provoke anxiety. The reduced arousal on the return trip then creates the difference in the perception of time.

To test this arousal hypothesis, people were shown either entertaining or boring videos. One set of participants were told that the upcoming video (from Saturday Night Live) is *"funny and is generally liked by most people who see it"* – creating greater anticipation and arousal. Other people were warned that the upcoming video (which was about accounting) *"is boring and is generally disliked by most people who see it"*. When asked how long it took for the videos to load before playing the respective films, the greater anticipation group (Saturday Night Live) felt that loading took longer, consistent with the idea that increased anticipation slowed the apparent passage of time (Chen et al., 2021).

Clearly, the causes of the return trip effect are not as simple as one might think. A number of factors appear to conspire to create the illusion that the return journey takes less time.

S Surprise and memory

Surprise stems from false expectations, which are drawn from memory. Take the one-liner *"Never trust atoms; they make up everything."* The joy of a good joke is not predicting the ingenious punchline. For the same reason, having to re-tell a joke is never a good idea.

Our memory plays a vital role in predicting the world about us, but surprises occur. These surprises are highly significant. The hugely influential Rescorla-Wagner Model (1972) of associative learning assumes that we learn fastest when events do not fit our expectations. The greater the difference between the predicted outcome and what actually happened (the prediction error), the greater the degree of learning. These expectations, based on past memory, exist because we constantly run simulations that predict the most likely next event and its outcome. Any anomaly with our predictions demands memory updating.

If this talk about prediction error sounds far removed from real life, you might be surprised to discover that the concept of a prediction error is now a cornerstone of cognitive neuroscience. This concept lies at the heart of many learning models, not to mention machine learning and Artificial Intelligence. It is now known that the difference between the predicted reward in a situation and the actual reward received (the reward prediction error) is signalled by the neurotransmitter dopamine. This neurotransmitter then helps to teach the learning system, including the hippocampus.

Surprise has other consequences. We try understand the cause of an anomaly. In doing so, we recruit more elaborative processing which, in turn, enhances memory encoding. The combined result is the better recall of surprising events. But we also need to determine just how much cognitive processing we should invest in resolving a surprising event. This calculation is needed because there are distinct degrees of surprise. Some unexpected events come ready-made with their explanations, while others are truly surprising, requiring an explanation from scratch. I might be surprised to see a rare vintage car on the road, but then that is where you expect to see cars. In contrast, my sighting of a full-size Dalek on a garage forecourt in Pontypridd defied everything I knew about both garages and Daleks. (Again, apologies if you have never seen 'Dr Who'.) Such challenging surprises are recalled more accurately. However, a totally bizarre, inexplicable statement is likely to be dismissed and poorly remembered.

Surprise is also inherent in the Von Restorff effect. Imagine hearing a list of words that all come from the same category (e.g., makes of cars), but then suddenly hearing the word 'chipmunk', before returning to the cars. 'Chipmunk' is likely to be recalled better than the surrounding car names. Likewise, a design that is radically different from its neighbours will stand out and be better remembered. In this way, an item that is 'isolated' from its neighbours will be better recalled. For this reason, current explanations of the Von Restorff effect centre on the added attention given to the item that seems out of context,

These same effects have been exploited in marketing, where attempts are made to make slogans or products that stand-out by being radically different from their competitors. During COVID-19 there were many signs about social distancing. One striking sign proclaimed, "Think Distance, Think Cow". Figure 19.8 shows an even more striking Australian version. These signs were effective as the combined image of a person and a cow (or three koalas) would be highly unusual and unexpected given the subject matter, while a cow length is something most of us can readily appreciate.

For many surprises there is an added emotional aspect, be it good or bad. Emotional arousal initiates a set of brain mechanisms involving the amygdala and hippocampus that boost memory. While I could not find any studies that have tested whether a surprise birthday party is especially memorable, there is a clear prediction that it would be.

T Truth serums

Understandably, there is much interest in whether 'truth serums' exist. The idea that a drug might make us so compliant that we willingly and accurately retrieve our memories is both fascinating and horrifying. Interest in truth drugs goes far back in time. The Roman

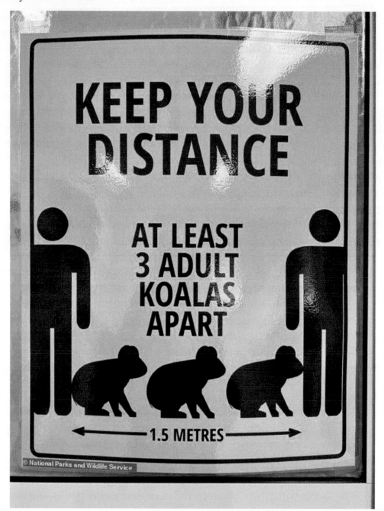

Figure 19.8 Australian sign explaining social distancing during COVID.

philosopher, Pliny the Elder, is reported as saying 'In vino veritas', or 'in wine there is truth'. In reality, alcohol would make a very poor 'truth drug' as it directly disrupts memory and further impedes recall by creating state-dependent effects, although it can reduce inhibition.

The first use of a supposed truth serum is often credited to the Texan obstetrician Robert House in 1922. He claimed that women in childbirth when given scopolamine (an acetyl choline antagonist) would become drowsy, yet still able to give accurate responses to questions, with some answers being surprisingly candid. House thought that scopolamine could help when interrogating reluctant suspects. Amazingly, he was permitted to give scopolamine to two prisoners in the Dallas County jail. Both men were believed to be guilty, both denied guilt under scopolamine, and both were eventually acquitted.

The use of scopolamine was subsequently rejected in a U.S. court case in 1926, which questioned both its scientific rationale and effectiveness. The rationale for scopolamine is indeed perplexing. Not only does the drug cause drowsiness, but it also causes memory loss (see Chapter 17, *Losing memory: Amnesias and simulated amnesias*). It has, for example, been used to create animal models of memory loss in aging and dementia. At higher doses it causes incapacitation and amnesia.

Nowadays, the term truth drug or truth serum is usually applied to barbiturates such as sodium pentothal (Figure 19.9). Other drugs that have been investigated include psychedelics, including LSD. The goal of these drugs is to reduce inhibition and increase talkativeness. For example, barbiturates were sometimes used after World War II to help those with post-traumatic stress disorder to recall painful memories. In 1947, the U.S. military first attempted to manufacture an effective truth serum when it initiated project Chatter, which was followed by a series of CIA projects, including MK Ultra and MK DELTA. Favoured drugs included barbiturates, which act as depressants. At the right dose, such drugs might leave someone less inhibited and more talkative. However, there is no evidence that this drug-induced state also improves recall accuracy, while there are legitimate concerns about heightened suggestibility.

Nowadays, most countries ban the use of such drugs in legal cases, citing both ethical concerns and their lack of proven effectiveness. For example, in 1963, the U.S. Supreme Court ruled that confessions due to the administration of a truth serum were unconstitutionally coerced and, therefore, inadmissible. It has, for example, been argued that truth serums violate the fifth amendment of the U.S. Constitution, the right to remain silent. Nevertheless, as part of the investigations in the assassination of John Kennedy (J.F.K.), Perry Russo was interrogated in 1967 when under the influence of sodium pentothal.

The 911 attacks in the U.S. and their aftermath resurrected interest in the potential use of truth drugs. More recently, India has occasionally sanctioned the use of barbiturates during interrogation. One apparent example concerned the terrorist Ajmal Kasab, who was captured by police in the 2008 attacks in Mumbai. Despite their suspected use in several countries, it is worth remembering that 'truth serums' lower the threshold of reporting both

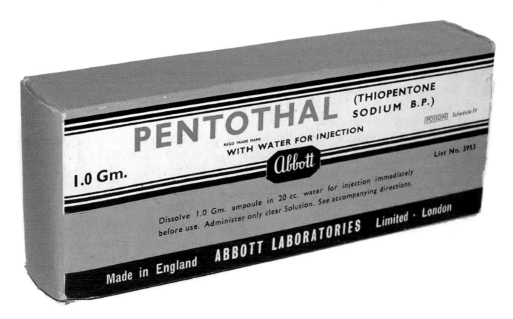

Figure 19.9 Sodium pentothal, one of the most famous drugs purported to be a truth serum.

true and false information. For this simple reason, they remain of no real value and may constitute a form of torture.

U Unconscious learning: Can you learn when anaesthetised?

In a dramatic study from 1965, with very dubious ethics, Dr Bernard Levinson staged a mock crisis during ten dental surgeries taking place under general anaesthesia. On each occasion, the anaesthetist exclaimed "*Just a moment! I don't like the patient's colour. Much too blue. His (or her) lips are very blue. I'm going to give a little more oxygen.*" Although none of the patients could explicitly recall these dramatic events, four subsequently provided detailed reports when under hypnosis (Levinson, 1965). This study has rightly been much criticised, and so please treat it with enormous scepticism. Nevertheless, it does capture the nightmarish possibility that we might remember being operated on, even though the surgeon believes you are unconscious.

While most people do not to remember anything from when under a general anaesthetic, a few claim that they can recall explicit details. Some of these rare cases stem from faulty anaesthesia, often associated with apparatus failure. These traumatic instances highlight the need to separate those patients who were truly unconscious and those who were lightly anaesthetised during the learning experience. Unfortunately, the depth of individual anaesthesia cannot be determined in many past studies.

Research into this question is typically opportunistic, taking advantage of surgical procedures that need to take place. The overall conclusion, you may be relieved to read, is that explicit memories are not formed when someone is correctly under general anaesthesia. Nevertheless, like sleep, implicit learning is possible. The implicit learning most often seen is priming. In a popular design, test words are given repeatedly during anaesthesia. This word exposure is followed by tests to see if that word has remained at the forefront of memory. In one such study, the word 'banana' was said multiple times. Following surgery, when patients were asked to generate an example of a fruit, the word 'banana' was offered more often than would be normal.

Other priming effects following surgery include stem completion. If you see the letters 'b a n' and asked to say the first word that comes into your mind, the word banana is likely to pop up if it has been said to you repeatedly during surgery. Conceptual priming, which implies accessing semantic knowledge, has also sometimes been observed following surgery, but is more associated with very light anaesthesia. It is safe to say that implicit learning during surgery is capricious, with about half of all studies finding any effects. Contributing factors probably include the type and depth of anaesthesia.

A different approach has been to implant suggestions during surgery, such as to touch your nose or your ear during the post-operative interview. There are inconsistent claims that such instructions can alter post-operative behaviour. Nevertheless, the few positive findings add to the possibility that comments made during surgery might affect later recovery. This intriguing possibility has been repeatedly tested but the findings are impressively inconclusive. To be on the safe side, it is probably best to focus on positive comments during surgery.

V Vegetative brain state, awareness, and new learning

Every now and then, a scientific discovery stops you in your tracks and causes you to look at things differently. One of those discoveries concerned patients in a 'vegetative state'. The term describes patients who show signs of wakefulness but remain entirely unaware of their surroundings. Consequently, they fail to display purposeful or voluntary behavioural responses to a host of stimuli yet maintain their sleep cycles, can show eye opening, and move spontaneously. Normal communication is not possible.

It was assumed that these patients were unaware of their environment. We now know that for some vegetative state patients this description is wrong. Not only does their brain activity reveal hidden levels of awareness but by voluntarily changing their own brain activity they can begin to communicate.

If you are asked to imagine playing tennis or imagine moving from room to room in a familiar house, two different patterns of fMRI brain activity are seen. The tennis scenario produces increased activity in motor and pre-motor areas, while moving between rooms increases activity in areas for spatial navigation. Astonishingly, when a young woman diagnosed as being in a vegetative state was asked to imagine these two different actions, her patterns of brain activity corresponded to those produced by people with normal awareness (Owen & Coleman, 2008). Consequently, her brain activity revealed an awareness of spoken commands, despite her diagnosis.

If nothing else, this remarkable demonstration, now repeated by others, highlights problems with the label 'vegetative state'. In response, the term 'cognitive motor dissociation' (CMD) has been introduced in the U.K. to describe those patients who behaviourally match the diagnosis of vegetative state but also show neuroimaging evidence of covert awareness. It is now thought that about one fifth of those patients diagnosed with prolonged disorders of consciousness are sufficiently aware to follow commands during a neuroimaging session.

There is, however more. Some vegetative state patients can use imagery to provide a neural 'word', for example, the word 'yes'. In this way a patient successfully answered the question "Is your father called Terry?" by imagining playing tennis (the signal for 'yes') when given the correct name. This ability not only requires covert awareness but learning the appropriate response for yes (thinking about tennis) and using working memory to decipher the question and then give the appropriate answer. These abilities raise any number of questions, including whether the patient could participate in making medical decisions.

Remarkably, a patient who emerged from a diagnosed vegetative state was able to report some memories from that time (Taylor et al., 2020). He was, for example, able to describe going into a brain scanner and could remember the name of one of his research team. This unique case highlights how someone who is behaviourally unresponsive might retain more cognitive abilities than expected from their diagnosis. The possibility of retained memory functions when in a vegetative state has obvious implications for both clinicians and family members when they are in the presence of the patient.

W White matter learning

Our brains have a lot of white matter. It makes up about one half of our brain's volume, and each adult has around 160,000 km of myelinated axons, should they ever be laid end to end. (That distance is the same as going around the world four times!) Instead, our axons often aggregate in parallel to create pathways that carry information across the brain. These pathways appear white because many axons have a fatty myelin sheath. Myelin creates an electrically insulated coat that speeds up nerve transmission. Faster transmission has enormous survival benefits, but that is not the only way in which white matter gives us an edge.

For many decades, neuroscientists studying memory mechanisms focussed on neuronal plasticity. Particular attention has been given to the synapse, the junction between neurons.

There is no doubt that synaptic changes are integral to new learning, but we now know that this far from the whole story. In recent years, white matter has come under the spotlight, aided by the development of non-invasive methods like diffusion imaging, which make it possible to measure the properties of our white matter (Figure 19.10).

Initial evidence that white matter changes contribute to learning came from the study of people who have spent thousands of hours learning specific sensorimotor skills. Both highly skilled musicians and professional ballet dancers display differences in the properties of those white matter tracts that support the demands of their respective careers. The question remains, however, whether those differences were a prerequisite to achieving exceptional performance or whether the thousands of hours of practice caused those white matter changes. To resolve this question, a longitudinal study was needed.

Heidi Johansen-Berg and her colleagues asked volunteers to practice juggling for six weeks. The researchers then showed that white matter pathways changed their properties in areas related to reaching and grasping (Scholz et al., 2009). This discovery was the gateway to subsequent studies showing how different types of learning can instigate changes in relevant white matter pathways. These studies also showed how quickly white matter changes can occur with training. For example, just two hours of training in a game that combined car racing and navigational skills affected the status of the fornix. The fornix is of particular interest as it is one the most important hippocampal pathways, being vital for normal navigation and memory.

In addition to learning motor skills, white matter changes can contribute to episodic memory. Adult participants received eight weeks of intensive verbal memory training in which they used the Method of Loci to help recall target words. Changes were found in anterior white matter regions that then correlated with memory performance, suggesting that these same changes made a real difference to performance levels. This conclusion has received added support from animal studies, where it is possible to closely regulate training and confirm any white matter changes.

There are many ways in which experience might influence our white matter, including the modification or production of more myelin, changes to its blood supply, glial cell

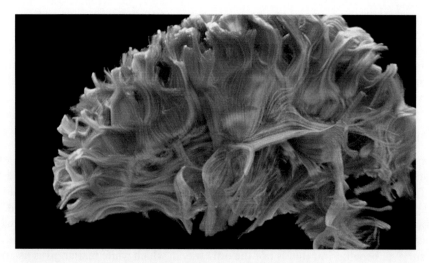

Figure 19.10 Reconstruction of the brain's white matter based on diffusion imaging.

Source: Derek Jones, Cardiff University, and Siemens Healthineers.

responses, as well as an increase or decrease in axonal diameter (Sampaio-Baptista & Johansen-Berg, 2017). In most diffusion imaging studies, training seems to increase myelin or increase the packing density of neurons. Curiously, some training studies produce the opposite pattern, for reasons that remain unclear. Nevertheless, it is firmly agreed that our white matter is responsive to experience. These white matter changes are presumed to help with the speed of information transfer and improve the signal to noise ratio.

Numerous factors affect white matter plasticity. Immature brains often have the most responsive white matter. Exercise is also thought to further promote white matter fitness, as does sleep quality. White matter health is yet another reason not to smoke, as smoking is strongly linked with both grey matter and white matter shrinkage. Alcohol also causes reductions in both grey and white matter. These brain changes begin to appear in those who consume only one to two units a day and increase as alcohol consumption increases. (A pint of a low-strength beer, lager, or cider contains about two units, while a small glass of wine is about 1.5 units). Unsurprisingly, aging affects our white matter. Alarmingly, estimates of total axon length reveal an astonishing decrease of about 45% from the age of 20 to 80. This equates to a 10% loss each decade. Clearly, the more we know about how to slow this decrease down, the better. There is a clear message – look after your white matter as it matters.

XX XY Sex differences and memory

Any discussion of sex differences is fraught with jeopardy and controversy. Reporting a statistical difference will have no meaningful bearing on the ability of any given individual. With enough subjects, even very small effects can become highly significant. There is, for example, an overall male advantage for visuospatial working memory, but to have a good chance of detecting this difference in an experiment you would probably need over 600 participants (Voyer et al., 2021). With such small effects, this section relies heavily on meta-analyses that help to identify those sex differences that emerge after combining the findings of many separate studies. These analyses are confined to adult participants. I have used the word sex as the term 'gender' is often applied to the social construct that need not be exclusive to men or women.

For verbal working memory, the pattern is rather mixed (Voyer et al., 2021). Large-scale analyses point to advantages for women on cued tests of working memory, while men may outperform women on complex span tasks. No overall sex differences are seen for simple span tasks (short-term memory), such as those involving serial recall. For visuospatial working memory, there is a small, overall male advantage across most, but not all, tasks. One of the more consistent differences is for mental spatial rotation tasks, though the explanation for the male advantage is much debated.

Sex differences for episodic memory are more consistent, as can be seen in a meta-analysis that combined data from 617 studies with over a million total participants (Asperholm et al., 2019). There was an overall female advantage for episodic memory. This advantage was present in all continents, apart from Africa, where any differences were small and unreliable. Furthermore, in studies of aging, it is repeatedly the case that elderly women outperform men on tests of episodic memory.

When different types of episodic memory tasks were considered there was a female advantage for verbal memory tasks, such as those involving single words, sentences, prose, or nameable images. This female advantage also extended to less obviously verbal tasks such as the memory for faces as well as sensory stimuli such as odours, tastes, and colours. Any male advantage was restricted to remembering routes and abstract images.

Current findings for semantic memory are based on much smaller samples and, hence, seem more preliminary. While females repeatedly perform better on tests of fluency, such as generating words from a starting letter or category, tests of general knowledge either indicate no sex difference or sometimes suggest a very modest male advantage.

Together, there is a repeating pattern. There is a female advantage for many aspects of verbal memory, set against a male advantage for aspects of spatial memory. This division has obvious similarities to the many anecdotal descriptions of sex differences in cognition. Navigation is a familiar example. A meta-analysis of navigation tests did, indeed, find that men outperformed women. Navigation is a complex problem that combines many cognitive skills. Tasks with sex differences included route selection, orienteering from compass directions, various map-based tasks, and the recall of navigational findings (Nazareth et al., 2019).

Understandably, there is considerable interest in why these sex difference occur. One explanation is that they reflect more general underlying differences in cognition that then feed into both working memory and episodic memory. For example, women outperform men on verbal tasks such as reading, comprehension, and verbal fluency, while men outperform women on some spatial tasks, including mental rotation. Although these same tasks should not directly tax episodic memory, they highlight sex differences in the ease and flexibility of processing different kinds of information. These processing advantages could then benefit episodic memory. Although this explanation feels plausible, it is incomplete as it fails to explain the origins of these same underlying cognitive differences. Possible causes include the actions of sex-related hormones on the brain, along with the consequences of stereotypical expectations, coupled with how life experiences differ across the sexes.

Support for this last explanation comes from an internet survey of navigational skills that attracted 2.5 million people from all over the globe (Coutrot et al., 2018). People from richer countries displayed better navigation skills on this video task than those from poorer countries. A likely part of the reason is that people in richer countries are more likely to drive than take public transport. While the anticipated sex difference was found, it was much affected by the level of gender inequality in the different countries. The greater the level of inequality, the bigger the apparent superiority of men. Conversely, in those countries with the least apparent gender inequalities, such as Finland and Norway, any differences on the navigational tasks between men and women were much reduced. Clearly, culture and the environment are playing a part.

Another approach is to compare female and male brains. An analysis of over 40,000 brain scans from the U.K. Biobank concluded that male brains are on average larger and that this difference is not entirely explained by body size (Williams et al., 2021). Likewise, counts of neurons in the neocortex gave lifetime averages of 19 billion neurons for female brains and 23 billion neurons for male brains. Again, this 16% difference could not fully be accounted for by differences in body size. After adjusting for total brain volume, sex differences appear to be widespread, being found in two thirds of 629 brain measures (Williams et al., 2021). Areas such as the left amygdala, thalamus, and temporal pole appeared relatively larger in men while parts of the cingulate, superior parietal, and lateral prefrontal cortices, along with the hippocampus, appear relatively larger in women. The cerebellum also displays sex differences as it is around 10% larger in males, again after adjusting for any differences in total brain volume. (Remember, this structure holds around 80% of all of the brain's neurons.)

Despite the size of the U.K. Biobank sample, there is inevitable debate about the reliability and implications of these findings. Furthermore, interpreting the causes and consequences of any volume differences remains conjecture. Volume changes are a key element of development, including the planned loss of neurons during gestation, followed by the pruning of synapses over successive years. These actions serve to streamline brain processing and, thereby, enhance capabilities. Big is not always better.

Y Y is money called money? The worship of memory

The addition of this unashamed piece of trivia hopefully falls into the 'quite interesting' category. There is a convoluted pathway from the word 'memory' to the origin of the word 'money'. The word memory comes from Roman Latin but has earlier roots in the ancient Greek word 'mnḗmē'. (Meme has been adopted to describe an image or an idea spread via the internet.) In Greek mythology, Mnemosyne was the goddess of memory. She was the mother of the nine muses (all fathered by Zeus on nine consecutive nights). After your death, if you drank from Mnemosyne's lake in the underworld you would remember your previous life, as she was the goddess of memory. But, if you drank from the river Lethe, your past life would be obliterated from memory. Words such as mnemonic and mnemonist derive from mnḗmē'/Mnemosyne.

The Roman counterpart to Mnemosyne was Moneta, her name being attached to one aspect of the goddess Juno. It was at or near the temple of Juno Moneta that the Romans first began minting coins. This link with Moneta gave rise to the word money. Her name was not completely forgotten. There was, for example, an image of Moneta on some $50 bills printed by the Confederate States of America.

Z Being at the end of the alphabet: Good or bad? (not to forget zebrafish)

My surname begins with the letter A, and I have always felt that this has given me an advantage. I came near the top of alphabetical lists at school as well as attendance lists at meetings, making my name more prominent. I hate to admit it, but the A may have benefited my scientific career. For one thing, lists of scientific references at the back of research papers or books are normally alphabetical. Those high in the list receive more attention, just ask Aardvark Trading Limited or AA Bike Hire (both real). Indeed, studies repeatedly show that in elections, those candidates placed alphabetically at the top of the list have an advantage. Additionally, U.S. stocks near the top of an alphabetical listing have about 5–15% higher trading activity and liquidity than the stocks that appear toward the bottom. Having a surname starting with an A may, indeed, raise your profile.

In a similar vein, an analysis of U.S. based scientific journals found that those papers whose first author had a surname earlier in the alphabet received more citations. (Scientists like citations as they are a measure of whether your research is having an impact.) There is an added advantage in those academic disciplines where the multiple authors of a study may be named in alphabetical order. This practice gives your name unfair prominence if it starts near the beginning of the alphabet. While most disciplines list authors by contribution, journals in some disciplines, including economics, would often list authors alphabetically.

These various advantages help to explain the findings from a survey of U.S. Economics departments. Those faculty members with earlier surname initials were more likely to receive tenure at the top ten economics departments and were significantly more likely to become fellows of the Econometric Society. But such alphabetic advantages can occur earlier in a career. For example, a 2010 report of Czech students applying to university found that the admissions process had a bias favouring those early in the alphabet.

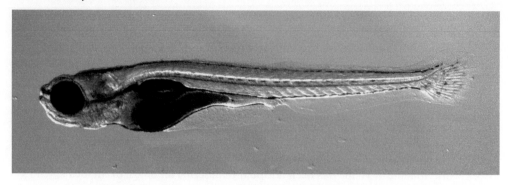

Figure 19.11 Zebrafish. A fish at 21 days-old showing its optical transparency that has made it so
popular with developmental biologists and geneticists.

There are, however, a few benefits of being near the end of the alphabet. A study involving thousands of invitations to review scientific papers in 2007 found that scientists with a surname beginning with the letter A received almost twice as many requests as those with a surname beginning with an S. Trust me, reviewing papers is very time consuming and largely thankless.

To conclude, I will briefly mention a scientific success story that does begin with the letter Z – zebrafish. Their story deserves mention as these fish are revealing new insights into just how memories are formed. Zebrafish, named after their striped appearance, are popular in aquariums. They are also popular with scientists. Not only has the zebrafish genome been completely sequenced, but the size and transparency of the fish when young offer astonishing opportunities to visualise brain development and neuronal activity (Figure 19.11). These fish are also very versatile. Zebrafish demonstrate classical conditioning and, based on their ability to associate an object's location with its context, they may display aspects of episodic memory.

The result is that the transparent larval zebrafish is an exceptional vertebrate model for studying the physiological and cellular mechanisms of memory storage. Astonishingly, it is possible in a one-to-two week old zebrafish to record simultaneously all the animal's neurons in the brain during behaviour. It is also possible to measure structural changes within and between synapses in the living fish. These features create new opportunities to study the development of brain-wide engrams and follow what happens next.

Finally, this information about zebrafish should make you question the myth about goldfish – that their memory lasts only up to three seconds. It is not clear where this myth came from, but the film 'Finding Nemo' does not help. Rest assured, goldfish can retain information about places or objects associated with food for weeks.

20 Naming the brain

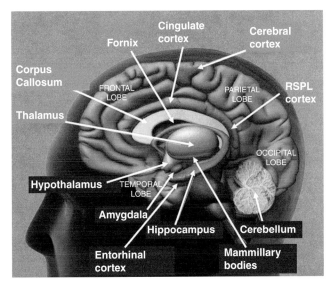

Figure 20.1 Side view of the human brain showing the location of key brain structures. The hippocampus and its tract, the fornix, are made distinct. RSPL, retrosplenial cortex.

Amygdala: The amygdala is a temporal lobe structure that sits in front of the hippocampus. Its name derives from the structure's fanciful resemblance to an 'almond'. (The Greek word for almond is amýgdalo.) While the term amygdalectomy describes the surgical removal of the amygdala, the same term also applies to the surgical removal of the tonsils, which are also almond shaped. Please never mix up these terms.

Cerebellum: The name, from Latin, means 'little brain' yet the cerebellum contains considerably more neurons than the rest of the brain. The cerebellum is part of the hindbrain, in humans sitting below the back of the cerebral cortex. It has important roles for movement and motor skills, but also makes much wider contributions in regulating cognition and emotion.

Cerebral cortex: The term 'cortex' means outer layer or rind. The cerebral cortex is the pinkish-grey tissue that covers much of the brain – imagine thick, pinkish grey porridge. It is composed of distinct layers of neurons. The cerebral cortex is divided into four lobes: frontal, parietal, temporal, and occipital.

DOI: 10.4324/9781003537649-20

Cingulate cortex: A large strip of cortex, close to the midline of the brain. It envelops much of the corpus callosum, hence its name, which means girdle.

Corpus callosum: This is the enormous white matter tract that connects the two cerebral hemispheres. Corpus means body, while callosum refers to its texture, which feels hard when compared to grey matter. You may be familiar with the term 'skin callus', which comes from the Latin word used for hard skin, 'callum'. (The term 'callous' has the same origin, meaning emotionally hardened.)

Diencephalon: The name diencephalon means 'between-brain' or 'interbrain', reflecting its importance as a mediating point between cortical and subcortical brain structures. It is principally composed of the thalamus and hypothalamus.

Entorhinal cortex: Part of the parahippocampal region, being a gateway into and out of the hippocampus. The name 'entorhinal' reflects how it is part of the rhinal (olfactory) cortex. The word 'rhinal' refers to the nose or olfaction (think rhinoceros).

Fornix: In Latin, this word means an arch, a shape that accurately reflect the appearance of this fibre tract as it links the hippocampus with many other brain sites. The Latin word for arch has also left us the English word fornicate. There are various questionable explanations as to how the Latin for arch takes us to this particular meaning.

Hippocampus: The hippocampus is the brain structure most often referred to in this book as it is vital for explicit memory. The hippocampus is named after its fanciful resemblance to a sea horse, the name being taken from the Greek for horse (hippos) and sea creature or sea monster (kámpos). A name more rarely used for the hippocampus is Ammon's Horn. Amun was the ram headed God of Egypt. (Tutankh*amun* took his name from this deity, as do fossil ammonites). If you were to remove just the hippocampus from a brain you will immediately see how it looks like a pair of ram's horns. (Ammon was the Greek form of Amun). Incidentally, if you dissect the hippocampus in a particular plane, you reveal a part that looks just like a row of molar teeth, hence the name 'dentate gyrus' for that hippocampal subregion.

Hypothalamus: 'Hypo' means less than or below (think hypodermic, below the skin), so the hypothalamus sits below the thalamus.

Mammillary bodies: At the back of the hypothalamus are the mammillary bodies. These structures are so named because of a superficial resemblance to the mammary glands. Astonishingly, a debate exists among neuroanatomists over whether they should be spelt 'mammillary' or 'mamillary'. As Ted Jones observed, the more obscure the debate the greater the heat generated. I am sure you will be relieved to know that I use the 'mammillary' spelling, as this is the original form.

Parietal lobe: The parietal lobe is one of the four lobes of the cerebral cortex. Its name comes from the parietal bone, which derives its name from the Latin 'paries', which means wall.

Prefrontal cortex: The frontal lobe is one of the four lobes of the cerebral cortex. While the motor cortex and premotor areas form the back of the frontal lobe, in front of those areas sits the prefrontal cortex.

Retrosplenial cortex: The name 'retrosplenial' derives from its location, being behind ('retro') the splenium (the most posterior portion of the corpus callosum, which looks like a medical splint – the Latin name for splint being splenium).

Temporal lobe: The temporal lobe is one of the four lobes of the cerebral cortex. In addition to its cortical areas, it contains the amygdala and hippocampus. The name temporal lobe has an intriguing origin. Its proximity to the temples on the upper side of our head matches its location. The 'temples' get their name from the Latin word for time, 'tempus'. Apparently, the appearance of grey hair, often initially around the temporal area, signifies the passage of time.

Thalamus: The word 'thalamus' means antechamber or bridal bed, the name arising from the attempt to compare the structure of the brain with the layout of a Greek house.

21 Twenty (plus one) ways to improve your memory

Tell me and I forget, teach me and I may remember, involve me and I learn
attributed to Benjamin Franklin

1 *Understanding:* The route to richer encoding and better recall is through understanding what you are trying to learn. This process creates active learning.
2 *Become involved with the information:* Try to work out how it how relates to other areas of knowledge. How might the concepts impact on you or others? Try to explain the information to another person.
3 *Mnemonics:* These can be ideal for some kinds of information, for example, lists of names. You are free to make up your own mnemonic, which may prove to be more effective than one given to you.
4 *Spaced rather than massed learning:* Schedule learning so that you can repeat it after an interval (distributed practice) and avoid cramming.
5 *Test yourself:* Spaced learning brings with it the opportunity for a retrieval test prior to follow-up further learning. Even if you make errors, this will help in the long run.
6 *Make sure you had the information right at the beginning:* Do not be embarrassed to ask someone to repeat information, such as their name or directions.
7 *Visual imagery:* Imagery is at the heart of so many mnemonics and learning aids. Do not be afraid to employ your powers of visualisation, which can help in multiple ways. It is no coincidence that pictorial aids are a mainstay of teaching, lectures, and seminars.
8 *External memory aids are good:* The camera on a mobile phone can be invaluable, for example, when confronted with a map on an information board. Diaries and calendars all have their place. Stick-it notes can be a great help for those with chronic memory problems.
9 *Elaborative processing:* Think about the material to be learnt in different ways and from different perspectives. Engage in deeper rather than superficial processing.
10 *Memory as problem-solving:* Turn learning into a puzzle. Self-discovery adds to the levels of interaction and creates Aha! moments. The resulting self-generation of information adds to its memorability. Encourage curiosity.
11 *The myth of multi-tasking:* Do one thing and do it properly. There is the misguided belief that multi-tasking creates greater overall efficiency. Alas, multi-tasking involves constant switching, which reduces performance. Figure 21.1 highlights the dangers of multi-tasking.
12 *Regular, quality sleep:* Sleep helps both future and past learning. The recommended amount of sleep each night for adults is between seven and ten hours. There is, however, an optimal 'Goldilocks' amount of sleep, not too little and not too much. A nap during the day can also help with learning. Beware the blue light from smartphones, TVs, and computer screens as it can upset sleep patterns.

DOI: 10.4324/9781003537649-21

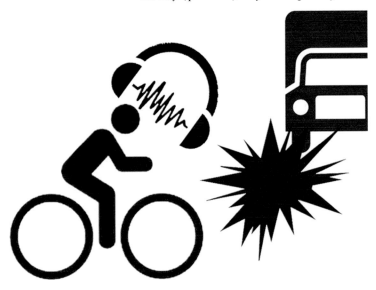

Figure 21.1 The myth of multi-tasking. Cycling and listening on headphones do not mix. Please don't ever be tempted.

13 *Imagery for perceptual-motor skills:* Mental practice and rehearsal is a great complement when refining a desired skill. You can employ both internal and external imagery.

14 *Avoid the illusion of mastery:* When you re-read familiar material it will often feel as though it has been mastered because you will process it more quickly. Your metamemory may also be prone to overconfidence. These are yet more reason why testing yourself or explaining to others is so useful in determining what you really do and do not know.

15 *Maintain a healthy brain:* Walking, other forms of exercise, social interactions, cognitive stimulation, and ample sleep are all good for the health of your brain. A well-balanced diet is also good, alcohol is not.

16 *Avoid distractions:* Distraction comes in many forms, but common sources include background conversations and music, the TV, smartphones, and running multiple computer screens. Distractions invariably hinder learning.

17 *Smart drugs are not a smart idea:* Resist any temptation to use unprescribed stimulants in the belief that they will boost your normal learning powers.

18 *Combat absent mindedness:* Always avoid using unusual places for safe keeping. Reserve set places for keys, glasses, passports, etc. As you lock a door think about the action in a way that sets it apart, so that you can later mentally confirm that you did indeed lock the car or the house.

19 *Become an expert:* As you acquire knowledge about a topic you gradually become an expert. This means that while initial learning may seem like hard work, acquiring subsequent information will become increasingly effective.

20 *Learning and remembering in the same context:* Do not be surprised if your recall is disrupted by changes in location from initial learning, along with any changes to your physical and emotional states (state-dependency).

21 *Re-read this book.*

References

Adolphus, K., Lawton, C. L., & Dye, L. (2019). Associations between habitual school-day breakfast consumption frequency and academic performance in British adolescents. *Frontiers in Public Health*, 7, 481259.

Alex, A., Abbott, K. A., McEvoy, M., Schofield, P. W., & Garg, M. L. (2020). Long-chain omega-3 polyunsaturated fatty acids and cognitive decline in non-demented adults: A systematic review and meta-analysis. *Nutrition Reviews*, *78*(7), 563–578.

Anderson, M. C., & Hulbert, J. C. (2021). Active forgetting: Adaptation of memory by prefrontal control. *Annual Review of Psychology*, *72*, 1–36.

Anderson, S. W., Rizzo, M., Skaar, N., Stierman, L., Cavaco, S., Dawson, J., & Damasio, H. (2007). Amnesia and driving. *Journal of Clinical and Experimental Neuropsychology*, *29*(1), 1–12.

Asperholm, M., Högman, N., Rafi, J., & Herlitz, A. (2019). What did you do yesterday? A meta-analysis of sex differences in episodic memory. *Psychological Bulletin*, *145*(8), 785.

Au, R.N., 2022. Neuro-doping, tDCS and Chess — are WADA's Regulations under Threat? *LSE Law Review*, *8*(1), 51–120.

Baddeley, A. (2012). Working memory: Theories, models, and controversies. *Annual Review of Psychology*, *63*, 1–29.

Baddeley, A. D., & Longman, D. J. A. (1978). The influence of length and frequency of training session on the rate of learning to type. *Ergonomics*, *21*(8), 627–635.

Banks, I. (1992). *The Crow Road*. New York, Scribner's.

Battleday, R. M., & Brem, A. K. (2015). Modafinil for cognitive neuroenhancement in healthy non-sleep-deprived subjects: A systematic review. *European Neuropsychopharmacology*, *25*(11), 1865–1881.

Bowles, B., Crupi, C., Pigott, S., Parrent, A., Wiebe, S., Janzen, L., & Köhler, S. (2010). Double dissociation of selective recollection and familiarity impairments following two different surgical treatments for temporal-lobe epilepsy. *Neuropsychologia*, *48*(9), 2640–2647.

Brady, T. F., Konkle, T., Alvarez, G. A., & Oliva, A. (2008). Visual long-term memory has a massive storage capacity for object details. *Proceedings of the National Academy of Sciences*, *105*(38), 14325–14329.

Bransford, J. D., & Johnson, M. K. (1972). Contextual prerequisites for understanding: Some investigations of comprehension and recall. *Journal of Verbal Learning and Verbal Behavior*, *11*(6), 717–726.

Brighetti, G., Bonifacci, P., Borlimi, R., & Ottaviani, C. (2007). "Far from the heart far from the eye": Evidence from the Capgras delusion. *Cognitive Neuropsychiatry*, *12*(3), 189–197.

Brown, M. W., Warburton, E. C., & Aggleton, J. P. (2010). Recognition memory: Material, processes, and substrates. *Hippocampus*, *20*(11), 1228–1244.

Campbell, B. A., & Campbell, E. H. (1962). Retention and extinction of learned fear in infant and adult rats. *Journal of Comparative and Physiological Psychology*, *55*(1), 1.

Carroll, L. (1871). *Through the Looking-Glass*. London, Macmillan Publishers.

Cepeda, N. J., Vul, E., Rohrer, D., Wixted, J. T., & Pashler, H. (2008). Spacing effects in learning: A temporal ridgeline of optimal retention. *Psychological Science*, *19*(11), 1095–1102.

Chase, W. G., & Simon, H. A. (1973). Perception in chess. *Cognitive Psychology*, *4*(1), 55–81.

Chen, Z., Hamilton, R., & Rucker, D. D. (2021). Are we there yet? An anticipation account of the return trip effect. *Social Psychological and Personality Science*, *12*(2), 258–265.

Collerton, D., & Perry, E. (2011). Dreaming and hallucinations–continuity or discontinuity? Perspectives from dementia with Lewy bodies. *Consciousness and Cognition, 20*(4), 1016–1020.

Collins, W. (1868). *The Moonstone*. London, Tinsley Brothers.

Conti, A. A., McLean, L., Tolomeo, S., Steele, J. D., & Baldacchino, A. (2019). Chronic tobacco smoking and neuropsychological impairments: A systematic review and meta-analysis. *Neuroscience & Biobehavioral Reviews, 96*, 143–154.

Cousins, J. N., Wong, K. F., Raghunath, B. L., Look, C., & Chee, M. W. (2019). The long-term memory benefits of a daytime nap compared with cramming. *Sleep, 42*(1), zsy207.

Coutrot, A., Silva, R., Manley, E., de Cothi, W., Sami, S., Bohbot, V. D., & Spiers, H. J. (2018). Global determinants of navigation ability. *Current Biology, 28*(17), 2861–2866.

Coveney, A. P., Switzer, T., Corrigan, M. A., & Redmond, H. P. (2013). Context dependent memory in two learning environments: The tutorial room and the operating theatre. *BMC Medical Education, 13*, 1–7.

Craik, F. I. (2002). Levels of processing: Past, present… and future?. *Memory, 10*(5–6), 305–318.

Curot, J., Busigny, T., Valton, L., Denuelle, M., Vignal, J. P., Maillard, L., … Barbeau, E. J. (2017). Memory scrutinized through electrical brain stimulation: A review of 80 years of experiential phenomena. *Neuroscience & Biobehavioral Reviews, 78*, 161–177.

Davies, S. J., Lum, J. A., Skouteris, H., Byrne, L. K., & Hayden, M. J. (2018). Cognitive impairment during pregnancy: A meta-analysis. *Medical Journal of Australia, 208*(1), 35–40.

DeCasien, A. R., Guma, E., Liu, S., & Raznahan, A. (2022). Sex differences in the human brain: A roadmap for more careful analysis and interpretation of a biological reality. *Biology of Sex Differences, 13*(1), 43.

Deary, I. J., & Der, G. (2005). Reaction time, age, and cognitive ability: Longitudinal findings from age 16 to 63 years in representative population samples. *Aging, Neuropsychology, and Cognition, 12*(2), 187–215.

Deary, I. J., Pattie, A., & Starr, J. M. (2013). The stability of intelligence from age 11 to age 90 years: The Lothian birth cohort of 1921. *Psychological Science, 24*(12), 2361–2368.

Dickens, C. (1853). *Bleak house*. London, Bradbury & Evans.

Doyle, A. C. (1891). *The adventures of sherlock holmes*. The Strand Magazine. George Newnes Ltd.

Dresler, M., Shirer, W. R., Konrad, B. N., Müller, N. C., Wagner, I. C., Fernández, G., Czisch, M., & Greicius, M. D. (2017). Mnemonic training reshapes brain networks to support superior memory. *Neuron, 93*(5), 1227–1235.

Dusoir, H., Kapur, N., Byrnes, D. P., McKinstry, S., & Hoare, R. D. (1990). The role of diencephalic pathology in human memory disorder: Evidence from a penetrating paranasal brain injury. *Brain, 113*(6), 1695–1706.

Ebbinghaus, H. (1885) *Memory: A contribution to experimental psychology*. Translated by H.A. Ruger & C.E. Bussenius (1913). Originally published by Teachers College, Columbia University.

Ellis, N.C. & Hennelly, R.A. (1980). A bilingual word-length effect: Implications for intelligence testing and the relative ease of mental calculation in Welsh and English. *British Journal of Psychology, 71*, 43–51.

Elward, R. L., & Vargha-Khadem, F. (2018). Semantic memory in developmental amnesia. *Neuroscience Letters, 680*, 23–30.

Ericsson, K. A., Delaney, P. F., Weaver, G., Mahadevan, R. (2004). Uncovering the structure of a memorists superior "basic" memory capacity. *Cognitive Psychology 49*, 191–237.

Ferguson, M. A., Lim, C., Cooke, D., Darby, R. R., Wu, O., Rost, N. S., Corbetta, M., Grafman, J., & Fox, M. D. (2019). A human memory circuit derived from brain lesions causing amnesia. *Nature Communications, 10*(1), 3497.

Finney, J. (1954). *The body snatchers*. Springfield, Ohio, Collier's Magazine

Fitzpatrick, C., Archambault, I., Janosz, M., & Pagani, L. S. (2015). Early childhood working memory forecasts high school dropout risk. *Intelligence, 53*, 160–165.

Foster, N. L., Was, C. A., Dunlosky, J., & Isaacson, R. M. (2017). Even after thirteen class exams, students are still overconfident: The role of memory for past exam performance in student predictions. *Metacognition and Learning, 12*, 1–19.

Freud, S. (1891). *The standard edition of the complete psychological works* (24 volumes). Hogarth Press, 1953–1974.

Freud, S. (1905) *Three essays on the theory of sexuality* (Trans. James Strachey). New York, Basic Books.

Franke, A. G., Gränsmark, P., Agricola, A., Schühle, K., Rommel, T., Sebastian, A., Ballo, H.E., Gorbulev, S., Gerdes, C., Frank, B., Ruckes, C., Tuscher, O., & Lieb, K. (2017). Methylphenidate, modafinil, and caffeine for cognitive enhancement in chess: A double-blind, randomised controlled trial. *European Neuropsychopharmacology*, *27*(3), 248–260.

Frankenberg, C., Knebel, M., Degen, C., Siebert, J. S., Wahl, H. W., & Schröder, J. (2022). Autobiographical memory in healthy aging: A decade-long longitudinal study. *Aging, Neuropsychology, and Cognition*, *29*(1), 158–179.

Gabriel, T. (2017). The day that went missing: A first-person account of transient global amnesia. *Cognitive and Behavioral Neurology*, *30*(1), 1–4.

Gathercole, S. E., Pickering, S. J., Ambridge, B., & Wearing, H. (2004). The structure of working memory from 4 to 15 years of age. *Developmental Psychology*, *40*(2), 177–190.

Gauthier, I., Skudlarski, P., Gore, J. C., & Anderson, A. W. (2000). Expertise for cars and birds recruits brain areas involved in face recognition. *Nature Neuroscience*, *3*(2), 191–197.

Gefen, T., Kawles, A., Makowski-Woidan, B., Engelmeyer, J., Ayala, I., Abbassian, P., Zhang, H., Weintraub, S., Flanagan, M. E., Mao, Q., Bigio, E. H., Rogalski, E., Mesulam, M. M., & Geula, C. (2021). Paucity of entorhinal cortex pathology of the Alzheimer's type in SuperAgers with superior memory performance. *Cerebral Cortex*, *31*(7), 3177–3183.

Geiselman, R. E., Fisher, R. P., MacKinnon, D. P., & Holland, H. L. (1985). Eyewitness memory enhancement in the police interview: Cognitive retrieval mnemonics versus hypnosis. *Journal of Applied Psychology*, *70*(2), 401.

Ghoneim, M. M., & Mewaldt, S. P. (1975). Effects of diazepam and scopolamine on storage, retrieval and organizational processes in memory. *Psychopharmacologia*, *44*, 257–262.

Godden, D. R., & Baddeley, A. D. (1975). Context-dependent memory in two natural environments: On land and underwater. *British Journal of Psychology*, *66*(3), 325–331.

Goldstein, R., Almenberg, J., Dreber, A., Emerson, J. W., Herschkowitsch, A., & Katz, J. (2008). Do more expensive wines taste better? Evidence from a large sample of blind tastings. *Journal of Wine Economics*, *3*(1), 1–9.

Goodwin, D. W., Othmer, E., Halikas, J. A., & Freemon, F. (1970). Loss of short term memory as a predictor of the alcoholic "blackout". *Nature*, *227*(5254), 201–202.

Gorbach, T., Pudas, S., Bartrés-Faz, D., Brandmaier, A. M., Düzel, S., Henson, R. N., … Nyberg, L. (2020). Longitudinal association between hippocampus atrophy and episodic-memory decline in non-demented APOE ε4 carriers. *Alzheimer's & Dementia: Diagnosis, Assessment & Disease Monitoring*, *12*(1), e12110.

Harding, A., Halliday, G., Caine, D., & Kril, J. (2000). Degeneration of anterior thalamic nuclei differentiates alcoholics with amnesia. *Brain*, *123*(1), 141–154.

Harrison, N. A., Johnston, K., Corno, F., Casey, S. J., Friedner, K., Humphreys, K., Jaldow, E.J., Pitkanen, M., & Kopelman, M. D. (2017). Psychogenic amnesia: Syndromes, outcome, and patterns of retrograde amnesia. *Brain*, *140*(9), 2498–2510.

Hasher, L., & Griffin, M. (1978). Reconstructive and reproductive processes in memory. *Journal of Experimental Psychology: Human Learning and Memory*, *4*(4), 318.

Hassabis, D., Kumaran, D., Vann, S. D., & Maguire, E. A. (2007). Patients with hippocampal amnesia cannot imagine new experiences. *Proceedings of the National Academy of Sciences*, *104*(5), 1726–1731.

Heck, P. R., Simons, D. J., & Chabris, C. F. (2018). Results of two nationally representative surveys. *PloS One*, *13*(7), e0200103.

Heishman, S. J., Kleykamp, B. A., & Singleton, E. G. (2010). Meta-analysis of the acute effects of nicotine and smoking on human performance. *Psychopharmacology*, *210*, 453–469.

Higgs, S., Williamson, A. C., Rotshtein, P., & Humphreys, G. W. (2008). Sensory-specific satiety is intact in amnesics who eat multiple meals. *Psychological Science*, *19*(7), 623–628.

Hoekzema, E., Barba-Müller, E., Pozzobon, C., Picado, M., Lucco, F., García-García, D., Soliva, J. C., Tobeña, A., Desco, M., Crone, E. A., Ballesteros, A., Carmona, S., & Vilarroya, O. (2017). Pregnancy leads to long-lasting changes in human brain structure. *Nature Neuroscience*, *20*(2), 287–296.

Holmes, J., & Gathercole, S. E. (2014). Taking working memory training from the laboratory into schools. *Educational Psychology*, *34*(4), 440–450.

Hughes, B., Sullivan, K. A., & Gilmore, L. (2020). Why do teachers believe educational neuromyths? *Trends in Neuroscience and Education*, *21*, 100145.

James W. (1890) *The principles of psychology*. Volume 1. Henry Holt & Company.

Johnson, S. (1759). Idler #74 (September 15, 1759) London, The Universal Chronicle.

Jonin, P. Y., Besson, G., La Joie, R., Pariente, J., Belliard, S., Barillot, C., & Barbeau, E. J. (2018). Superior explicit memory despite severe developmental amnesia: In-depth case study and neural correlates. *Hippocampus*, *28*(12), 867–885.

Juster, N. (1961). *The Phantom Tollbooth*. Epstein & Carrol Associates Inc.

Kafka, F. (1915). *Metamorphosis*. Leipzig, Die Weissen Blätter.

Kerchner, G. A., Racine, C. A., Hale, S., Wilheim, R., Laluz, V., Miller, B. L., & Kramer, J. H. (2012). Cognitive processing speed in older adults: Relationship with white matter integrity. *PloS One*, *7*(11), e50425.

Kirschner, P. A. (2017). Stop propagating the learning styles myth. *Computers & Education*, *106*, 166–171.

Kirwan, C. B., Bayley, P. J., Galván, V. V., & Squire, L. R. (2008). Detailed recollection of remote autobiographical memory after damage to the medial temporal lobe. *Proceedings of the National Academy of Sciences*, *105*(7), 2676–2680.

Kreitewolf, J., Wöstmann, M., Tune, S., Plöchl, M., & Obleser, J. (2019). Working-memory disruption by task-irrelevant talkers depends on degree of talker familiarity. *Attention, Perception, & Psychophysics*, *81*, 1108–1118.

Kuch, K., & Cox, B. J. (1992). Symptoms of PTSD in 124 survivors of the Holocaust. *American Journal of Psychiatry*, *149*(3), 337–340.

Lamport, D. J., Christodoulou, E., & Achilleos, C. (2020). Beneficial effects of dark chocolate for episodic memory in healthy young adults: A parallel-groups acute intervention with a white chocolate control. *Nutrients*, *12*(2), 483.

Lenton, A. P., Blair, I. V., & Hastie, R. (2001). Illusions of gender: Stereotypes evoke false memories. *Journal of Experimental Social Psychology*, *37*(1), 3–14.

LePort, A. K., Mattfeld, A. T., Dickinson-Anson, H., Fallon, J. H., Stark, C. E., Kruggel, F., Cahill, L., & McGaugh, J. L. (2012). Behavioral and neuroanatomical investigation of highly superior autobiographical memory (HSAM). *Neurobiology of Learning and Memory*, *98*(1), 78–92.

LePort, A. K., Stark, S. M., McGaugh, J. L., & Stark, C. E. (2016). Highly superior autobiographical memory: Quality and quantity of retention over time. *Frontiers in Psychology*, *6*, 172904.

Levinson, B. W. (1965). States of awareness during general anaesthesia: Preliminary communication. *British Journal of Anaesthesia*, *37*(7), 544–546.

Levy, B. R., Zonderman, A. B., Slade, M. D., & Ferrucci, L. (2012). Memory shaped by age stereotypes over time. *Journals of Gerontology: Series B*, *67*(4), 432–436.

Lilienfeld, S. O., Lynn, S. J., Ruscio, J., & Lilenfield B. (2009). *50 Great myths of popular psychology: Shattering widespread misconceptions about human behavior*. John Wiley and Sons Ltd.

Liu, J., Wu, L., Um, P., Wang, J., Kral, T. V., Hanlon, A., & Shi, Z. (2021). Breakfast consumption habits at age 6 and cognitive ability at age 12: A longitudinal cohort study. *Nutrients*, *13*(6), 2080.

Loftus, E. F., & Pickrell, J. E. (1995). The formation of false memories. *Psychiatric Annals*, *25*(12), 720–725.

Mackes, N. K., Golm, D., Sarkar, S., Kumsta, R., Rutter, M., Fairchild, G., & ERA Young Adult Follow-up team. (2020). Early childhood deprivation is associated with alterations in adult brain structure despite subsequent environmental enrichment. *Proceedings of the National Academy of Sciences*, *117*(1), 641–649.

Macready, A. L., Kennedy, O. B., Ellis, J. A., Williams, C. M., Spencer, J. P., & Butler, L. T. (2009). Flavonoids and cognitive function: A review of human randomized controlled trial studies and recommendations for future studies. *Genes & Nutrition*, *4*(4), 227–242.

Mandler, G. (1980). Recognizing: The judgment of previous occurrence. *Psychological Review*, *87*(3), 252–271.

McDermott, K. B., Gilmore, A. W., Nelson, S. M., Watson, J. M., & Ojemann, J. G. (2017). The parietal memory network activates similarly for true and associative false recognition elicited via the DRM procedure. *Cortex*, *87*, 96–107.

McFarland, M. J., Hauer, M. E., & Reuben, A. (2022). Half of US population exposed to adverse lead levels in early childhood. *Proceedings of the National Academy of Sciences*, *119*(11), e2118631119.

Merckelbach, H., Dekkers, T., Wessel, I., & Roefs, A. (2003). Amnesia, flashbacks, nightmares, and dissociation in aging concentration camp survivors. *Behaviour Research and Therapy*, *41*(3), 351–360.

Miller, G. A. (1956). The magical number seven, plus or minus two: Some limits on our capacity for processing information. *Psychological Review, 63*(2), 81.

Milner, B., Corkin, S., & Teuber, H. L. (1968). Further analysis of the hippocampal amnesic syndrome: 14-year follow-up study of HM. *Neuropsychologia, 6*(3), 215–234.

Morone, G., Ghanbari Ghooshchy, S., Pulcini, C., Spangu, E., Zoccolotti, P., Martelli, M., Spitoni, G. F., Russo, V., Ciancerelli, I., Paolucci, S. & Iosa, M. (2022). Motor Imagery and Sport Performance: A Systematic Review on the PETTLEP Model. *Applied Sciences, 12*(19), 9753.

Morgan, C.L. (1903). *An Introduction to Comparative Psychology*. London, W. Scott Publishing Co.

Moscovitch, M., Cabeza, R., Winocur, G., & Nadel, L. (2016). Episodic memory and beyond: The hippocampus and neocortex in transformation. *Annual Review of Psychology, 67*, 105–134.

Nader, K., Schafe, G. E., & Le Doux, J. E. (2000). Fear memories require protein synthesis in the amygdala for reconsolidation after retrieval. *Nature, 406*(6797), 722–726.

Nazareth, A., Huang, X., Voyer, D., & Newcombe, N. (2019). A meta-analysis of sex differences in human navigation skills. *Psychonomic Bulletin & Review, 26*, 1503–1528.

Neale, C., Camfield, D., Reay, J., Stough, C., & Scholey, A. (2013). Cognitive effects of two nutraceuticals Ginseng and Bacopa benchmarked against modafinil: A review and comparison of effect sizes. *British Journal of Clinical Pharmacology, 75*(3), 728–737.

Nelson, K. (Ed.) (2006). *Narratives from the Crib*. Harvard University Press.

Nicholson, P., Mayho, G., Sharp, C. (2015). *Cognitive enhancing drugs and the workplace*. British Medical Association.

Noonan, M. (2013). Mind maps: Enhancing midwifery education. *Nurse Education Today, 33*(8), 847–852.

Nyberg, L., Lövdén, M., Riklund, K., Lindenberger, U., & Bäckman, L. (2012). Memory aging and brain maintenance. *Trends in Cognitive Sciences, 16*(5), 292–305.

Open Science Collaboration. (2015). Estimating the reproducibility of psychological science. *Science, 349*(6251), aac4716.

Owen, A. M., & Coleman, M. R. (2008). Functional neuroimaging of the vegetative state. *Nature Reviews Neuroscience, 9*(3), 235–243.

Park, K. C., Jin, H., Zheng, R., Kim, S., Lee, S. E., Kim, B. H., & Yim, S. V. (2019). Cognition enhancing effect of panax ginseng in Korean volunteers with mild cognitive impairment: A randomized, double-blind, placebo-controlled clinical trial. *Translational and Clinical Pharmacology, 27*(3), 92–97.

Parker, E. S., Cahill, L., & McGaugh, J. L. (2006). A case of unusual autobiographical remembering. *Neurocase, 12*(1), 35–49.

Patihis, L., Ho, L. Y., Loftus, E. F., & Herrera, M. E. (2021). Memory experts' beliefs about repressed memory. *Memory, 29*(6), 823–828.

Patterson, K., & Ralph, M. A. L. (2016). The hub-and-spoke hypothesis of semantic memory. In G. Hickock & S. Small (Eds.), *Neurobiology of language* (pp. 765–775). Academic Press.

Penfield, W. (1968). Engrams in the Human Brain: Mechanisms of Memory. *Proceedings of the Royal Society of Medicine, 61*, 831–840).

Penfield, W. (1969). Consciousness, memory, and man's conditioned reflexes. In K. Pribram (Ed.), *On the biology of learning* (pp. 129–168). Harcourt, Brace & World.

Phipps, C. J., Murman, D. L., & Warren, D. E. (2021). Stimulating memory: Reviewing interventions using repetitive transcranial magnetic stimulation to enhance or restore memory abilities. *Brain Sciences, 11*(10), 1283.

Picard-Deland, C., & Nielsen, T. (2022). Targeted memory reactivation has a sleep stage-specific delayed effect on dream content. *Journal of Sleep Research, 31*(1), e13391.

Ponce, H. R., Mayer, R. E., & Méndez, E. E. (2022). Effects of learner-generated highlighting and instructor-provided highlighting on learning from text: A meta-analysis. *Educational Psychology Review, 34*(2), 989–1024.

del Pozo Cruz, B., Ahmadi, M., Naismith, S. L., & Stamatakis, E. (2022). Association of daily step count and intensity with incident dementia in 78 430 adults living in the UK. *JAMA Neurology, 79*(10), 1059–1063.

Pratchett, T. (1992). *Lords and ladies*. Victor Gollancz Ltd.

Pratchett, T. (2008). Terry Pratchett: I'm slipping away a bit at a time... and all I can do is watch it happen | *Daily Mail* Online,7th October

Proust, M. (1913). *À la Recherche du Temps Perdu*. Paris: Éditions Gallimard.

Pyszora, N. M., Barker, A. F., & Kopelman, M. D. (2003). Amnesia for criminal offences: A study of life sentence prisoners. *The Journal of Forensic Psychiatry, 14*(3), 475–490.

Quiroga, R. Q., Reddy, L., Kreiman, G., Koch, C., & Fried, I. (2005). Invariant visual representation by single neurons in the human brain. *Nature, 435*(7045), 1102–1107.

Rauscher, F. H., Shaw, G. L., & Ky, K. N. (1995). Listening to Mozart enhances spatial-temporal reasoning: Towards a neurophysiological basis. *Neuroscience Letters, 185*(1), 44–47.

Redshaw, J., & Suddendorf, T. (2020). Temporal junctures in the mind. *Trends in Cognitive Sciences, 24*(1), 52–64.

Repantis, D., Schlattmann, P., Laisney, O., Heuser, I. (2010). Modafinil and methylphenidate for neuroenhancement in healthy individuals: A systematic review. *Pharmacological Research, 62,* 187–206.

Roberts, C. A., Jones, A., Sumnall, H., Gage, S. H., & Montgomery, C. (2020). How effective are pharmaceuticals for cognitive enhancement in healthy adults? A series of meta-analyses of cognitive performance during acute administration of modafinil, methylphenidate and D-amphetamine. *European Neuropsychopharmacology, 38,* 40–62.

Roediger, H. L., & McDermott, K. B. (1995). Creating false memories: Remembering words not presented in lists. *Journal of Experimental Psychology: Learning, Memory, and Cognition, 21*(4), 803–814.

Rosenbaum, R. S., Köhler, S., Schacter, D. L., Moscovitch, M., Westmacott, R., Black, S. E., Gao, F., & Tulving, E. (2005). The case of KC: Contributions of a memory-impaired person to memory theory. *Neuropsychologia, 43*(7), 989–1021.

Sala, G., & Gobet, F. (2020). Cognitive and academic benefits of music training with children: A multilevel meta-analysis. *Memory & Cognition, 48*(8), 1429–1441.

Sampaio-Baptista, C., & Johansen-Berg, H. (2017). White matter plasticity in the adult brain. *Neuron, 96*(6), 1239–1251.

Scarf, D., Smith, C., & Stuart, M. (2014). A spoon full of studies helps the comparison go down: A comparative analysis of Tulving's spoon test. *Frontiers in Psychology, 5,* 108572.

Schacter, D. L. (2022). The seven sins of memory: An update. *Memory, 30*(1), 37–42.

Schacter, D. L., & Addis, D. R. (2007). The cognitive neuroscience of constructive memory: Remembering the past and imagining the future. *Philosophical Transactions of the Royal Society B: Biological Sciences, 362*(1481), 773–786.

Schacter, D. L., Wang, P. L., Tulving, E., & Freedman, M. (1982). Functional retrograde amnesia: A quantitative case study. *Neuropsychologia, 20*(5), 523–532.

Scholz, J., Klein, M. C., Behrens, T. E., & Johansen-Berg, H. (2009). Training induces changes in white-matter architecture. *Nature Neuroscience, 12*(11), 1370–1371.

Seehagen, S., Schneider, S., Sommer, K., La Rocca, L., & Konrad, C. (2021). State-dependent memory in infants. *Child Development, 92*(2), 578–585.

Shaw, J., & Porter, S. (2015). Constructing rich false memories of committing crime. *Psychological Science, 26*(3), 291–301.

Simons, D. J., Boot, W. R., Charness, N., Gathercole, S. E., Chabris, C. F., Hambrick, D. Z., & Stine-Morrow, E. A. (2016). Do "brain-training" programs work? *Psychological Science in the Public Interest, 17*(3), 103–186.

Simons, D. J., & Chabris, C. F. (1999). Gorillas in our midst: Sustained inattentional blindness for dynamic events. *Perception, 28*(9), 1059–1074.

Simons, D. J., & Chabris, C. F. (2011). What people believe about how memory works: A representative survey of the U.S. population. *PLoS One,* 6(8), e22757.

Slaughter, V. (2021). Do newborns have the ability to imitate? *Trends in Cognitive Sciences, 25*(5), 377–387.

Smeets, T., Telgen, S., Ost, J., Jelicic, M., & Merckelbach, H. (2009). What's behind crashing memories? Plausibility, belief and memory in reports of having seen non-existent images. *Applied Cognitive Psychology: The Official Journal of the Society for Applied Research in Memory and Cognition, 23*(9), 1333–1341.

Smith, C. N., Frascino, J. C., Kripke, D. L., McHugh, P. R., Treisman, G. J., & Squire, L. R. (2010). Losing memories overnight: A unique form of human amnesia. *Neuropsychologia, 48*(10), 2833–2840.

Snitz, B. E., O'Meara, E. S., Carlson, M. C., Arnold, A. M., Ives, D. G., Rapp, S. R., Saxton, J., Lopez, O. L., Dunn, L. O., Sink, K. M., & Dekosky, S. T. (2009). Ginkgo biloba for preventing cognitive decline in older adults: A randomized trial. *JAMA, 302*(24), 2663–2670.

Snowdon, D. (2002). *Aging with grace: What the nun study teaches us about leading longer, healthier, and more meaningful lives.* Bantam.

Spanò, G., Pizzamiglio, G., McCormick, C., Clark, I. A., De Felice, S., Miller, T. D., ... Maguire, E. A. (2020). Dreaming with hippocampal damage. *elife*, *9*, e56211.

Squire, L. R., Clark, R. E., & Knowlton, B. J. (2001). Retrograde amnesia. *Hippocampus*, *11*(1), 50–55.

Stephenson, J. (2009). Best practice? Advice provided to teachers about the use of Brain Gym® in Australian schools. *Australian Journal of Education*, *53*(2), 109–124.

Stevenson, R.L. (1886). *Kidnapped*. London, Cassell and Co.

Stojanoski, B., Wild, C. J., Battista, M. E., Nichols, E. S., & Owen, A. M. (2021). Brain training habits are not associated with generalized benefits to cognition: An online study of over 1000 "brain trainers". *Journal of Experimental Psychology: General*, *150*(4), 729.

Stracciari, A., Ghidoni, E., Guarino, M., Poletti, M., & Pazzaglia, P. (1994). Post-traumatic retrograde amnesia with selective impairment of autobiographical memory. *Cortex*, *30*(3), 459–468.

Taylor, N., Graham, M., Delargy, M., & Naci, L. (2020). Memory during the presumed vegetative state: Implications for patient quality of life. *Cambridge Quarterly of Healthcare Ethics*, *29*(4), 501–510.

Teuber, H. L., Milner, B., & Vaughan Jr, H. G. (1968). Persistent anterograde amnesia after stab wound of the basal brain. *Neuropsychologia*, *6*(3), 267–282.

Thomas, D. (1952) *A child's Christmas in Wales*, New York: Published by Holiday House, 1985.

Thompson, R., Smith, R. B., Karim, Y. B., Shen, C., Drummond, K., Teng, C., & Toledano, M. B. (2022). Noise pollution and human cognition: An updated systematic review and meta-analysis of recent evidence. *Environment International*, *158*, 106905.

Tsivilis, D., Vann, S. D., Denby, C., Roberts, N., Mayes, A. R., Montaldi, D., & Aggleton, J. P. (2008). A disproportionate role for the fornix and mammillary bodies in recall versus recognition memory. *Nature Neuroscience*, *11*(7), 834–842.

Twain, M. (1907). Mark Twain's Own Autobiography, *North American Review*, 1 March. 1907.

Tulving, E. (2005). Episodic memory and autonoesis: Uniquely human. In H. Terrace & J. Metcalfe (Eds.), *The missing link in cognition* (pp. 4–56). Oxford University Press, New York.

Vallotton, C. (2011). Babies open our minds to their minds: How "listening" to infant signs complements and extends our knowledge of infants and their development. *Infant Mental Health Journal*, *32*(1), 115–133.

Vann, S. D., Tsivilis, D., Denby, C. E., Quamme, J. R., Yonelinas, A. P., Aggleton, J. P., Montaldi, M., & Mayes, A. R. (2009). Impaired recollection but spared familiarity in patients with extended hippocampal system damage revealed by 3 convergent methods. *Proceedings of the National Academy of Sciences*, *106*(13), 5442–5447.

van de Ven, N., van Rijswijk, L., & Roy, M. M. (2011). The return trip effect: Why the return trip often seems to take less time. *Psychonomic Bulletin & Review*, *18*(5), 827–832.

Voyer, D., Saint Aubin, J., Altman, K., & Gallant, G. (2021). Sex differences in verbal working memory: A systematic review and meta-analysis. *Psychological Bulletin*, *147*(4), 352.

Wagenaar, W. A. (1986). My memory: A study of autobiographical memory over six years. *Cognitive Psychology*, *18*(2), 225–252.

Wagenaar, W. A., & Groeneweg, J. (1990). The memory of concentration camp survivors. *Applied Cognitive Psychology*, *4*(2), 77–87.

Wearing, D. (2005). *Forever today: A memoir of love and amnesia*. London, Random House.

Weiskrantz, L., & Warrington, E. K. (1979). Conditioning in amnesic patients. *Neuropsychologia*, *17*(2), 187–194.

Wesnes, K. A., Brooker, H., Watson, A. W., Bal, W., & Okello, E. (2017). Effects of the Red Bull energy drink on cognitive function and mood in healthy young volunteers. *Journal of Psychopharmacology*, *31*(2), 211–221.

Wilde, O. (1895). *The importance of being earnest*. New York: Dover Publications, 1990.

Williams, C. M., Peyre, H., Toro, R., & Ramus, F. (2021). Neuroanatomical norms in the UK Biobank: The impact of allometric scaling, sex, and age. *Human Brain Mapping*, *42*(14), 4623–4642.

Woollett, K., & Maguire, E. A. (2011). Acquiring "the Knowledge" of London's layout drives structural brain changes. *Current Biology*, *21*(24), 2109–2114.

Yonelinas, A. P. (2002). The nature of recollection and familiarity: A review of 30 years of research. *Journal of Memory and Language*, *46*(3), 441–517.

Yonelinas, A. P., Ranganath, C., Ekstrom, A. D., & Wiltgen, B. J. (2019). A contextual binding theory of episodic memory: Systems consolidation reconsidered. *Nature Reviews Neuroscience*, *20*(6), 364–375.

Züst, M. A., Ruch, S., Wiest, R., & Henke, K. (2019). Implicit vocabulary learning during sleep is bound to slow-wave peaks. *Current Biology*, *29*(4), 541–553.

Index

absent mindedness 66–68, 257
acetyl choline 197, 244
Agatha Christie 188–189
aging 30–38; brain changes 33–35, 37; brain reserve 35–36; cognitive reserve 33, 36–37, 204, 215; episodic memory 31; lifestyle factors 35–36; priming 30, 32; reaction times 32–33; semantic memory 31, 33; terminal decline 37–38; working memory 31, 33
alcohol 11, 81, 195, 206, 244, 249
alcoholic blackout 194–196
alphabet position 251
Alzheimer's disease 198–207; amyloid 200–204, 206; apolipoprotein E (APOE) 207; diagnosis 200–202; genetic factors 206; lifestyle factors 204–206, 214, 218; Mild Cognitive Impairment 80, 116, 118, 202–203, 207, 215; nun study 204–205; pathology 200–203; progression 202–203
amnesia 166–167; anterograde amnesia 167–178; Clive Wearing 167; Confabulation 168, 175; crime and amnesia 192–194; developmental amnesia 184–186; diencephalic 173–176; dreaming 126; drug-induced 194–197; explicit vs implicit memory 169–171, 178; faking amnesia 191–194; fugue 188; functional amnesia 166, 188; future memory 129; infantile amnesia 21–27; neuropathology 171–177; psychogenic amnesia 167, 187–190, 193; recognition memory 141–143; retrograde amnesia 167, 178–184; simulating amnesia 190–194; temporal lobe amnesia 173–174; Transient Global Amnesia 186–187
amphetamine 107–109
amygdala 190, 253
amyloid 200–207
anterior thalamic nuclei 175–176
anterograde amnesia 167–178
aphantasia: people who lack imagery 93, 212–213
Attention Deficit Hyperactivity Disorder (ADHD) 12, 107

autism 12, 88, 90–93
autobiographical memory 5, 31, 167, 181, 213

background sounds 160
Bacopa 116
benzodiazepines 196–197
bias 60–63, 74–76
bilingualism 213–215
birds 58–59, 131, 149, 240
blocking 68–69
brain development 11–12, 15–17, 28
Brain Gym® 234
brain training 215–216
brain volume 15, 20, 28, 30, 250
breakfast 114

caffeine 81
capacity of memory 1–2
Capgras delusion 216–217
central executive 159, 161
cerebellum 11, 20, 250, 253
cerebral cortex 16, 20, 34, 253
change blindness 63–65
chess 58, 109
childhood amnesia 21–27
children's memory 12–29; episodic memory 14–15, 17; false memories 49; first memories 21–27; forked-tube test 135; imitation 12, 14; self-awareness 14, 24; semantic memory 14, 18; signing 14; spoon test 133; working memory 18–19
chimpanzees 132
chocolate 114
cingulate cortex 254
classical conditioning 5–6, 10, 13, 39–40, 170, 219–221
cocaine 107
cognitive enhancers 106–120, 257; drugs 106–112; electrical brain stimulation 118–120; food supplements 112–118
computerised brain training 215–216
concussion 179–180, 191, 205
conditioned taste aversion 219–221

conditioning *see* classical conditioning
confabulation 168, 175, 223
confirmation bias 61, 74
consciousness 247
consistency bias 76
conspiracy theorists 74–76
consolidation 16
context dependent memory 23, 78–83, 257
continuity errors 64
corpus callosum 233–236, 254
Corsi block task 152
critical period 16
curiosity 240–241, 256

Dead or Alive Test 178, 192
default mode network 128
déjà vu 143
delusions 130
dementia 198–211; Alzheimer's disease 198–207;
    frontotemporal 209–211; Lewy body
    dementia 207–209; semantic dementia
    210–211; vascular dementia 209
development amnesia 184–186
diencephalic amnesia 171–177
diencephalon 170–171, 254
digit span 18, 151–152, 154–155, 158, 162
directed forgetting 66, 76–77
direct transcranial current stimulation 119
distributed practice 228–231
divers 78–79
dreams 123, 125–126, 129, 213
driving 170, 203, 228–230
Down's syndrome 206
dual-code theory 98
dual-process models of recognition 140–143
duplicates 216–217
dyslexia 235–236

Ebbinghaus 69–70, 154
echoic memory 6, 147–150
eidetic memory 92–93
Einstein 19, 93–94
emotion 190, 193
encoding specificity hypothesis 82
encoding variability 231
energy drinks 113–114
engram 40–43, 45–46, 71, 252
entorhinal cortex 254
epigenetics 28–29
episodic buffer 159, 161
episodic foresight 129–135
episodic memory 2, 6, 17, 40, 129, 131, 170, 181,
    203, 210, 214, 249
exercise 204–205, 217–218, 249
expert knowledge 57–60, 84, 257
explicit (declarative) memory 2–3, 6, 26, 170
eyewitness testimony 44–45, 48–49, 61, 72, 82

face recognition 59
false confessions 73
false memories 47–50, 72
familiarity based liking 221
feeling of knowing 68, 227
feigning amnesia 190–194
flavonoids 114–115
flicker fusion frequency 147
foetal learning 10–12
food preferences 11, 219–221
forgetting 66–83; absent mindedness 66–68; bias
    74–76; context effects 78–83; directed
    forgetting 66, 76–77; interference 69–70;
    misattribution 71; persistence 76; seven sins
    66; suggestibility 72–73; transience 69
forgetting curve 69–70
fornix 35, 141, 176–177, 248, 254
Fregoli syndrome 217
frontotemporal dementia 209–211
fugue 188–189
future memory 128–131

gambling 227
generation effect 221–223, 241
ginkgo 115
ginseng 115–116
glucose 112–114
gorillas 65
grandmother cells 225–226

habituation 6, 13, 40
halo effect 63
haptic memory 6, 150–151, 155
highlighting text 223–225
Highly Superior Autobiographical Memory
    (HSAM) 88–89
Hippocampus 170, 254; aging 36; amnesia 129,
    171, 174, 184–186; brain development 16, 25,
    250; consolidation 59, 182–184; exercise 217;
    neurogenesis 26, 51, 114, 131, 204, 217; place
    cells 131, 177; replay 123, 132, 177; sleep 123,
    126; stimulation 225–226
H.M. 152–153, 168–169, 173, 182
humour and memory 58
hyperphantasia 212
hypnosis: memory recall 44–46; legalities 45,
    223; regression 27
hypothalamus 171, 173, 254

iconic memory 6, 145–147
illusions of memory 223–225, 257
imagery and memory 95–104, 212–213, 256–257
imagery and sport 102–105
imitation 12, 14, 220
implicit memory 2–4, 6, 14, 168
improving your memory 95–105, 107–120,
    256–257

inattentional blindness 46–65
incidental learning 56–57
infantile amnesia *see* childhood amnesia
intentional forgetting 66, 76–77
interference 70–71, 153; proactive 70–71; retroactive 70–71
interrogation 73–74
irrelevant speech (sound) effect 160–161

jamais vu 143
Jennifer Aniston neurons 225–226
Jorvik Viking Centre 80
Jost's law 69

Kim Peek 91–92
Korsakoff syndrome 169, 172–175, 181

language learning 12, 14–15, 23–24, 213–215, 230
learner drivers 228–230
learning: distributed (spaced) practice 228–231; incidental learning 56; levels of processing 52–57; mnemonics 95–101; repetition *see* parrot learning
learning styles 234
left vs right brain 233–236
levels of processing 52–60, 163, 214
Lewy Body dementia 207–209
Lloyd-Morgan's canon 134
link system mnemonics 96–97
lion's mane 117
long-term memory 6

mammillary bodies 171, 173, 175–176, 254
mammillothalamic tract 171, 175–176
massed learning 228–231, 256
memory capacity 1–2, 51, 153–155, 161–162
memory champions 1, 85, 87, 95
memory permanence 39–51
memory recovery 43
memory span 18, 84–85, 87
mental time travel 128–135
metacognition 226
metamemory 225–228
method of loci 95–96, 248
methylphenidate (Ritalin) 108–109, 118
Mild Cognitive Impairment 80, 116, 118, 202–203, 207, 215
mind maps 97–98
mirror neurons 108
MMSE (Mini Mental Status Examination) 116, 118, 200, 202, 209, 214
mnemonics 85, 95–101, 256
mnemonists 84–87
Modafinil 108–109, 118
mood congruency 82
motivated forgetting 76–77, 86
motor learning 102–105, 228–229, 233–234, 248

Mozart effect 231–233
multiple trace theory 183–184
music 160, 231–233
myelin 247–248

names–remembering 100–101
n-back task 158
neuroenhancers: caffeine 112–114; methylphenidate (Ritalin) 108–109, 118; Modafinil 108–109, 118; nicotine 81–82, 110–112; Piracetam 110
neurogenesis 26, 51, 114, 131, 204, 217
neuromyths 233–236
nicotine 81, 110–112
NonREM sleep (NREM) 122–123
nootropics *see* neuroenhancers
nuns 204
nutritional supplements 106, 114–118

odour *see* olfaction
olfaction 11, 79–80, 155
omega-3 fats 116
openness in science 236
operant learning 13
overconfidence 227

parietal lobe 254
Parkinson's disease 207–208
parrot learning *see* rote learning
parrots–language 240
peg-word mnemonics 97
Penfield, Wilder 41–43, 45, 144
perceptual learning 60
phonological loop 159–162
piracetam 110
place cells 131, 177
plagiarism 72
post-traumatic stress disorder (PTSD) 51, 76–77, 80, 197
prefrontal cortex 20, 25, 31–32, 50, 77, 138, 164–165, 184, 217, 254
pregnancy and memory 8–9
priming 6–7, 30, 32, 40, 143, 169
proactive interference 70–71
procedural learning 6–7, 123
prospective memory 136–138, 202
psychogenic amnesia 167, 187–190, 193

rapid eye movement (REM) sleep 122–123, 126, 209
reaction time 32–33, 112–113, 116
recognition memory 79, 139–144, 185, 191; amnesia and recognition 141–143, 185; context 79; dual-process models 140; familiarity-based 140; forced-choice tests 191; priming 143; recollective-based 140; single process models 141

recollection 52–53
reconsolidation 50–51, 183
reconstructive memory 47, 50
repetition and learning 238–240
replicability in science 236–238
reproducibility in science 236–238
Rescorla-Wagner model 242–243
retrieval 7; brain mechanisms 182–184; context
    23, 43–44, 78–83, 257; cue based 40, 44;
    mode 184; reconstructive 47
retrograde amnesia 167, 178–184; assessment
    178–179; causes 178, 184; concussion
    179–180; consolidation model 182–183;
    multiple trace theory 183–184; neuropathol-
    ogy 180–181; Ribot's law 181–182
retrosplenial cortex 254
return trip effect 241–242
Ribot's law 181–182, 210
Ritalin 108–109, 118
robustness in science 236–238
rote learning 238–240

savants 90–93
schemas 17, 52–53
scopolamine 197, 244
semantic dementia 210–211
semantic memory 2, 7, 169, 210–211, 240
sensory memory 7, 145–150
sex differences and memory 249–251
Shereshevsky 85–86
short-term memory 6–7, 151–155; capacity 151,
    153–155; memory span 152; visuo-spatial
    152, 155
singing 36, 60
skilled memory theory 86, 101
sleep 121–127, 205, 209, 256; consolidation 123;
    dream content 123, 125, 129, 213; dream recall
    125–126; implicit memory 127; learning while
    asleep 126–127; napping 125; problem solving
    123–124; procedural learning 123, 125
smart drugs *see* cognitive enhancers
smell *see* olfaction
sodium pentobarbital 245
song learning 238
sound localisation 148
spaced learning 228–231, 256
spatial memory 203, 249–250
state-dependent learning 14, 47, 81–82, 109,
    113, 193

stereotypes and memory 60–63
super-recognisers 89–90
surprise and memory 52, 221–222, 242–243
synaesthesia 85
synapses 11, 16, 19

tactile memory *see* haptic memory
taste aversions 219–221
taste preferences 11, 219–221
taxi drivers 59–60
temporal lobe 128, 171, 173–174, 254
thalamus 171, 255
theory-of-mind 134
time: estimation 137, 169, 241–242; monitoring
    137, 169; time travel 128–135
tip-of-the-tongue 68–69, 227, 240
trace decay 70
transcranial magnetic stimulation (TMS)
    118–119
Transient Global Amnesia 186–187
traumatic memories 187–188
truth serums 47, 243–246

unconscious learning 246
understanding and memory 52, 256

vaping *see* nicotine
vascular dementia 209
vegetative brain state 246–247
visual-paired comparison 13
visuospatial scratchpad *see* working memory
von Restorff effect 243

walnuts 116
Wearing, Clive 167–168
Wernicke's disease 173
white matter: aging 33, 35, 249; development 20,
    247–249; plasticity 9, 36
wine 60, 114
World Memory Championships 1, 85, 87, 95
working memory 6–7, 153, 156–165, 203, 213,
    215, 249; aging 41–42; central executive
    159–161; childhood 18–19, 156, 162;
    complex span 158; episodic buffer 159, 161;
    phonological loop 159–162; visuospatial
    sketchpad 159, 161, 249; word length effect
    162

zebrafish 252

For Product Safety Concerns and Information please contact our
EU representative GPSR@taylorandfrancis.com Taylor & Francis
Verlag GmbH, Kaufingerstraße 24, 80331 München, Germany